T0259596

# Pediatric Pharmacology and Drug Therapy

*Editor*

JACOB V. ARANDA

# PEDIATRIC CLINICS OF NORTH AMERICA

www.pediatric.theclinics.com

*Consulting Editor*
BONITA F. STANTON

December 2017 • Volume 64 • Number 6

**ELSEVIER**

1600 John F. Kennedy Boulevard • Suite 1800 • Philadelphia, Pennsylvania, 19103-2899

http://www.theclinics.com

**THE PEDIATRIC CLINICS OF NORTH AMERICA Volume 64, Number 6**
**December 2017 ISSN 0031-3955, ISBN-13: 978-0-323-55290-5**

Editor: Kerry Holland
Developmental Editor: Casey Potter

*The Pediatric Clinics of North America* (ISSN 0031-3955) is published bimonthly by Elsevier Inc., 360 Park Avenue South, New York, NY 10010-1710. Months of issue are February, April, June, August, October, and December. Periodicals postage paid at New York, NY and additional mailing offices. Subscription prices are $208.00 per year (US individuals), $589.00 per year (US institutions), $281.00 per year (Canadian individuals), $784.00 per year (Canadian institutions), $338.00 per year (international individuals), $784.00 per year (International institutions), $100.00 per year (US students and residents), and $165.00 per year (international and Canadian residents and students). To receive students/resident rare, orders must be accompanied by name of affiliated institution, date of term, and the signature of program/residency coordinator on institution letterhead. Orders will be billed at individual rate until proof of status is received. Foreign air speed delivery is included in all *Clinics* subscription prices. All prices are subject to change without notice. **POSTMASTER:** Send address changes to *The Pediatric Clinics of North America*, Elsevier Health Sciences Division, Subscription Customer Service, 3251 Riverport Lane, Maryland Heights, MO 63043. **Customer Service: 1-800-654-2452 (US and Canada). From outside of the US and Canada: 1-314-447-8871. Fax: 1-314-447-8029. For print support, E-mail: JournalsCustomerService-usa@elsevier.com. For online support, E-mail: JournalsOnlineSupport-usa@elsevier.com.**

*Reprints.* For copies of 100 or more, of articles in this publication, please contact the Commercial Reprints Department, Elsevier Inc., 360 Park Avenue South, New York, NY 10010-1710. Tel.: 212-633-3874; Fax: 212-633-3820; E-mail: reprints@elsevier.com.

*The Pediatric Clinics of North America* is also published in Spanish by McGraw-Hill Inter-americana Editores S.A., Mexico City, Mexico; in Portuguese by Riechmann and Affonso Editores, Rua Comandante Coelho 1085, CEP 21250, Rio de Janeiro, Brazil; and in Greek by Althayia SA, Athens, Greece.

*The Pediatric Clinics of North America* is covered in *MEDLINE/PubMed (Index Medicus)*, *Excerpta Medica*, *Current Contents*, *Current Contents/Clinical Medicine*, *Science Citation Index*, *ASCA*, *ISI/BIOMED*, and *BIOSIS*.

## PROGRAM OBJECTIVE

The goal of the *Pediatric Clinics of North America* is to keep practicing physicians and residents up to date with current clinical practice in pediatrics by providing timely articles reviewing the state-of-the-art in patient care.

## TARGET AUDIENCE

All practicing pediatricians, physicians and healthcare professionals who provide patient care to pediatric patients.

## LEARNING OBJECTIVES

Upon completion of this activity, participants will be able to:
1. Review guidelines for pediatric pharmacology.
2. Discuss emerging drug therapies for pediatric conditions such as diabetes and inflammatory bowel disease, among others.
3. Recognize developing drug therapies for newborns.

## ACCREDITATION

The Elsevier Office of Continuing Medical Education (EOCME) is accredited by the Accreditation Council for Continuing Medical Education (ACCME) to provide continuing medical education for physicians.

The EOCME designates this enduring material for a maximum of 15 *AMA PRA Category 1 Credit*(s)™. Physicians should claim only the credit commensurate with the extent of their participation in the activity.

All other healthcare professionals requesting continuing education credit for this enduring material will be issued a certificate of participation.

## DISCLOSURE OF CONFLICTS OF INTEREST

The EOCME assesses conflict of interest with its instructors, faculty, planners, and other individuals who are in a position to control the content of CME activities. All relevant conflicts of interest that are identified are thoroughly vetted by EOCME for fair balance, scientific objectivity, and patient care recommendations. EOCME is committed to providing its learners with CME activities that promote improvements or quality in healthcare and not a specific proprietary business or a commercial interest.

**The planning committee, staff, authors and editors listed below have identified no financial relationships or relationships to products or devices they or their spouse/life partner have with commercial interest related to the content of this CME activity:**
William C. Anderson III, MD; Jacob V. Aranda, MD, PhD, FRCPC; Jeff Barrett, PhD; Dirk Bassler, MD, MSc; Kay D. Beharry, BS; Vivian L. Chin, MD; Louis T. Dang, MD, PhD; Anjali Fortna; Densley Francois, PharmD; Tsuyoshi Fukuda, PhD; Roy Gerona, PhD; Margaret R. Hammerschlag, MD; Kerry Holland; Aditi Khokhar, MBBS; Catherijne A.J. Knibbe, PharmD, PhD; Mary W. Lenfestey, MD; Leah Logan; Susan McCune, MD; Naomi Miyazawa, MS, PA-C; Yeruk (Lily) Mulugeta, PharmD; Sheila Perez-Colon, MD; Claudette L. Poole, MD; Mihai Puia Dumitrescu, MD, MPH; Hari Cheryl Sachs, MD; Roopali Sharma, PharmD; Faye S. Silverstein, MD; Vikram Sinha, PhD; Susan C. Smolinske, PharmD; Elizabeth A. Spencer, MD; Anita Paula Tataru, MSc (Pharm), PharmD; Vatcharapan Umpaichitra, MD; Gloria B. Valencia, MD; John van den Anker, MD, PhD; Alexander A. Vinks, PharmD, PhD, FCP; Vignesh Viswanathan; Brandon J. Warrick, MD; Ye Xiong, PhD; Lynne Yao, MD; Guy Young, MD; Anne Zajicek, PharmD, MD.

**The planning committee, staff, authors and editors listed below have identified financial relationships or relationships to products or devices they or their spouse/life partner have with commercial interest related to the content of this CME activity:**
**Marla C. Dubinsky, MD** is a consultant/advisor for AbbVie Inc; Boehringer Ingelheim GmbH; Celgene Corporation; Genentech, a Member of the Roche Group; Janssen Global Services, Inc; Pfizer Inc; Prometheus; Salix Pharmaceuticals; Shire; Takeda Pharmaceutical Company Limited; and UCB, Inc.
**Robert L. Findling, MD, MBA** receives or has received research support, acted as a consultant and/or served on a speaker's bureau for Akili Interactive Labs; Alcobra Pharma; Amerex Corporation; American Academy of Child & Adolescent Psychiatry; American Psychiatric Association Publishing; Bracket; ePharmaSolutions; Forest Laboratories; Genentech, a Member of the Roche Group; Ironshore Inc; KemPharm, Inc; Lundbeck; Aevi Genomic Medicine, Inc., formerly Medgenics, Inc; the National Insitutes of Health; Neurim Pharmaceuticals; Otsuka; Aevi Genomic Medicine, Inc.; Pfizer Inc; Physicians Postgraduate Press, Inc; F. Hoffmann-La Roche Ltd; SAGE Therapeutics; Shire; Sunovion Pharmaceuticals Inc., a U.S. subsidiary of Sumitomo Dainippon Pharma Co., Ltd.; Supernus Pharmaceuticals; Syneurx International Corp;

Takeda Pharmaceutical Company Limited; Teva Pharmaceutical Industries Ltd; Touchpoint, a Publicis Health Company; Tris Pharma; and Validus Holdings, Ltd.

**Melanie C. Gleason, MS, PA-C** has research support from GlaxoSmithKline plc and Colorado Department of Public Health and Environment.

**David W. Kimberlin, MD** has research support from Alios, a Johnson & Johnson Services, Inc company.

**P. Brian Smith, MD, MPH, MHS** is a consultant/advisor for Nutricia, and has research support from Medela LLC and Infant Bacterial Therapeutics AB.

**Fabrizio Salomone, PhD** has an employment affiliation with CHIESI Farmaceutici S.p.A.

**Josef Neu, MD** is a consultant/advisor for Purdue and Astellas Pharma US, Inc.

**Etaterina Stepanova, MD, PhD** has research support from Psychnostics, LLC.

**Stanley J. Szefler, MD** is a consultant/advisor for AstraZeneca; Aerosene; Genentech, a Member of the Roche Group; GlaxoSmithKline plc; Novartis Global; F. Hoffmann-La Roche Ltd; and Teva Pharmaceutical Industries Ltd; and has stock ownership in GlaxoSmithKline plc.

## UNAPPROVED/OFF-LABEL USE DISCLOSURE

The EOCME requires CME faculty to disclose to the participants:

1. When products or procedures being discussed are off-label, unlabelled, experimental, and/or investigational (not US Food and Drug Administration [FDA] approved); and
2. Any limitations on the information presented, such as data that are preliminary or that represent ongoing research, interim analyses, and/or unsupported opinions. Faculty may discuss information about pharmaceutical agents that is outside of FDA-approved labelling. This information is intended solely for CME and is not intended to promote off-label use of these medications. If you have any questions, contact the medical affairs department of the manufacturer for the most recent prescribing information.

## TO ENROLL

To enroll in the *Pediatric Clinics of North America* Continuing Medical Education program, call customer service at 1-800-654-2452 or sign up online at http://www.theclinics.com/home/cme. The CME program is available to subscribers for an additional annual fee of USD 290.

## METHOD OF PARTICIPATION

In order to claim credit, participants must complete the following:

1. Complete enrolment as indicated above.
2. Read the activity.
3. Complete the CME Test and Evaluation. Participants must achieve a score of 70% on the test. All CME Tests and Evaluations must be completed online.

## CME INQUIRIES/SPECIAL NEEDS

For all CME inquiries or special needs, please contact elsevierCME@elsevier.com.

# Contributors

## CONSULTING EDITOR

**BONITA F. STANTON, MD**
Founding Dean, School of Medicine, Professor of Pediatrics, Seton Hall-Hackensack
Meridian School of Medicine University, South Orange, New Jersey, USA

## EDITOR

**JACOB V. ARANDA, MD, PhD, FRCPC**
Professor of Pediatrics and Ophthalmology, Director of Neonatology and the New York
Pediatric Developmental Pharmacology Research Center, SUNY Downstate Medical
Center, Brooklyn, New York, USA

## AUTHORS

**WILLIAM C. ANDERSON III, MD**
Section of Allergy and Immunology, Assistant Professor, Department of Pediatrics,
University of Colorado School of Medicine, Children's Hospital Colorado, Aurora,
Colorado, USA

**JACOB V. ARANDA, MD, PhD, FRCPC**
Professor of Pediatrics and Ophthalmology, Director of Neonatology and the New York
Pediatric Developmental Pharmacology Research Center, SUNY Downstate Medical
Center, Brooklyn, New York, USA

**JEFF BARRETT, PhD**
Vice President and Global Head of the Interdisciplinary Program in
Pharmacometrics Program (IPP) and Global Head of Pediatric Clinical Pharmacology,
Sanofi Pharmaceuticals, Swiftwater, Pennsylvania, USA

**DIRK BASSLER, MD, MSc**
Professor, Department of Neonatology, University of Zurich, Head, Department of
Neonatology, University Hospital Zurich, Zurich, Switzerland

**KAY D. BEHARRY, BS**
Assistant Professor and Director of Neonatal Pharmacology Translational Lab, SUNY
Downstate Medical Center, Brooklyn, New York, USA

**VIVIAN L. CHIN, MD**
Assistant Professor, Department of Pediatrics, Division of Pediatric Endocrinology,
SUNY Downstate Medical Center and Kings County Hospital Center, Brooklyn,
New York, USA

**LOUIS T. DANG, MD, PhD**
Clinical Lecturer, Division of Pediatric Neurology, Department of Pediatrics, University of
Michigan, C.S. Mott Children's Hospital, Ann Arbor, Michigan, USA

**MARLA C. DUBINSKY, MD**
Chief, Pediatric Gastroenterology and Hepatology, Professor, Department of Pediatrics,
Co-director, The Susan and Leonard Feinstein Inflammatory Bowel Disease Clinical
Center, Icahn School of Medicine at Mount Sinai, Mount Sinai Hospital, New York,
New York, USA

**ROBERT L. FINDLING, MD, MBA**
The Johns Hopkins University School of Medicine, Baltimore, Maryland, USA

**DENSLEY FRANCOIS, PharmD**
Departments of Pharmacy and Pediatrics, SUNY Downstate Medical Center, Brooklyn,
New York, USA

**TSUYOSHI FUKUDA, PhD**
Associate Professor, Division of Clinical Pharmacology, University of Cincinnati College of
Medicine, Cincinnati Children's Hospital Medical Center, Department of Pediatrics,
University of Cincinnati College of Medicine, Cincinnati, Ohio, USA

**ROY GERONA, PhD**
Clinical Toxicology and Environmental Biomonitoring Lab, University of California San
Francisco, San Francisco, California, USA

**MELANIE C. GLEASON, MS, PA-C**
Senior Instructor, Department of Pediatrics, University of Colorado School of Medicine,
Breathing Institute, Children's Hospital Colorado, Aurora, Colorado, USA

**MARGARET R. HAMMERSCHLAG, MD**
Department of Pediatrics, Division of Pediatric Infectious Diseases, SUNY Downstate
Medical Center, Brooklyn, New York, USA

**ADITI KHOKHAR, MBBS**
Division of Pediatric Endocrinology, Department of Pediatrics, State University of
New York Upstate Medical University, Syracuse, New York, USA

**DAVID W. KIMBERLIN, MD**
Professor, Department of Pediatrics, The University of Alabama at Birmingham,
Birmingham, Alabama, USA

**CATHERIJNE A.J. KNIBBE, PharmD, PhD**
Department of Clinical Pharmacy, Professor of Individualized Drug Treatment,
St Antonius Hospital, Nieuwegein, The Netherlands; Division of Pharmacology, Leiden
Academic Center for Drug Research, Faculty of Science, Leiden University, Leiden,
The Netherlands

**MARY W. LENFESTEY, MD**
Postdoctoral Fellow, Division of Pediatric Gastroenterology, University of Florida,
Gainesville, Florida, USA

**SUSAN McCUNE, MD**
Director, Office of Pediatric Therapeutics, US Food and Drug Administration, Silver
Spring, Maryland, USA

**NAOMI MIYAZAWA, MS, PA-C**
Senior Instructor, Department of Pediatrics, University of Colorado School of Medicine,
Breathing Institute, Children's Hospital Colorado, Aurora, Colorado, USA

**YERUK (LILY) MULUGETA, PharmD**
Clinical Reviewer, Division of Pediatric and Maternal Health, CDER, US Food and Drug Administration, Silver Spring, Maryland, USA

**JOSEF NEU, MD**
Professor, Department of Pediatrics, University of Florida, Gainesville, Florida, USA

**SHEILA PEREZ-COLON, MD**
Assistant Professor of Pediatrics, Division of Pediatric Endocrinology, Department of Pediatrics, SUNY Downstate Medical Center and Kings County Hospital Center, Brooklyn, New York, USA

**CLAUDETTE L. POOLE, MD**
Fellow of Pediatric Infectious Disease, Department of Pediatrics, The University of Alabama at Birmingham, Birmingham, Alabama, USA

**MIHAI PUIA-DUMITRESCU, MD, MPH**
Department of Pediatrics, Division of Neonatal-Perinatal Medicine, Duke University Medical Center, Duke Clinical Research Institute, Durham, North Carolina, USA

**HARI CHERYL SACHS, MD**
US Food and Drug Administration, Silver Spring, Maryland, USA

**FABRIZIO SALOMONE, PhD**
Neonatology and Pulmonary Rare Disease Unit, Head, Corporate Pre-Clinical R and D, Chiesi Farmaceutici S.p.A, Parma, Italy

**ROOPALI SHARMA, PharmD**
Department of Pharmacy Practice, Touro College of Pharmacy, New York, New York, USA; Department of Medicine, SUNY Downstate Medical Center, Brooklyn, New York, USA

**FAYE S. SILVERSTEIN, MD**
Professor, Division of Pediatric Neurology, Departments of Pediatrics and Neurology, University of Michigan, Ann Arbor, Michigan, USA

**VIKRAM SINHA, PhD**
Associate Vice President & Head, Quantitative Pharmacology and Pharmacometrics, Merck & Co., Inc, North Wales, Pennsylvania, USA

**P. BRIAN SMITH, MD, MPH, MHS**
Professor, Department of Pediatrics, Division of Neonatal-Perinatal Medicine, Duke University Medical Center, Duke Clinical Research Institute, Durham, North Carolina, USA

**SUSAN C. SMOLINSKE, PharmD, DABAT**
Director, New Mexico Poison and Drug Information Center, Professor, Pharmacy Practice and Administration, The University of New Mexico, Albuquerque, New Mexico, USA

**ELIZABETH A. SPENCER, MD**
Department of Pediatrics, The Susan and Leonard Feinstein Inflammatory Bowel Disease Clinical Center, Icahn School of Medicine Mount Sinai, Mount Sinai Hospital, New York, New York, USA

**EKATERINA STEPANOVA, MD, PhD**
The Johns Hopkins University School of Medicine, Baltimore, Maryland, USA

**STANLEY J. SZEFLER, MD**
Professor, Department of Pediatrics, University of Colorado School of Medicine, Breathing Institute, Children's Hospital Colorado, Aurora, Colorado, USA

**ANITA PAULA TATARU, MSc (Pharm), PharmD**
Faculty of Pharmaceutical Sciences, The University of British Columbia, British Columbia, Canada

**VATCHARAPAN UMPAICHITRA, MD**
Assistant Professor, Division Director, Division of Pediatric Endocrinology, Department of Pediatrics, SUNY Downstate Medical Center and Kings County Hospital Center, Brooklyn, New York, USA

**GLORIA B. VALENCIA, MD**
Professor of Pediatrics, Director of NICU, SUNY Downstate Medical Center, Brooklyn, New York, USA

**JOHN VAN DEN ANKER, MD, PhD**
Division of Paediatric Pharmacology and Pharmacometrics, University Children's Hospital, Basel, Switzerland; Division of Clinical Pharmacology, Children's National Health System, Washington, DC, USA

**ALEXANDER A. VINKS, PharmD, PhD, FCP**
Cincinnati Children's Research Foundation Endowed Chair, Professor of Pediatrics and Pharmacology, Scientific Director, Pharmacy Research in Patient Services, Director, Division of Clinical Pharmacology, University of Cincinnati College of Medicine, Cincinnati Children's Hospital Medical Center, Director, Pediatric Clinical Pharmacology Fellowship Program, Department of Pediatrics, University of Cincinnati College of Medicine, Cincinnati, Ohio, USA

**BRANDON J. WARRICK, MD**
The University of New Mexico, Albuquerque, New Mexico, USA

**YE XIONG, PhD**
Division of Clinical Pharmacology, Research Fellow, Cincinnati Children's Hospital Medical Center, Cincinnati, Ohio, USA

**LYNNE YAO, MD**
Director, Division of Pediatric and Maternal Health, CDER US Food and Drug Administration, Silver Spring, Maryland, USA

**GUY YOUNG, MD**
Director, Hemostasis and Thrombosis Center, Children's Hospital Los Angeles, Professor of Pediatrics, Keck School of Medicine of University of Southern California, Los Angeles, California, USA

**ANNE ZAJICEK, PharmD, MD**
Chief, Obstetric and Pediatric Pharmacology and Therapeutics Branch, Eunice Kennedy Shriver National Institute of Child Health and Human Development, Bethesda, Maryland, USA

# Contents

> Pediatric legislation has generated information about the efficacy, safety, and dosing of more than 600 products in children. Extrapolation of adult efficacy data has been an integral part of pediatric drug development. Advances in our understanding of physiology and pharmacology have improved the approach to pediatric dose selection. However, a high percentage of pediatric trials do not meet their primary efficacy endpoint. Delays in initiating completing pediatric studies persist. This article describes these advances and provides innovative approaches to optimize pediatric drug development.

> As new therapies for pediatric asthma are approved by the Food and Drug Administration, clinicians should be aware of their benefits and limitations. Accompanying these therapies are potential obstacles, including the delivery of inhaled therapies and age-specific issues regarding implementation and adherence. New insights are being added to well-established controller medications, including inhaled corticosteroids and long-acting β-agonists, whereas new medications previously approved in adults, including tiotropium and biologics, are now being evaluated for use in children. These drugs can be useful additive therapies to treat patients who are currently not responding to guidelines-based therapy.

> Bipolar disorder is a debilitating illness that often leads to functional impairment when untreated. Monotherapy with mood stabilizers is preferable, although combination therapy may be necessary in refractory cases. Most studies focus on the use of lithium, anticonvulsants, and second-generation antipsychotics in the treatment of acute manic or depressive phases, as well as maintaining adequate response after the episode. More research is needed in the area of psychopharmacology of pediatric bipolar disorder to bridge the gap between clinical needs and the available data.

New psychoactive substances (NPS), namely cannabinoids, cathinones, and opioids, have surged in popularity among adults and school-age children, resulting in serious morbidity and mortality globally. In the past decade, there has been a rapid evolution of NPS resulting in hundreds of new compounds. Little to no evidence for clinical use is available on most compounds. The clinical presentations of patients intoxicated with cannabinoids and cathinones are highly variable, but most commonly present with a sympathomimetic toxidrome, for example, agitation, delirium, and tachycardia. Those with opioids present with a classic opioid toxidrome: coma, dilated pupils, and respiratory failure.

High-quality systematic reviews of use of herbal or homeopathic remedies in children often suffer from design flaws, such as not following PRISMA guidelines, inconsistent outcome measurements, and paucity of high-quality studies. Herbal remedies have modest demonstrated benefits with insufficient evidence to recommend any particular supplement. Homeopathic remedies have no role in treatment of pediatric conditions, and have been associated with great harm in infants given homeopathic teething products. Two types of herbal supplements are associated with high risk in adolescents: energy drinks and adulterated weight-loss products. Parents should be counseled about risks of these products.

Venous thromboembolism is occurring with increasing frequency in children, resulting in the more widespread use of anticoagulation in pediatrics. Antithrombotic drugs in children can be divided into the standard and alternative agents. This article discusses standard and alternative anticoagulants. Because standard anticoagulants have significant limitations, including variable pharmacokinetics, issues with therapeutic drug monitoring, frequency of administration, efficacy, and adverse effects, it is expected that the use of alternative anticoagulants will increase over time. With their improved properties and recent prospective clinical trial data, the current and future use of these agents will likely slowly replace of the standard anticoagulants.

Microbes and humans have been closely associated throughout evolution; this symbiotic and/or commensal relationship is crucial for normal development and health. The use of probiotics has been the topic of intense investigation in the past couple of decades because they have the capability to promote health. Based on these studies, it can be debated whether they are being used to promote overall health or to treat and prevent diseases. This article provides an overview and analysis of evidence about what is currently known about the health benefits of these agents that are marketed for use in children and neonates.

The mainstay of treatment of childhood epilepsy is to administer antiepileptic drugs (AEDs). This article provides an overview of the clinical approach to drug treatment of childhood epilepsy, focusing on general principles of therapy and properties of recently introduced medications. Initiation and cessation of therapy, adverse medication effects, drug interactions, indications for the various AEDs, and off-label use of AEDs are reviewed. The distinct challenges in treatment of epileptic spasms and neonatal seizures are addressed. Finally, ideas for the future of drug treatment of childhood epilepsy are presented, with particular attention to precision medicine.

Clinical trials for the most effective drugs in the armamentarium of medications for inflammatory bowel disease (IBD) have shown only a 50% to 60% response rate, and this drops to 30% in maintenance. However, therapeutic drug monitoring (TDM) to adjust dosing to account for patient-specific characteristics, which has been shown to improve outcomes, was not used in these trials. This article details the development of TDM within the IBD space as it evolved from thiopurines to biologics and continues to evolve with loftier treat-to-target goals and more sophisticated dashboard systems.

Non-steroidal anti-inflammatory drugs (NSAIDs) and acetaminophen are used in young infants and newborns for pain and fever control, patent ductus closure, prevention of intraventricular hemorrhage, and potentially for prevention of retinopathy of prematurity. These drugs inhibit cyclooxygenase 1 (COX-1), COX-2, and peroxidases, thus blocking prostaglandin (PG) synthesis. PGs are eicosanoids that regulate several physiologic, pathologic, and cellular processes, including vasomotor tone, platelet aggregation, sensitization of neurons to pain, and many molecular events critical to physiologic homeostasis. NSAIDs inhibit caspases and cell death. Increasing knowledge of these molecular entities may allow targeted drug development to prevent or minimize neonatal morbidities.

With the increasing incidence of childhood obesity, clinicians need to understand its comorbidities and their management. The American Diabetes Association recommends pediatricians screen high-risk overweight and obese children. Identifying and treating prediabetic children and adolescents can help to reduce the burden of type 2 diabetes. Lifestyle interventions are pivotal. Metformin is the only oral medication approved for diabetes treatment in children. It has been studied in clinical trials in nondiabetic children and has been shown to have beneficial effects on body weight. Effects on diabetes prevention have not been studied and long-term data are limited in the pediatric population.

All definitions of bronchopulmonary dysplasia (BPD) have limitations, and a new definition for the purpose of clinical research, benchmarking, and prognostic prediction is needed. Different inhaled and systemic drugs are currently used to prevent or treat BPD. Despite some positive effects on BPD, more information about the effects of inhaled corticosteroids is required to assess overall efficacy and associated risks. One needs to balance the risks of neurodevelopmental impairment owing to systemic corticosteroids against those of BPD itself. Future studies should, therefore, focus on infants with a very high risk of developing BPD and include pharmacokinetics and long-term developmental outcomes.

Several new antimicrobial agents, daptomycin, ceftaroline, telavancin, dalbavancin, and tedizolid, have been approved for the treatment of staphylococcal infections, including methicillin-resistant *Staphylococcus aureus* (MRSA), in adults. Ceftaroline and daptomycin have been approved by the US Food and Drug Administration for use in children. Ceftaroline, a beta-lactam antibiotic with activity against MRSA, has been approved for treatment of community-acquired bacterial pneumonia and complicated skin and skin structure infections. Daptomycin has been approved for treatment of complicated skin and skin structure infections. In this article, we review the pharmacokinetics and pharmacodynamics of these antibiotics and available data on use in children.

Invasive fungal infections are a significant cause of morbidity and mortality in infants and children. Early diagnosis is critical, and treatment with the appropriate drug and dose should be initiated promptly. Although an increasing number of studies have examined dosing of antifungals in this population, pediatric safety and efficacy data are lacking.

This article focuses on the clinically relevant approved antiviral medications available for the treatment of infants and children. A brief overview of drug categories, mechanism of action, resistance, pharmacokinetics, and side effects is provided for the more commonly prescribed antivirals. The patient categories addressed are treatment and prophylaxis of influenza, neonatal herpes simplex virus and congenital cytomegalovirus, treatment and prophylaxis of viral disease in the immunocompromised host, and a brief introduction to the antivirals available to treat hepatitis B and hepatitis C in children.

With the alarming increase of obesity in children, pediatricians are increasingly being confronted with difficult dosing decisions. Many drug labels do not provide specific dosing instructions for children who are obese. In this article, we describe the physiologic parameters altered by obesity and their influences on drug disposition and effect. We review the principles of allometry, and the key pharmacokinetic parameters that can be used to derive age-appropriate dosing regimens. Last, we illustrate how appropriate weight descriptors can be selected, and how important pharmacokinetic parameters can be extrapolated for dosing in obese children when pediatric pharmacokinetic information is available.

# PEDIATRIC CLINICS OF NORTH AMERICA

# Preface
# Evolution of Pharmacotherapeutics and Pharmacotoxidromes in Newborns and Children: Progress and Challenges

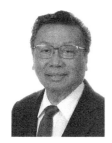

Jacob V. Aranda, MD, PhD, FRCPC
*Editor*

*The dose makes the poison ("sola dosis facit venenum") or the remedy.*
*Alle Dinge sind Gift, und nichts ist ohne Gift, allein die Dosis macht dass ein Ding*
*kein Gift ist. (All things are poison, and nothing is without poison, the dosage alone*
*makes it so a thing is not a poison).*
— *Paracelsus (Philippus von Hohenheim): 1493-1541*

Drugs can heal and can kill! Knowledge and familiarity of the pharmacologic actions and clinical pharmacology profiles of drugs used in newborns and children may determine whether these drugs may cure or may harm. This issue of the *Pediatric Clinics of North America* focuses on the evolution and the substantial advances in drug therapies in newborns and children. Many drug tragedies in the past, which led to the deaths of vulnerable sick newborns, infants, and children, occurred due to ignorance and knowledge gaps. In the era of neonatal pharmacoempericism (circa 1940 to 1970), newborns and infants were considered miniature adults. Thus, drugs like chloramphenicol to treat neonatal sepsis were given as scaled-down doses based on the assumption that newborns and children were miniature adults, leading to tragedies like the chloramphenicol gray baby syndrome and death. The problems in pediatric drug dose selection, dose extrapolations, and progress in pediatric drug development are detailed in the first article by Mulugeta and colleagues. The article discusses the advances in developmental pharmacology and therapeutics and the recent legislative and regulatory

Pediatr Clin N Am 64 (2017) xv–xvii
https://doi.org/10.1016/j.pcl.2017.09.002
0031-3955/17/© 2017 Published by Elsevier Inc.

**pediatric.theclinics.com**

initiatives as well as the collective efforts of the research and regulatory agencies (eg, National Institute of Child Health and Human Development, US Food and Drug Administration [FDA]), pharmaceuticals, and academics that led to substantial increase in pediatric drug studies and labeling. The authors also discuss the role of modelling and simulation studies, the need for more data sharing and collaboration among investigators, and the on-going initiatives to facilitate and further advance pediatric drug development.

Updates on the current and rapidly evolving drug therapies in asthma, bipolar disorders, seizures, inflammatory bowel diseases, obesity, and bronchopulmonary dysplasia are provided. The pharmacotherapeutic management of childhood asthma is rapidly evolving and thus requires timely revisions of the management guidelines. Inhaled corticosteroids and long-acting β-adrenergic agonists are the principal controller therapies for persistent asthma with newer formulations improving drug delivery. In addition, controller therapies previously approved for adult asthma, including tiotropium and biologics (eg, omalizumab), are now being investigated and used in younger children. This issue also reminds the pediatric health care provider that pharmacotherapy of children and adolescents with bipolar disorder remains challenging. Until recently, very limited data pertaining to the pharmacologic management of pediatric bipolar disorder were available. Once again, children were essentially treated as "small adults" with clinicians adapting information from clinical trials in adults despite apparent differences in the efficacy and safety profiles of these pharmacologic interventions in youth and adults. This issue of *Pediatric Clinics of North America* discusses drugs currently approved by the FDA for the treatment of bipolar disorder and summarizes studies directly comparing monotherapy options as well as combinations of different classes of medications. This issue also provides a much needed update on the pharmacologic agents for seizure management in children. The evolving role and increasing importance of therapeutic drug monitoring (TDM) for the management of inflammatory bowel disease (IBD) in children is also provided in this issue. TDM allows individualized or personalized drug therapy that optimizes or maximizes benefit while minimizing or avoiding toxicity. From its origin with thiopurines and now the monoclonal antibodies to TNF-α, interleukin, or integrin, TDM has been utilized in IBD to maximize patient outcomes and minimize adverse events.

The advances in anticoagulant therapy and probiotics for newborns and children and the clinical pharmacology of nonsteroidal anti-inflammatory drugs in newborns and children are also highlighted in this issue. Moreover, novel antimicrobials for gram-positive infections as well as antifungals and antiviral drugs for newborns and children are also reviewed. The sinister and increasing problem of pharmacotoxidromes (toxic syndromes) due to abuse of designer drugs, such as the new psychoactive substances, particularly among school children and young adults is extensively reviewed here. The diagnostic tools as well as guidelines to assist the pediatric health care giver to better recognize, manage, and obtain timely consults for these children suspected of drug abuse are discussed. Similarly, the dietary supplements that are commonly used in children despite lack of evidence of their usefulness and appropriate pharmacologic evaluation are discussed. The increasing problem of obesity in the pediatric population not only raises the question of how best to provide the appropriate effective and safe drug dose to these obese children but also calls for more studies in this area.

Drugs, to cure or to comfort, form one of the major pillars of patient care in newborns, children, and adolescents. This issue of the *Pediatric Clinics of North America* attempted to provide a broad albeit selected evolving and advancing knowledge base in neonatal and pediatric pharmacotherapies and pharmacotoxidromes to help clinicians choose and use drugs wisely, rationally, safely, and effectively.

Jacob V. Aranda, MD, PhD, FRCPC
New York Pediatric Developmental Pharmacology Research Center
State University of New York
Downstate Medical Center
Brooklyn, NY 11203, USA

*E-mail address:*
Jacob.aranda@downstate.edu

# Development of Drug Therapies for Newborns and Children

## The Scientific and Regulatory Imperatives

Yeruk (Lily) Mulugeta, PharmD[a],*, Anne Zajicek, PharmD, MD[b],
Jeff Barrett, PhD[c], Hari Cheryl Sachs, MD[a], Susan McCune, MD[a],
Vikram Sinha, PhD[d], Lynne Yao, MD[a]

## KEYWORDS

• Pediatric • Neonatal • Research • Extrapolation • Dosing • Regulations

## KEY POINTS

- Pediatric drug development laws have improved labeling of products, including off-patent products, for use in pediatric patients.
- Extrapolation of efficacy data from adults relies on the understanding of the disease and response to therapy in adults and application to pediatric patients.
- Dose selection in pediatric patients, including neonates, should be based on understanding the influence of growth and development on pharmacokinetics and pharmacodynamics.
- Data on age- and disease-appropriate biomarkers in pediatric patients are critically lacking.
- Tremendous strides are being made in establishing consortia and clinical research infrastructure to facilitate drug development in pediatric patients, including neonates.

Disclaimer: This article reflects the views of the authors and should not be construed to represent views or policies of the US Food and Drug Administration.
Disclosures: No direct financial interest in the subject matter or materials discussed in the article for any of the authors.
[a] Division of Pediatric and Maternal Health, CDER US Food and Drug Administration, 10903 New Hampshire Avenue, Silver Spring, MD 20903, USA; [b] Obstetric and Pediatric Pharmacology and Therapeutics Branch, Eunice Kennedy Shriver National Institute of Child Health and Human Development, 6710B Rockledge Drive Room 2334, MSC 7002, Bethesda, MD 20817, USA; [c] Sanofi Pharmaceuticals, Discovery Drive, Swiftwater, PA 18370, USA; [d] Merck & Co., Inc, PO Box 1000, UG4D-48, North Wales, PA 19454, USA
* Corresponding author. US Food and Drug Administration, 10903 New Hampshire Avenue, Building 22/5483, Silver Spring, MD 20903.
E-mail address: yeruk.mulugeta@fda.hhs.gov

Pediatr Clin N Am 64 (2017) 1185–1196
http://dx.doi.org/10.1016/j.pcl.2017.08.015
0031-3955/17/© 2017 Elsevier Inc. All rights reserved.

## INTRODUCTION

Pediatric advocacy and legislative initiatives have propelled pediatric drug development forward. There still remain significant challenges, including lack of basic science knowledge of disease mechanism for some conditions affecting neonates and children, application of extrapolation and dose-ranging studies to pediatric populations, and incorporation of Good Clinical Practice guidance into clinical trials. This paper will discuss these and other topics from a regulatory, industry, and academic/NIH point of view.

## PEDIATRIC LEGISLATION AND IMPACT

For new medications to be marketed in the United States, they must be approved under the Food, Drug, and Cosmetic (FD&C) Act. Under the FD&C Act, drug manufacturers must demonstrate the effectiveness of their products through the conduct of adequate and well-controlled studies to obtain marketing approval. During the review of the marking application, the US Food and Drug Administration (FDA) must assess whether the drug is safe and effective in its proposed use(s), and whether the benefits of the drug outweigh the risks. Pediatric disasters such as the sulfanilamide tragedy (where sulfanilamide was dissolved in an elixir flavored with diethylene glycol and resulted in 100 fatalities) prompted many of the FDA's current regulations that require drugs to be safe and effective, as well as pure. Despite this, in 1968 Dr Harry Shirkey published an editorial in the *Journal of Pediatrics* in which he stated, "By an odd and unfortunate twist of fate, infants and children are becoming therapeutic or pharmaceutical orphans."[1] His editorial noted that most drugs approved by FDA, including drugs that were commonly used in infants and children, were not approved for children and product labeling contained no information about the efficacy or safety of the drug when used in children.

Indeed, many pharmaceutical manufacturers were reluctant to study drugs in children owing to ethical and financial constraints or trial design challenges. Medications were often administered to children empirically, assuming that they were "little adults." This simplistic and often erroneous assumption resulted in pediatric dosing recommendations derived solely as fractions of adult dosing rather than on intrinsic factors based on known differences in growth and development (eg, volume of distribution and maturation of the metabolic and excretory pathways). Safety and efficacy were also simply assumed to be the same in the pediatric and the adult populations, and did not take into account both known and potential safety and efficacy differences that may be present in a growing and developing pediatric patient.[2]

Efforts to increase the availability of clinical data to support evidence of efficacy and safety of drugs used in infants and children were made over the next 20 years, but it was not until congress passed the first incentives for conducting pediatric studies in the Food and Drug Modernization Act of 1997 that drug development began to include children more consistently. This provision allowed the FDA to issue a Written Request outlining the studies needed on a specific drug for 1 or more conditions or indications, including indications not approved in adults. The FDA can grant 6 months of marketing exclusivity to sponsors who complete the voluntary pediatric studies included in a Written Request. The incentives first authorized under the Food and Drug Modernization Act of 1997 were reauthorized in 2002 in the Best Pharmaceuticals for Children Act (BPCA). BPCA was permanently reauthorized for FDA in 2012 under the FDA Safety and Innovation Act. Additionally, the ability to obtain pediatric exclusivity was extended to biologic products under the Patient Protection and Affordable Care Act of 2010. The BPCA also established a partnership between the FDA and the National Institutes of Health (NIH) to conduct studies on older drugs (eg, off-patent products) used in children for which pediatric information is lacking.

In addition to incentives to conduct pediatric studies under the BPCA, congress also passed legislation to require pediatric studies for certain drugs and biologics approved in adults. The Pediatric Research Equity Act (PREA), first enacted in 2003, requires pediatric assessments of new drugs for all new active ingredients, indications, dosage forms, dosing regimens, and routes of administration. The pediatric assessment must include data adequate to assess the dosing, safety, and effectiveness of the product for the claimed indications in all relevant pediatric subpopulations. PREA works in conjunction with the BPCA but, unlike the BPCA, PREA applies only to those drugs developed for diseases and/or conditions that occur in both the adult and pediatric populations. PREA, like the BPCA, was also permanently reauthorized in 2012 under FDA Safety and Innovation Act.

## EVIDENCE TO SUPPORT APPROVAL AND PEDIATRIC EXTRAPOLATION

For new medications to be marketed in the United States, they must be approved under the FD&C Act. Under the FD&C Act, drug manufacturers must demonstrate the effectiveness of their products through the conduct of adequate and well-controlled studies to obtain marketing approval. In certain cases, the effectiveness of an approved drug product may be demonstrated adequately without additional adequate and well-controlled studies. Pediatric extrapolation is an approach that allows for effectiveness to be established in pediatric populations without controlled clinical trials and relies on a series of evidence-based assumptions. Two fundamental assumptions are that there are similar disease progressions and similar responses to intervention in the adult and pediatric populations.

Pediatric extrapolation has evolved as an approach to maximize the use of available data and to minimize the exposure of children to unnecessary clinical trials.[3,4] When pediatric extrapolation is considered, the appropriate design of pediatric studies is determined based on the level of uncertainty in the prior data and therefore the level of extrapolation (**Table 1**). The degree of uncertainty in the prior data relies on the understanding of the similarity in the natural history, pathophysiology, clinical characteristics, and outcome measures between the target pediatric population and adults. In addition, knowledge of developmental changes related to the drug target as well as on the similarity in outcomes in adults and for other drugs or biological products evaluated for the same indication provides support for leveraging prior data.

The use of pediatric extrapolation in pediatric drug development has been previously reviewed by the FDA.[5] Among 366 studies submitted to the FDA between 1998 and 2008, 1 or more adequate and well-controlled studies were required in almost 60% of the cases reviewed, suggesting that there were limitations in the available data to support extrapolation of efficacy from adult data. The FDA review also revealed that a rigorous and consistent approach to defining and establishing disease and response similarity (or lack thereof) is still missing. As the approach to pediatric extrapolation evolves, there is increasing interest in the application of Bayesian statistical methods to provide more scientific rigor and consistency when pediatric extrapolation is used. Similar to pediatric extrapolation, the ability to "borrow" adult data using Bayesian statistics relies on the understanding of degree of disease and response similarity between the 2 populations.[6] To date, there has been limited application of formal Bayesian strategies in pediatric product development. However, increased use of Bayesian strategies may improve the interpretability of data generated from pediatric studies when extrapolation of efficacy from adults is justified.

**Table 1**
Examples of extrapolation approaches and study designs

| Level of Uncertainty (Similarity of Disease, Response Similarity and/or Exposure-Response Between Adults and Pediatric Patients) | Design of Pediatric Studies | Examples with Pediatric Labeling Updates (2015–2017) |
|---|---|---|
| Low uncertainty | PK and safety study | Partial onset seizures (perampanel), asthma in adolescents (omalizumab, reslizumab), GERD (dexlansoprazole, omeprazole), cIAIs (moxifloxacin), ABSSI and CAPB (ceftaroline) |
| Some uncertainly around one of the assumptions | PK/PD studies | Regional anesthesia (tetracaine/oxymetazoline), control of serum phosphorus in chronic kidney disease (sevelamer), HIV (emtricitabine, tenofovir alafenamide), treatment of anemia (darbepoetin) |
| | Dose-controlled efficacy/safety study | Ulcerative colitis (mesalamine), |
| | Uncontrolled efficacy/safety study | Medical imaging (gadobutrol, sulfur hexafluoride/Lumason, |
| High uncertainly | Adequate and well-controlled efficacy/safety study | Type 2 diabetes, multiple sclerosis, migraine (topiramate, zolmitriptan, sumatriptan/naproxen), pain in infants (intravenous acetaminophen, oxycodone), fibromyalgia (pregabalin), chemotherapy induced nausea/vomiting (aprepitant), attention deficit hyperactivity disorder (methylphenidate-Aptensio XR), schizophrenia (asenapine), Lennox Gastaut (rufinamide), plaque psoriasis (etanercept) |

Abbreviations: ABSSI, acute bacterial skin and skin structure infections; CAPB, community-acquired bacterial pneumonia; cIAIs, complicated intraabdominal infections; GERD, gastroesophageal reflux disease; HIV, human immunodeficiency virus; PD, pharmacodynamics; PK, pharmacokinetics.

## PEDIATRIC DOSE SELECTION

Drug development in children is complicated by a relatively high trial failure rate. A recent review by the FDA showed that 42% of pediatric trials for drugs that were granted pediatric exclusivity failed to result in a pediatric indication.[7] Challenges with dose selection have been reported as important contributing factors to trial failures in children.[8,9] Therefore, understanding the effect of growth and maturation on pharmacokinetic (PK) and pharmacodynamic (PD) variability is critical for the design of pediatric trials.[10,11]

Ultimately, the goal of research and development of new medicines is to identify and confirm safe and effective dosing tailored to the target pediatric population for the intended indication. Historically, dosing in children has been viewed as a scaling exercise with a simple normalization of bodyweight or body surface area applied to the adult dose:

$$Dose_P = dose_A \times \frac{BW_P}{BW_A}$$

Where $P$ is pediatric, $A$ is adult, and BW is bodyweight.

With this equation, the developing child is ignored and the approach relies on linear scaling of body weight to adjust dose. This approach underpredicts dose requirements across the pediatric continuum though it is not equally flawed in all age and weight ranges. Substituting body surface area for bodyweight in a similar manner is used extensively in pediatric oncology settings. Again, there is sufficient experience to know that this linear scaling method underpredicts infant and neonate dosing requirements.[12]

Although the knowledge supporting dosing for older children down to infants has improved,[13] neonates and the complexities of their age, weight, and maturity continue to create a mostly empiric practice. The issue of size has been rigorously examined,[10] although the mathematical explanations defining the nonlinear relationships that govern how dosing should (or could) be optimized often confuse the caregiver and more simplistic approaches prevail.

Two primary factors drive dosing considerations for the neonate—namely, size and maturation (development stage). The issue of size is complicated by the confounding of 2 measured physiologic variables, body weight and age. In older children (>2 years of age), weight-adjusted dosing via allometric relationship or staggered by age groups (linear scaled within a common age group and then adjusted across age groups) is sufficient to address size. This is not the case for neonates. Body composition in the neonate is a dynamic variable, changing with time. Depending on the attributes of the drug itself (molecular weight, lipophilicity, permeability, etc), the impact of these shifts on drug disposition may be projected, but this effect must be balanced against what would happen owing to absorption (depending on route of administration) and elimination (based on the specific clearance mechanisms).

Allometric or power models are used in various biological settings to adjust for size dependencies of growing and developing systems. The value of the exponent varies with the type of biologic variable and there is certainly no consensus on the numeric validity of these generalized constants.

$$Y = a \times BW^b \begin{cases} b = 0.25, & \text{time} - \text{related variables} \\ b = 0.75, & \text{metabolic variables} \\ b = 1, & \text{anatomic variables} \end{cases}$$

Where $Y$ is the body part being measured in relationship to size, $a$ is the initial growth index, $b$ is the scaling exponent, and BW is bodyweight.

Systemic clearance (CL) as a key population parameter from which both maturation (MF) and organ function (OF) require consideration when adjusting for pediatric populations:

$$CL_P = CL_A \times \left(\frac{BW}{70}\right)^{0.75} \times MF \times OF$$

Maturation is generally considered a continuous function that achieves an asymptote at the adult value (MF = 1) at some finite point in development. Usually the MF is derived from a time index related to birth. Expressions for MF based on postconceptual age, postmenstrual age, postnatal age, and gestational age have been considered.[10]

Inconsistent use of terminology has limited the accurate interpretation of data on health outcomes for newborn infants, especially for those born preterm or conceived using assisted reproductive technology.[14] See Figure 1 in the article "Age Terminology During the Perinatal Period" (http://pediatrics.aappublications.org/content/114/5/1362.long) where Engle illustrates the relationship between the various age indices. These relationships are critical for the refinement of dosing considerations in the neonate and infants. Likewise, the construction of these relationships depends on the design of pediatric clinical trials, particularly the collection of within patient data in the developing neonate and infant.

## DESIGNS OF PEDIATRIC PHARMACOKINETIC AND PHARMACOKINETIC/ PHARMACODYNAMIC STUDIES

The design of PK and PK/PD studies in pediatric patients should be based on the understanding of the impact of developmental changes on PK and PD. In patients 2 years of age and older, given that most metabolic and excretory pathways are mature, PK data may be collected in a small cohort of patients as a lead-in phase to an efficacy/safety study or in some cases (adolescents) using sparse sampling during the phase III trials rather than conducting a separate PK study. In addition, age cohorts can be enrolled simultaneously rather than sequentially by age unless there are specific PK and/or safety data needed from older cohorts. A sequential design is often justified in infants and neonates where PK and/or safety data from older infants may be used for dose selection in subsequent cohorts. "Caution" alone does not justify a sequential approach, because it leads to significant delay in the completion of PK studies in pediatric patients.

The rich prior data in pediatric drug development coupled with the small population to study make the use of adaptive designs a necessity. Seamless phase II/III design is a form of adaptive design that has high relevance to pediatric development. Similar to other adaptive designs, this design provides an opportunity to adapt (eg, drop or add dose arm[s]) based on data from the early phase of study (typically PK/PD) and reduces overall sample size. As such, a seamless phase II/III design achieves within a single trial objectives that are normally achieved through 2 trials: a separate PK/PD and subsequent efficacy trial, avoiding delays from having to complete one trial before starting another. The suitability of this approach ultimately depends on many factors, including PK/PD in adults, the disease state, the safety of the product, and the age group under consideration. Furthermore, modeling and simulation can be used to predict PK and select the initial dose(s).

## ROLE OF BIOMARKERS

The need for efficient and feasible pediatric drug development programs has stimulated interest in the development of biomarkers that may substitute for clinical endpoints or optimize clinical trials. A biomarker is "a defined characteristic that is measured as an indicator of normal biological processes, pathogenic processes, or responses to an exposure or intervention, including therapeutic interventions." Molecular, histologic, radiographic, or physiologic characteristics are types of biomarkers. A biomarker is not an assessment of how an individual feels, functions, or survives. Categories of bio-markers include susceptibility/risk, diagnostic, monitoring, prognostic, predictive, PD/response, and safety. Owing to the frequent confusion about identification and qualifi-cation among researchers, the FDA–NIH Joint Leadership Council developed a resource called the BEST Resource (Biomarkers, EndpointS, and other Tools).[15]

To date, there are a limited number of validated biomarkers for use in the pediatric population.[16] In the absence of pediatric data, adult biomarkers are often applied directly to children. This approach may not take into consideration the pathophysi-ology of the pediatric disease and developmental impacts on the biomarker. Age-related changes in biologic surrogates are illustrated by the use of systolic blood pressure in antihypertensive drug trials. Blood pressure in adults is not only a biomarker, but also a surrogate marker of risk for myocardial infarction and stroke in adults. After the passage of the BPCA, the FDA issued several Written Requests to industry sponsors to perform pediatric studies for antihypertensive drugs. Contrary to findings in adults, most pediatric studies failed to show a significant reduction in systolic blood pressure. A secondary analysis of these data was performed by the FDA,[9] showing that the reason for the primary outcome failing was multifactorial (lack of dose ranging and pediatric formulations, etc) and revealed that use of diastolic blood pressure rather than systolic blood pressure reduction would have been an age-appropriate PD/response biomarker.

Biomarker development is even more challenging in neonates given that most dis-eases are unique to the neonatal age group and may not have a close correlate in older pediatric patients or adults. Pediatric trials should therefore be designed to collect and analyze biomarker data and assess PK–biomarker or biomarker–clinical endpoint re-lationships when applicable. Where there is an adult correlate, these data may inform the ability to extrapolate adult efficacy data to children using a biomarker endpoint in future trials.

## ROLE OF MODELING AND SIMULATION

In addition to innovative trial designs and development of biomarkers, modeling and simulation is increasingly used to optimize pediatric drug development. Modeling and simulation is a useful tool to systemically evaluate existing data and integrate knowledge across trials and populations. The experience with the use of model-based analysis to support regulatory decisions in pediatric drug development has been previously described and includes optimization of dose selection; substantiation of trial design; and description of dose–exposure and exposure–response relation-ships to support extrapolation of efficacy from adult data.[17–19]

As science and technology continue to advance, in silico and other alternative modeling study methods may be developed that can provide preliminary data to inform the design and conduct of PK/PD studies for investigational drugs in pediatric populations including term and preterm infants. For example, the development of a physiologically based PK in silico model that integrates drug-dependent parameters (eg, renal clearance, metabolic pathways) and system-dependent parameters (eg, non–drug parameters such as blood flow rate, protein binding, and enzyme and transporter activities) is a possible approach. Physiologically based PK has been used in pediatric drug development programs for (a) planning for a first-in-pediatric PK study, (b) optimizing the study design, (c) verifying the model in specific age groups, (d) recommending starting doses, (e) informing enzyme ontogeny using a benchmark drug, and (f) facilitating covariate analysis for the effects of organ dysfunction or drug interactions in pediatric patients.[19] The model selected should incorporate in vivo PK/PD data obtained in other groups of pediatric and adult patients as well as healthy human volunteer studies, as appropriate.

Clinical trial simulations can be performed to integrate PK, PD, disease progression, and study design considerations to help guide a pediatric drug development program. In term and preterm infants, owing to constraints related to enrollment and blood sampling, clinical trial simulations can be particularly helpful to assess sample size considerations and design a trial that is both feasible and can adequately evaluate drug exposure, effectiveness, and safety in this population.

## NEED FOR DATA SHARING AND COLLABORATION

Data sharing and cross-collaboration among investigators have been mandated by the NIH for several years,[20] but true access to raw data has been difficult to achieve. This is due to many factors, including lack of uniformity in data collection methods and data fields across investigators. Several NIH initiatives have sought to fix this, with the use of common data bases such as i2b2, and common data elements. The Eunice Kennedy Shriver National Institute of Child Health and Human Development has developed the Data and Specimen Hub,[21] which stores raw data from clinical trials in an accessible format for data manipulation.

The challenges with conducting clinical trials in the pediatric population require innovative approaches leveraged from the rare disease experience. It is imperative that the pediatric community work collaboratively to develop and label drugs for pediatric diseases including neonatal diseases. In 2014, the FDA worked with the Critical Path Institute to determine if there was sufficient interest in developing a neonatal consortium. Based on the identification of a significant number of stakeholders, the International Neonatal Consortium (INC) was launched in May 2015.[22] INC is composed of stakeholders from academia, industry, regulatory agencies, other government agencies, neonatal/parent advocacy groups, and neonatal nurses. INC has created a forum for the global neonatal community to share data, knowledge, and expertise to advance medical innovation and regulatory science for neonates to maximize opportunities to label drugs for use in neonates. Initial priorities for INC include a master protocol for the treatment of neonatal seizures, as well as white papers on neonatal clinical pharmacology white paper,[23] long-term outcome measures, classification of adverse events, and endpoints for therapeutic trials in bronchopulmonary dysplasia. New working groups have been established to discuss hemodynamic adaption, retinopathy of prematurity, necrotizing enterocolitis, and communications.

Adequately developed clinical research infrastructure is essential to address operational challenges in pediatric drug development. In 2011, the European Network of Pediatric Research at the European Medicines Agency was established as a network of research networks to enable collaboration between academia and the pharmaceutical industry, both within and outside the European Union.[24] In 2017, Institute for Advanced Clinical Trials for Children (available: https://www.iactc.org/) was launched as a new nonprofit using public–private collaboration to "optimize pediatric study designs, protocols, best practices, training and engagement of patients and parents to advance clinical trials to improve children's health."[25] These collaborative trial networks will provide the foundation to support the increase in pediatric trials that will be needed in the future.

## EXPERIENCE WITH DRUG DEVELOPMENT FOR OFF-PATENT DRUGS

Under the BPCA, funding can be granted through the NIH to studies to obtain pediatric-specific labeling information in off-patent drugs. Under this program, the Eunice Kennedy Shriver National Institute of Child Health and Human Development has been tasked to develop a program for pediatric drug development, prioritize drugs and therapeutic areas in need of study, sponsor clinical trials, and submit the data to FDA for review and potential labeling changes. The National Institute of Child Health and Human Development has sponsored more than 2 dozen pediatric clinical trials under the BPCA program resulting in more than 7 drug or device labeling changes. The experience since 2002 indicates that (a) there is a paucity of investigators with the capabilities to design and perform pediatric clinical trials, (b) there is likewise a lack of pharmacometricians with pediatric expertise, (c) incorporation of data from other sources, such as electronic health record, can provide needed real-world data that can augment prospective clinical trials, and (d) investigators must become familiar and adhere to cGCP guidance to attain FDA labeling, the highest bar for data quality.

## OPPORTUNITIES AND CHALLENGES

The implementation of the BPCA and PREA has led to the addition of specific pediatric information in more than 650 drugs and biological products (1997–2016, **Fig. 1**). Pediatric-specific product development plans are now more commonly incorporated into overall product development. However, despite the successes over the last 20 years, many challenges and opportunities remain. More than 50% of drugs commonly used in pediatrics are not labeled for pediatric use.[26] In addition, the

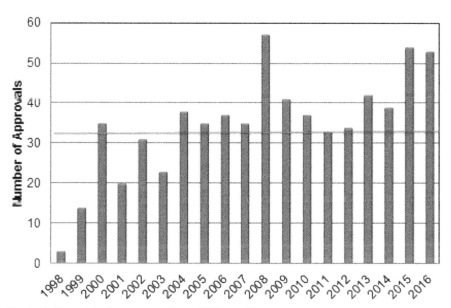

**Fig. 1.** Pediatric labeling changes from 1998 to 2016.

development of therapies for pediatric-specific diseases (eg, neonatal diseases, pediatric cancer) has lagged behind development of other pediatric diseases, in part because the requirements for conducting pediatric studies under PREA generally pertain to drugs and indications that are developed for adults. The FDA can issue Written Requests under the BPCA to encourage drug manufacturers to conduct studies for pediatric-specific diseases; however, this process is voluntary.

Despite an increasing understanding of PK, PD, and clinical conditions, clinical trials in children continue to pose practical and ethical challenges. Phenotypic variability, poorly understood natural history, maturational changes related to PK and PD, and the lack of biomarkers, outcome measures, and endpoints underscore the need to optimize the collection, analysis, and interpretation of data on PK, PD, safety, and efficacy in children.

In addition, there are clinical and operational challenges that can affect the efficiency of pediatric product development. For example, some pediatric product development programs face feasibility issues, including a small number of eligible children for clinical research. Current standards of care can influence physician and patient treatment choices that may impact pediatric clinical trial design. Alternative approaches may provide opportunities to address these issues when structured and integrated into the development program. Innovative clinical trial designs that can increase feasibility while obtaining necessary information to support the efficacy and the safety of the product for use in all relevant pediatric populations should be considered. Successful pediatric product development programs rely on the ability to recruit and retain pediatric patients. Strategies that foster input from children, their caregivers, and the advocacy communities can facilitate participation, recruitment, and acceptability of a clinical study. Finally, many pediatric product development programs are multiregional and must adhere to regional regulatory requirements. Therefore, the development of a scientific approach that is aligned across regulatory authorities can improve the efficiency and success of pediatric clinical trials.

Despite the overall advances in therapeutics development for children, there remains, on average, an 8-year lag between the time of a drug's initial approval in adults and the addition of pediatric-specific labeling information.[17] During this time, prescribers are forced to use products off-label in their pediatric patients. Many studies have shown that off-label drug use in pediatrics is associated with significantly increased risk for developing adverse drug reactions.[27,28]

Finally, pediatric-specific safety data, including long-term safety, are often not available at the time of approval. Therefore, the development of strategies to systematically capture and evaluate long-term effects in a disease or condition, and increase data interpretability should be considered. Such strategies have included patient registries that prospectively collect safety data and can include both untreated patients and patients treated with different products (eg, multiproduct and disease-based registries). The use of larger data sources, such as electronic health records systems may also be useful, if appropriate data collection methods can be standardized and consistently applied.

Meeting these challenges and opportunities will hopefully guide the future direction of pediatric therapeutics development.

## REFERENCES

1. Shirkey H. Editorial comment: therapeutic orphans. Pediatrics 1999; 104(Supplement 3):583–4.

2. Roberts R, Rodriguez W, Murphy D, et al. Pediatric drug labeling: improving the safety and efficacy of pediatric therapies. JAMA 2003;290:905–11.

3. U.S. Food and Drug Administration (FDA). Draft guidance for industry. Exposure-response relationships — Study design, data analysis, and regulatory applications 2003.
4. U.S. Food and Drug Administration (FDA). Draft guidance for industry. General clinical pharmacology considerations for pediatric studies for drugs and biological products 2014.
5. Dunne J, Rodriguez WJ, Murphy MD, et al. Extrapolation of adult data and other data in pediatric drug-development programs. Pediatrics 2011;128(5):e1242–9.
6. Gamalo-Siebers M, Savic J, Basu C, et al. Statistical modeling for Bayesian extrapolation of adult clinical trial information in pediatric drug evaluation. Pharm Stat 2017;16(4):232–49.
7. Wharton GT, Murphy MD, Avant D, et al. Impact of pediatric exclusivity on drug labeling and demonstrations of efficacy. Pediatrics 2014;134:e512–8.
8. Benjamin DK Jr, Smith PB, Jadhav P, et al. Pediatric antihypertensive trial failures: analysis of end points and dose range. Hypertension 2008;51:834–40.
9. Momper JD, Mulugeta Y, Burckart GJ. Failed pediatric drug development trials. Clin Pharmacol Ther 2015;98:245–51.
10. Anderson BJ, Holford NH. Understanding dosing: children are small adults, neonates are immature children. Arch Dis Child 2013;98(9):737–44.
11. Kearns GL, Abdel-Rahman SM, Alander SW, et al. Developmental pharmacology—drug disposition, action, and therapy in infants and children. N Engl J Med 2003;349(12):1157–67.
12. Johnson TN. The problems in scaling adult drug doses to children. Arch Dis Child 2008;93(3):207–11.
13. Zhang Y, Wei X, Bajaj G, et al. Challenges and considerations for development of therapeutic proteins in pediatric patients. J Clin Pharmacol 2015;55(S3):S103–15.
14. Engle WA. Age terminology during the perinatal period. Pediatrics 2004;114(5):1362–4.
15. US Food and Drug Administration (FDA)–National Institutes of Health (NIH) Biomarker Working Group. BEST (Biomarkers, EndpointS, and other Tools) resource. Available at: https://www.ncbi.nlm.nih.gov/books/NBK326791. Accessed December 5, 2017.
16. Savage WJ, Everett AD. Biomarkers in pediatrics: children as biomarker orphans. Proteomics Clin Appl 2010;4(12):915–21.
17. Mehrotra N, Bhattaram A, Earp JC, et al. Role of quantitative clinical pharmacology in pediatric approval and labeling. Drug Metab Dispos 2016;44(7):924–33.
18. Bhattaram VA, Bonapace C, Chilukuri DM, et al. Impact of pharmacometric reviews on new drug approval and labeling decisions-a survey of 31 new drug applications submitted between 2005 and 2006. Clin Pharmacol Ther 2007;81(2):213–21.
19. Leong R, Vieira ML, Zhao P, et al. Regulatory experience with physiologically based pharmacokinetic modeling for pediatric drug trials. Clin Pharmacol Ther 2012;91(5):926–31.
20. National Institutes of Health (NIH). FINAL NIH statement on sharing research data. Available at: https://grants.nih.gov/grants/guide/notice-files/NOT-OD-03-032.html. Accessed December 5, 2017.
21. Data and Specimen hub (DASH). Welcome to DASH. Available at: https://dash.nichd.nih.gov/. Accessed December 5, 2017.
22. Critical Path Institute (C-PATH). International Neonatal Consortium. Available at: https://c-path.org/programs/inc/. Accessed December 5, 2017.

23. Ward RM, Benjamin D, Barrett JS, et al, International Neonatal Consortium. Safety, dosing, and pharmaceutical quality for studies that evaluate medicinal products (including biological products) in neonates. Pediatr Res 2017;81(5): 692–711.

24. European Medicines Agency (EMA). European Network of Paediatric Research at the European Medicines Agency (Enpr-EMA). Available at: http://www.ema.europa.eu/ema/index.jsp?curl=pages/partners_and_networks/general/general_content_000303.jsp. Accessed December 5, 2017.

25. The Catalyst. New nonprofit – I-ACT for Children – launches to promote innovative medicines development for young patients in need. Available at: http://catalyst.phrma.org/new-nonprofit-i-act-for-children-launched-to-promote-innovative-medicines-development-for-young-patients-in-need. Accessed December 5, 2017.

26. Sachs AN, Avant D, Lee CS, et al. Pediatric information in drug product labeling. JAMA 2012;307(18):1914–5.

27. Neubert A, Dormann H, Weiss J, et al. The impact of unlicensed and off-label drug use on adverse drug reactions in paediatric patients. Drug Saf 2004; 27(13):1059–67.

28. Turner S, Nunn AJ, Fielding K, et al. Adverse drug reactions to unlicensed and off-label drugs on paediatric wards: a prospective study. Acta Paediatr 1999; 88(9):965–8.

# Approaching Current and New Drug Therapies for Pediatric Asthma

William C. Anderson III, MD[a],*, Melanie C. Gleason, MS, PA-C[b],
Naomi Miyazawa, MS, PA-C[b], Stanley J. Szefler, MD[b]

## KEYWORDS

- Drug development • Drug delivery • Adherence • Inhaled corticosteroids
- Long-acting β-agonists • Tiotropium • Biologics • Omalizumab

## KEY POINTS

- Extrapolation for the management of childhood asthma from adult pharmaceutical studies is limited, emphasizing the imperative for pediatric specific drug trials and indications.
- Families should be educated on the appropriate delivery technique for inhaled therapies, and new delivery devices that overcome technique obstacles should be considered.
- Age-specific challenges must be considered before choosing or escalating therapy, including appropriate diagnosis, family and school engagement, adherence, and psychosocial comorbidities.
- Inhaled corticosteroids (ICSs) and long-acting β-agonists (LABAs) are the principal controller therapies for persistent asthma, with new ICS formulations improving delivery and recent studies supporting the safety of LABAs.
- Controller therapies previously approved for adult asthma, including tiotropium and biologics, are now being investigated in younger children with associated clinical benefits.

Disclosure Statement: SJ Szefler is supported by the Colorado Department of Public Health and Environment 15 FLA 65765, 16 FHLA 76546 and 17FHLA87312, Caring for Colorado Foundation, the McCormick Foundation and Glaxo Smith Kline FLV116794. Also supported by NHLBI AsthmaNet U10 HL098075 and supported in part by Colorado CTSA Grant UL1 RR025780 from NCRR/NIH and UL1 TR000154 from NIH/NCATS.
MC Gleason is supported by Colorado Department of Public Health and Environment 15 FLA 65765, 16 FHLA 76546 and 17FHLA87312, Caring for Colorado Foundation, the McCormick Foundation and GlaxoSmithKline FLV116794.
[a] Section of Allergy and Immunology, Department of Pediatrics, University of Colorado School of Medicine, Children's Hospital Colorado, 13123 East 16th Avenue, Aurora, CO 80045, USA;
[b] The Breathing Institute, Department of Pediatrics, University of Colorado School of Medicine, Children's Hospital Colorado, 13123 East 16th Avenue, Aurora, CO 80045, USA
* Corresponding author.
E-mail address: william.anderson@childrenscolorado.org

## INTRODUCTION: PEDIATRIC ASTHMA DRUG DEVELOPMENT

A gap exists between the imperative need for novel pharmaceutical therapies for children and their development. A recent review demonstrated that despite children being responsible for almost half of the disease burden from asthma in high-income countries, less than 20% of asthma trials during that time had a pediatric focus.[1] Interventions have been made to spur pediatric drug development. The Best Pharmaceuticals for Children Act allows an additional 6 months of market exclusivity if the sponsor voluntarily includes pediatric studies.[2,3] The Pediatric Research Equity Act mandates that new drug studies include children if there is the potential for the drug to be used in the pediatric population.[2,3] Collectively, the Best Pharmaceuticals for Children Act and Pediatric Research Equity Act successfully resulted in more than 500 pediatric labeling changes since their inception.[4] Nonetheless, drugs for asthma are still frequently prescribed off-label in children, primarily secondary to age limits, with 24% to 45% of short-acting β-agonists (SABAs) and 26% to 80% of ICSs used off-label.[5]

The extrapolation of efficacy findings from adults to the pediatric population has streamlined the developmental process in adolescents and older children.[6] This strategy cannot be used in neonates, infants, and children given differences in respiratory function, immunology, and disease pathogenesis,[7] creating a substantial unmet need. Without evidence to support this off-label use, patients may be exposed to potential unintended harms.[3] Trying to extrapolate from adult studies to design pediatric studies can lead to study failure and subsequent lack of pediatric labeling, secondary to a lack of efficacy, inability to use the delivery device, limited drug dosing ranges, or safety concerns.[8]

This review highlights the forefront of pharmacologic therapies for the management of asthma in children, with a focus on their implications for clinicians in practice and potential limitations.

## DELIVERY DEVICES

Inhaled medications, especially ICSs and ICSs/long-acting β-agonists (LABAs), are the mainstay of treatment of the management of pediatric asthma.[9] The inhaled route for delivery of asthma medication is preferred to oral administration due to advantages associated with local delivery, including lower dosage, fewer systemic side effects, and quick onset of action.[10] The downside of inhaled therapy is the difficulty some patients, especially children, may have in applying appropriate inhaler technique, emphasizing the attention that must be paid to technique and delivery device when choosing a therapy.[11]

A metered-dose inhaler (MDI) with an add-on valve holding chamber (VHC), with or without a mask, is the principal delivery device in the pediatric population, improving delivery of medication to the lower respiratory tract.[12] When caregivers of children with asthma were surveyed, however, fewer than 4% were able to perform all the essential steps to correctly use an MDI with a VHC.[13] Technique should be checked and reinforced at every health care visit, and trainers, if available, should be used to assess adequate technique before dispensing. Families may feel nebulizers are an alternative to MDIs; however, studies using MDIs with spacers for SABAs found MDIs noninferior and more cost-effective than nebulizers.[14,15] Dry powder, breath-actuated devices are successful at removing some of the coordination barriers with MDI with VHC, but patients, including children, may have difficulty generating the appropriate inspiratory force to utilize these devices.[11]

Recently, new medication delivery devices with pediatric indications have been introduced to enhance optimal deposition into the lower respiratory tract and ease delivery. RespiClick (Teva Respiratory, Petach Tikva, Israel) is a dry powder form of SABA that does not require a VHC, which is Food and Drug Administration (FDA) approved down to 4 years old.[16] Respimat Soft Mist Inhaler (Bohringer Ingelheim, Ingelheim am Rhein, Germany), which is FDA approved for patients 6 years and older, combines the advantages of an MDI and a nebulizer to aerosolize propellant free-drug solutions as a soft mist, acting by way of a tension spring.[10] Aerospan (Meda, Somerset, New Jersey) is an ICS that has a built-in spacer, eliminating the need for patients to use a separate VHC.[17]

## AGE-SPECIFIC CHALLENGES TO ASTHMA THERAPY

National Heart, Lung, and Blood Institute (NHLBI) guidelines categorize asthma management by age group: 0 to 4 years, 5 years to 11 years, and greater than 12 years.[9] Beyond the problems with drug delivery (discussed previously) that can affect all ages, within each of these populations unique age-specific challenges exist that have an impact on drug development and clinical implementation.

### Young Children: 0 to 4 Years Old

Although wheezing with viral illness is common in young children, most tend to have transient wheezing, with episodes only 2 to 3 times per year.[18,19] Therefore, one of the treatment challenges for this age group is identifying which child with recurrent wheeze will benefit from routine use of a controller asthma medication. Current guidance from the Global Initiative for Asthma (GINA) recommends a probability-based approach, using frequency and severity of symptoms to guide treatment decisions, with a therapeutic trial of a controller medication for 2 months to 3 months.[18,20] As patterns of symptoms emerge over time for in individual child, the diagnosis and need for a controller medication should be reviewed regularly.[20] Treatment failure despite good adherence and correct technique should prompt early referral to rule out alternative diagnosis.[18,19]

Another commonly used approach for predicting likelihood of transient wheeze versus emerging asthma is to apply the Asthma Predictive Index to assess children with 4 or more wheezing episodes.[21] The Asthma Predictive Index takes into consideration the presence of atopy, adding additional support for predicting which children are more likely to have persistent wheezing.[21] This tool has a high negative predictive value in children with recurrent wheezing.[21] Lack of atopy does not rule out asthma, making it equally important to identify and treat children with nonallergic asthma.[18]

### School-Aged Children: 5 Years Old to 11 Years Old

The social environment of children 5 years old to 11 years old, consisting of family and peer networks at school, affect medication choice and adherence.[22] Although these children are learning to be more independent, they still require adult supervision for their medications, making both the attitudes from these caregivers and their own state of health strong determinants of medication adherence in these children.[22,23] For an optimal outcome and improved adherence, the provider should establish a practice of good education, child and parent communication, and standardization of care through established guidelines and standardized asthma control questionnaires.[24] Although parent engagement is paramount, the children also should be engaged in the clinic visit as they are beginning to understand their asthma, triggers, and basic medications, learning more detail as they get older.

At school, children in this age group want to belong and not be stigmatized by their peers for taking medications.[22] Taking medications at school and missing out or being limited in their participation with activities can affect a child's emotional state and contribute to poor adherence and school attendance.[25] Involving the school nurse or designated personnel with the monitoring and facilitation of medications during school has been shown to improve adherence, attendance, and participation.[26]

### Adolescents: 12 Years Old to 18 Years Old

Adolescents benefit from their grouping with adults in terms of their asthma management per NHLBI guideline recommendations,[9] often being the first group of pediatric-aged patients to gain FDA approval for new medications, such as omalizumab[27] and mepolizumab,[28] before younger populations. When prescribing or researching new drugs in adolescents, psychosocial challenges must be addressed that are unique to this population.[29,30] It is imperative to address these issues because adolescents have a higher morbidity and mortality from asthma than younger children but are less likely to seek medical treatment either routinely or in an emergency department.[29]

A primary obstacle to care in adolescents is poor medication adherence.[29–31] According to a telephone survey, based on parental report, adolescents assume 75% of their daily controller medication responsibility by age 15% and 100% of the responsibility by age 19,[32] underscoring the potential substantial impact of nonadherence in adolescents. The etiologies of this nonadherence in adolescents are multifactorial, including changes in cognitive development, desire for peer approval, anxiety and depression, and risk-taking behavior.[29–31,33–36] Before a clinician prescribes escalating therapies in adolescents, these conditions should be explored for potential reasons for poor control or medication nonadherence.

## UPDATES ON PHARMACEUTICAL THERAPIES

NHLBI and GINA provide guideline-based therapy for the management of asthma, which the authors believe are an invaluable resource for clinicians.[9,18] As therapies progress, new analysis should be paid toward the formulations and safety of mainstays of therapy, including ICSs, leukotriene receptor agonists (LTRAs), and LABAs, as well as the potential incorporation of new controller medications, which have recently been established in adults.

### Inhaled Corticosteroids

ICSs are an effective anti-inflammatory treatment and are still considered first-line therapy in the treatment of persistent asthma in children.[9,18] The formulation and subsequent delivery of ICSs are evolving. The new propellant hydrofluoroalkane (HFA) has led to smaller particle size steroids.[37] Lung deposition has significantly improved with the smaller particle size to approximately 50% to 60% compared with 20% with the larger particle size.[37] The smaller particle size has also improved administration discoordination effects typically seen with other large particle size ICS due their longer suspension within a VHC.[37] A Cochrane review comparing 3 HFA ICSs, ciclesonide, beclomethasone, and fluticasone propionate, in the treatment of chronic asthma in children less than 18 years of age for 12 weeks concluded that there was no 1 ICS that was superior in terms of safety, efficacy, and lung function outcomes.[38] In a historical matched cohort study of children 5 years old to 11 years old with asthma, children prescribed small-particle HFA ICSs had greater odds of asthma control and lower severe exacerbation rates when used as initial controller therapy or step-up therapy compared with standard-sized particle ICS.[39] Stepped-up small-particle HFA ICS dose had similar efficacy as ICS/LABA combination therapy.[39]

The bioavailability of HFA formulations combine oral and pulmonary vasculature absorption and therefore potentially have direct impact on the overall safety of these drugs.

Previous studies have shown concern for growth suppression from use of ICS in growing children, with long-term effects of a 1.2-cm reduction in overall adult mean height.[40] Systemic adverse effects on linear growth and hypothalamic-pituitary-adrenal axis suppression vary on formulations and are certainly dose dependent, but several studies have shown that ciclesonide, an HFA, compared with budesonide and fluticasone propionate, showed less growth suppression and little to no effect on hypothalamic-pituitary-adrenal axis function.[41–43]

### Leukotriene Modifiers

LTRAs have proved effective in exercise-induced asthma, allergic asthma, obese patients with asthma, and asthmatics who smoke as well as children exposed to tobacco smoke, aspirin-exacerbated respiratory disease, and preschool-aged patients with viral-induced wheezing.[44,45] Montelukast, the most widely used, studied, and tolerated LTRA, has been approved down to age 12 months.[46] Montelukast may be a favorable alternative for some patients who prefer not to use ICSs due its generic availability and once-daily dosing; however, they are not the preferred treatment of the management of persistent asthma per NHLBI guidelines.[9]

LTRAs have been generally well tolerated, with a good safety profile, but there has been some conflicting evidence with the use of montelukast and neuropsychiatric events.[44] LTRAs are associated with a higher incidence of eosinophilic granulomatosis with polyangiitis, previously known as Churg-Strauss syndrome, but its causality has yet to be proved.[47]

### Long-Acting β-Agonists

LABAs, administered in the form of a fixed-dose ICS/LABA combination therapy, are the preferred step-up treatment of moderate to severe persistent asthmatic patients who remain uncontrolled on ICS alone.[9,18] Although commonly used in the pediatric age group, this class of medication carries a black box warning, focused on an increased risk of severe asthma exacerbations and asthma-related death, and has a strong recommendation to transition to ICS monotherapy once asthma control is attained.[48]

Due to these safety concerns, the FDA mandated large postmarketing safety clinical trials to assess serious adverse effects in both pediatric and adult populations.[49] The pediatric study, which enrolled more than 6200 participants, demonstrated that ICS/LABA combination therapy, fluticasone propionate/salmeterol, had a risk of serious asthma-related events similar to the risk of fluticasone alone, and there were no asthma-related deaths.[49,50] The study in adolescents and adults had a similar finding in regard to serious asthma-related events.[50] Although not a primary safety endpoint, the number of pediatric patients who had a severe asthma exacerbation was 25% lower in the group who remained on fixed-dose combination therapy compared with those who were transitioned to ICS monotherapy.[49] This finding may have implications that should be considered when switching from ICS/LABA combination therapy to ICS alone. At the time of this writing, the FDA has not yet removed the black box warning on any of the currently available asthma medications that contain an LABA as a component, even in fixed combination with an ICS.

### Tiotropium

As with most new therapeutics moving into the pediatric population, initial studies on the benefit of tiotropium add-on therapy focused on adolescents. In patients 12 years old to 17 years old with moderate symptomatic asthma requiring ICS controller therapy with or without an LTRA, but without an LABA, the addition of tiotropium via the Respimat inhaler improved their lung function, including peak and trough forced expiratory volume in the first second of expiration ($FEV_1$) and morning and evening peak expiratory flow.[51,52] These lung function improvements, however, were not observed when tiotropium was added to high-dose ICS with 1 or more controllers, including LABA or LTRA, or medium-dose ICS with 2 or more controllers.[53] The study investigators posited that lack of efficacy may be secondary to a pronounced placebo response, poor treatment adherence, and short trial duration.[53]

Few data have been published on the use of tiotropium in younger children. In children 6 years old to 11 years old with symptomatic asthma requiring medium-dose ICS with or without LTRA, the addition of tiotropium similarly improved peak and trough $FEV_1$ and morning peak expiratory flow compared with placebo.[54] Despite this benefit, there was no statistically significant improvement in asthma control scores.[54] As the use of long-acting anticholinergics as add-on therapy to asthma management in children continues, several questions remain unanswered, including evidence on the long term-safety, the efficacy of tiotropium compared with LABAs and LTRA individually as add-on therapy, and biomarkers to predict treatment response.[55]

### Oral Steroids for Acute Exacerbations

Over the past 5 years to 10 years, there has been increasing use of dexamethasone in lieu of prednisone for the treatment of acute asthma in emergency departments. Dexamethasone is favored in the acute setting due to its shorter course of treatment, less need for repeat doses, and better taste resulting in less vomiting.[56,57] Compared with prednisone or prednisolone, dexamethasone is a long-acting corticosteroid with a half-life of 36 hours to 72 hours, which, when administered as a single dose or 2 doses over a 2-day period, is equivalent to a 5-day course of prednisone.[58] As opposed to dexamethasone, many patients prescribed several-day courses of prednisone were not adherent in filling their prescription, thus leading to a return to an emergency department.[57–59] In the inpatient setting, dexamethasone reduced overall length of stay for exacerbations compared with prednisone, and there was no significant difference between dexamethasone and prednisone in all-cause readmission rates.[56]

### Biologics

Biologics represent a new advance in individualized, precision medicine for the treatment of severe pediatric asthma that has failed to respond to the standards of care (discussed previously). The biologic with the most experience in the pediatric population is omalizumab, an anti-IgE monoclonal antibody, which has recently been approved by the FDA down to the age of 6 years.[27] Omalizumab has been reported to reduce asthma exacerbation rates, symptom days, hospitalizations, urgent physician visits, missed school days, and daily rescue medication use in children with persistent allergic asthma as young as 6 years old.[60]

In inner-city children 6 years old to 20 years old, the addition of omalizumab to guideline-based therapy decreased the number of days with asthma symptoms, reduced the proportion of participants with exacerbations, and allowed for a greater reduction of ICS and LABA controller therapy compared with placebo.[61] Omalizumab blunted the seasonal spring and fall asthma exacerbations typically seen in this population.[61] Extending from this ability of omalizumab to prevent fall exacerbations, a study of asthmatic children 6 years to 17 years of age with at least 1 recent exacerbation found that the addition of omalizumab 4 weeks to 6 weeks prior to return to school in the fall reduced the exacerbation rate, with the greatest benefit found in those requiring NHLBI step 5 care and those with an exacerbation during the run-in period.[62]

Mepolizumab, an anti–interleukin 5 monoclonal antibody, has been approved for adolescents with eosinophilic asthma as young as 12 years old.[28] Mepolizumab as an add-on therapy has been associated with a reduction in asthma exacerbations, improved $FEV_1$, asthma control scores, and reduced maintenance daily oral corticosteroid dose.[60,63] Because mepolizumab is used more in adolescents, special attention should be paid to its effectiveness and potential side-effect profiles, because the clinical trials to gain FDA approval included proportionally few adolescents.[63,64]

A practical limitation to the use of these biologics is their associated financial cost. When comparing GINA steps 4 and 5 treatment escalation options, the addition of omalizumab resulted in a more than $20,000 increase in annual health care expenditures compared with $2000 to $3000 with the use of oral corticosteroids or high-dose ICS.[65]

## SUMMARY

This review focuses on new information related to the management of childhood asthma, much of it over the past 5 years. Detailed information on asthma management, including in children, is contained in GINA. GINA is profiled as an asthma strategy rather than a guideline because countries differ by the availability, regulatory approval, and cost of medications.[18] Countries are, therefore, encouraged to develop their own set of local guidelines based on those individual parameters. Asthma guidelines, however, take a significant amount of time and resources to update. The US NHLBI asthma guidelines, as an example, are currently in the process of being revised after a 10-year period of time.[9]

As described in this review, many things can happen over a very short period of time, and thus guidelines need to be revised frequently. In particular, new developments involve the introduction of new medications, aspects of prevention of asthma exacerbations, and even prevention of the onset of the disease. Furthermore, new directions are taking place to link biomarkers, patient characteristics, and genetics to medication responses in an effort to individualize treatments.[66] This effort will help to bring the right medication to the right patient at the right period of time in the evolution of asthma.

As the new biologics are evaluated in children, especially young children, a shift may be seen in the treatment paradigm to use these medications at the early onset of disease rather than the very late stages. This approach occurred with the management of rheumatoid arthritis more than 15 years ago and played a significant role in altering the course of the disease and served to prevent irreversible changes in joint structure. A similar approach with asthma could serve to prevent deleterious long term adverse adult outcomes of childhood respiratory disease, such as chronic obstructive pulmonary disease.[67] It is apparent that this work is moving rapidly along and more changes in the management of childhood asthma over the next 10 years can be expected.

## REFERENCES

1. Bourgeois FT, Murthy S, Pinto C, et al. Pediatric versus adult drug trials for conditions with high pediatric disease burden. Pediatrics 2012;130(2):285–92.
2. England A, Wade K, Smith PB, et al, Best Pharmaceuticals for Children Act - Pediatric Trials Network Administrative Core Committee. Optimizing operational efficiencies in early phase trials: the pediatric trials network experience. Contemp Clin Trials 2016;47:376–82.

3. Bourgeois FT, Hwang TJ. The pediatric research equity act moves into adolescence. J Am Med Assoc 2017;317(3):259–60.

4. Frattarelli DA, Galinkin JL, Green TP, et al. Off-label use of drugs in children. Pediatrics 2014;133(3):563–7.

5. Silva D, Ansotegui I, Morais-Almeida M. Off-label prescribing for allergic diseases in children. World Allergy Organ J 2014;7(1):4.

6. Vinks AA, Emoto C, Fukuda T. Modeling and simulation in pediatric drug therapy: application of pharmacometrics to define the right dose for children. Clin Pharmacol Ther 2015;98(3):298–308.

7. Szefler SJ, Chmiel JF, Fitzpatrick AM, et al. Asthma across the ages: knowledge gaps in childhood asthma. J Allergy Clin Immunol 2014;133(1):3–13 [quiz: 14].

8. Momper JD, Mulugeta Y, Burckart GJ. Failed pediatric drug development trials. Clin Pharmacol Ther 2015;98(3):245–51.

9. National Asthma Education and Prevention Program. Expert panel report 3 (EPR-3): guidelines for the diagnosis and management of asthma - sumary report 2007. J Allergy Clin Immunol 2007;120(5 Suppl):S94–138.

10. Ibrahim M, Verma R, Garcia-Contreras L. Inhalation drug delivery devices: technology update. Med Devices (Auckl) 2015;8:131–9.

11. Braido F, Chrystyn H, Baiardini I, et al. "Trying, But Failing" - The role of inhaler technique and mode of delivery in respiratory medication adherence. J Allergy Clin Immunol Pract 2016;4(5):823–32.

12. Shaw N, Le Souef P, Turkovic L, et al. Pressurised metered dose inhaler-spacer technique in young children improves with video instruction. Eur J Pediatr 2016;175(7):1007–12.

13. Reznik M, Silver EJ, Cao Y. Evaluation of MDI-spacer utilization and technique in caregivers of urban minority children with persistent asthma. J Asthma 2014; 51(2):149–54.

14. Dhuper S, Chandra A, Ahmed A, et al. Efficacy and cost comparisons of bronchodilatator administration between metered dose inhalers with disposable spacers and nebulizers for acute asthma treatment. J Emerg Med 2011;40(3):247–55.

15. Leversha AM, Campanella SG, Aickin RP, et al. Cost and effectiveness of spacer versus nebulizer in young children with moderate and severe acute asthma. J Pediatr 2000;136(4):497–502.

16. Teva. ProAir RespiClick: FDA prescribing information. 2016. Available at: http://proair.com/respiclick/library/docs/PI.pdf. Accessed May 15, 2017.

17. Meda. Aerospan: FDA Prescribing information. 2015. Available at: http://aerospanrx.com/pdf/aerospan-pi.pdf. Accessed May 15, 2017.

18. Global Initiative for Asthma. Global strategy for asthma management and prevention, 2017. Available at: www.ginasthma.org. Accessed May 17, 2017.

19. Ren CL, Esther CR Jr, Debley JS, et al. Official American thoracic society clinical practice guidelines: diagnostic evaluation of infants with recurrent or persistent wheezing. Am J Respir Crit Care Med 2016;194(3):356–73.

20. Reddel HK, Bateman ED, Becker A, et al. A summary of the new GINA strategy: a roadmap to asthma control. Eur Respir J 2015;46(3):622–39.

21. Castro-Rodriguez JA, Holberg CJ, Wright AL, et al. A clinical index to define risk of asthma in young children with recurrent wheezing. Am J Respir Crit Care Med 2000;162:1403–6.

22. Costello RW, Foster JM, Grigg J, et al. The seven stages of man: the role of developmental stage on medication adherence in respiratory diseases. J Allergy Clin Immunol Pract 2016;4(5):813–20.

23. Grossoehme DH, Szczesniak RD, Britton LL, et al. Adherence determinants in cystic fibrosis: cluster analysis of parental psychosocial, religious, and/or spiritual factors. Ann Am Thorac Soc 2015;12(6):838–46.

24. Okelo SO, Eakin MN, Riekert KA, et al. Validation of parental reports of asthma trajectory, burden, and risk by using the pediatric asthma control and communication instrument. J Allergy Clin Immunol Pract 2014;2(2):186–92.

25. Schneider J, Wedgewood N, Llewellyn G, et al. Families challenged by and accommodating to the adolescent years. J Intellect Disabil Res 2006;50(Pt 12): 926–36.

26. Keeton V, Soleimanpour S, Brindis CD. School-based health centers in an era of health care reform: building on history. Curr Probl Pediatr Adolesc Health Care 2012;42(6):132–56 [discussion: 157–8].

27. Genentech. Xolair: FDA prescribing information. 2016. Available at: https://www.gene.com/download/pdf/xolair_prescribing.pdf. Accessed May 8, 2017.

28. GlaxoSmithKline. Nucala: FDA prescribing information. 2017. Available at: https://www.gsksource.com/pharma/content/dam/GlaxoSmithKline/US/en/Prescribing_Information/Nucala/pdf/NUCALA-PI-PIL.PDF. Accessed May 8, 2017.

29. Couriel J. Asthma in adolescence. Paediatric Respir Rev 2003;4(1):47–54.

30. Bitsko MJ, Everhart RS, Rubin BK. The adolescent with asthma. Paediatr Respir Rev 2014;15(2):146–53.

31. Stukus DR, Nassef M, Rubin M. Leaving home: helping teens with allergic conditions become independent. Ann Allergy Asthma Immunol 2016;116(5):388–91.

32. Orrell-Valente JK, Jarlsberg LG, Hill LG, et al. At what age do children start taking daily asthma medicines on their own? Pediatrics 2008;122(6):e1186–1192.

33. American Academy of Pediatrics, American Academy of Family Pediatrics, American College of Pediatrics, Transitions Clinical Report Authoring Group, Cooley WC, Sagerman PJ. Supporting the health care transition from adolescence to adulthood in the medical home. Pediatrics 2011;128(1):182–200.

34. Srivastava SA, Elkin SL, Bilton D. The transition of adolescents with chronic respiratory illness to adult care. Paediatr Respir Rev 2012;13(4):230–5 [quiz: 235].

35. Bender BG. Risk taking, depression, adherence, and symptom control in adolescents and young adults with asthma. Am J Respir Crit Care Med 2006;173(9): 953–7.

36. Lu Y, Mak KK, van Bever HP, et al. Prevalence of anxiety and depressive symptoms in adolescents with asthma: a meta-analysis and meta-regression. Pediatr Allergy Immunol 2012;23(8):707 16.

37. Leach C, Colice GL, Luskin A. Particle size of inhaled corticosteroids: does it matter? J Allergy Clin Immunol 2009;124(6 Suppl):S88–93.

38. Kramer S, Rottier BL, Scholten RJ, et al. Ciclesonide versus other inhaled corticosteroids for chronic asthma in children. Cochrane Database Syst Rev 2013;(2):CD010352.

39. van Aalderen WM, Grigg J, Guilbert TW, et al. Small-particle inhaled corticosteroid as first-line or step-up controller therapy in childhood asthma. J Allergy Clin Immunol Pract 2015;3(5):721–31.e16.

40. Kelly HW, Sternberg AL, Lescher R, et al. Effect of inhaled glucocorticoids in childhood on adult height. N Engl J Med 2012;367(10):904–12.

41. Gentile DA, Skoner DP. New asthma drugs: small molecule inhaled corticosteroids. Curr Opin Pharmacol 2010;10(3):260–5.

42. Agertoft L, Pedersen S. Lower-leg growth rates in children with asthma during treatment with ciclesonide and fluticasone propionate. Pediatr Allergy Immunol 2010;21(1 Pt 2):e199–205.

43. von Berg A, Engelstatter R, Minic P, et al. Comparison of the efficacy and safety of ciclesonide 160 microg once daily vs. budesonide 400 microg once daily in children with asthma. Pediatr Allergy Immunol 2007;18(5):391–400.

44. Marcello C, Carlo L. Asthma phenotypes: the Intriguing selective intervention with Montelukast. Asthma Res Pract 2016;2:11.

45. Pyasi K, Tufvesson E, Moitra S. Evaluating the role of leukotriene-modifying drugs in asthma management: are their benefits 'losing in translation'? Pulm Pharmacol Ther 2016;41:52–9.

46. Merck. Singulair: FDA Prescribing information. 2012. Available at: https://www.accessdata.fda.gov/drugsatfda_docs/label/2012/021409s036lbl.pdf. Accessed May 16, 2017.

47. Choby GW, Lee S. Pharmacotherapy for the treatment of asthma: current treatment options and future directions. Int Forum Allergy Rhinol 2015;5(Suppl 1): S35–40.

48. Butler MG, Zhou EH, Zhang F, et al. Changing patterns of asthma medication use related to US Food and Drug Administration long-acting beta2-agonist regulation from 2005-2011. J Allergy Clin Immunol 2016;137(3):710–7.

49. Stempel DA, Szefler SJ, Pedersen S, et al. Safety of adding salmeterol to fluticasone propionate in children with asthma. N Engl J Med 2016;375(9):840–9.

50. Bush A, Frey U. Safety of long-acting beta-agonists in children with asthma. N Engl J Med 2016;375(9):889–91.

51. Vogelberg C, Engel M, Moroni-Zentgraf P, et al. Tiotropium in asthmatic adolescents symptomatic despite inhaled corticosteroids: a randomised dose-ranging study. Respir Med 2014;108(9):1268–76.

52. Hamelmann E, Bateman ED, Vogelberg C, et al. Tiotropium add-on therapy in adolescents with moderate asthma: a 1-year randomized controlled trial. J Allergy Clin Immunol 2016;138(2):441–50.e8.

53. Hamelmann E, Bernstein JA, Vandewalker M, et al. A randomised controlled trial of tiotropium in adolescents with severe symptomatic asthma. Eur Respir J 2017; 49(1) [pii:1601100].

54. Vogelberg C, Moroni-Zentgraf P, Leonaviciute-Klimantaviciene M, et al. A randomised dose-ranging study of tiotropium Respimat(R) in children with symptomatic asthma despite inhaled corticosteroids. Respir Res 2015;16:20.

55. Vogelberg C. Emerging role of long-acting anticholinergics in children with asthma. Curr Opin Pulm Med 2016;22(1):74–9.

56. Parikh K, Hall M, Mittal V, et al. Comparative effectiveness of dexamethasone versus prednisone in children hospitalized with asthma. J Pediatr 2015;167(3): 639–44.e1.

57. Keeney GE, Gray MP, Morrison AK, et al. Dexamethasone for acute asthma exacerbations in children: a meta-analysis. Pediatrics 2014;133(3):493–9.

58. Andrews AL, Wong KA, Heine D, et al. A cost-effectiveness analysis of dexamethasone versus prednisone in pediatric acute asthma exacerbations. Acad Emerg Med 2012;19(8):943–8.

59. Cronin J, Kennedy U, McCoy S, et al. Single dose oral dexamethasone versus multi-dose prednisolone in treatment of acute exacerbations of asthma in children who attend the emergency department: study protocol for a randomized controlled trial. Trials 2012;13:141.

60. Federico MJ, Hoch HE, Anderson WC 3rd, et al. Asthma management for children: risk identification and prevention. Adv Pediatr 2016;63(1):103–26.

61. Busse WW, Morgan WJ, Gergen PJ, et al. Randomized trail of omalizumab (anti-IgE) for asthma in inner-city children. N Engl J Med 2011;364:1005–15.

62. Teach SJ, Gill MA, Togias A, et al. Preseasonal treatment with either omalizumab or an inhaled corticosteroid boost to prevent fall asthma exacerbations. J Allergy Clin Immunol 2015;136(6):1476–85.

63. Anderson WC 3rd, Szefler SJ. New and future strategies to improve asthma control in children. J Allergy Clin Immunol 2015;136(4):848–59.

64. Huffaker MF, Phipatanakul W. Pediatric asthma: guidelines-based care, omalizumab, and other potential biologic agents. Immunol Allergy Clin North Am 2015; 35(1):129–44.

65. Sullivan PW, Campbell JD, Ghushchyan VH, et al. Outcomes before and after treatment escalation to global initiative for asthma steps 4 and 5 in severe asthma. Ann Allergy Asthma Immunol 2015;114(6):462–9.

66. Fitzpatrick AM, Jackson DJ, Mauger DT, et al. Individualized therapy for persistent asthma in young children. J Allergy Clin Immunol 2016;138(6):1608–18.e12.

67. McGeachie MJ, Yates KP, Zhou X, et al. Patterns of growth and decline in lung function in persistent childhood asthma. N Engl J Med 2016;374(19):1842–52.

# Psychopharmacology of Bipolar Disorders in Children and Adolescents

Ekaterina Stepanova, MD, PhD[a],*, Robert L. Findling, MD, MBA[b]

## KEYWORDS

- Bipolar disorder • Pharmacotherapy • Children • Adolescents • Pediatric

## KEY POINTS

- Bipolar disorder is a chronic condition that oftentimes requires pharmacologic intervention.
- There are limited medication data available.
- Most studies targeted short-term treatment.

## INTRODUCTION

Bipolar disorder is a chronic and debilitating illness that often begins early in life, with the first episode frequently occurring in adolescence.[1,2] Compared with adults, youth diagnosed with bipolar disorder experience more severe symptoms and have poorer prognosis.[3] Bipolar disorder is estimated to be the fourth leading source of disability in individuals of 10 to 24 years of age.[4]

The recommended treatment for bipolar disorder includes a combination of psychopharmacological and psychosocial interventions.[5] Until recently, very limited data pertaining to pharmacologic management of pediatric bipolar disorder were available, and children were essentially treated as "small adults," with clinicians adapting

Disclosure Statement: Dr R.L. Findling receives or has received research support, acted as a consultant and/or served on a speaker's bureau for Actavis, Akili, Alcobra, American Academy of Child & Adolescent Psychiatry, American Psychiatric Press, Bracket, CogCubed, Cognition Group, Coronado Biosciences, Elsevier, Epharma Solutions, Forest, Genentech, GlaxoSmithKline, Guilford Press, Ironshore, Johns Hopkins University Press, KemPharm, Lundbeck, Medgenics, Merck, NIH, Neurim, Novartis, Otsuka, PCORI, Pfizer, Physicians Postgraduate Press, Purdue, Rhodes Pharmaceuticals, Roche, Sage, Shire, Sunovion, Supernus Pharmaceuticals, Syneurx, Takeda, Teva, Tris, Validus, and WebMD. Dr E. Stepanova receives research support from PsychNostics, LLC.

[a] Johns Hopkins University School of Medicine, Childrens' Mental Health Center, 401 North Caroline Street, Baltimore, MD 21231, USA; [b] Department of Psychiatry, Division of Child and Adolescent Psychiatry Johns Hopkins University School of Medicine, 1800 Orleans Street, Baltimore, MD 21287, USA
* Corresponding author.
*E-mail address:* estepan2@jhmi.edu

information from clinical trials on adults. However, the efficacy and safety profiles of pharmacologic interventions appear to be different in youth and adults.[6]

Pharmacotherapy of youth with bipolar disorder can be challenging. The choice of medication mostly depends on the phase of illness (manic, depressive, or maintenance treatment). In this review, we examine the current evidence for pharmacologic management of bipolar disorder in youth based on the phase of illness. In addition, we discuss medications currently approved by the Food and Drug Administration (FDA) for the treatment of bipolar disorder (**Table 1**), and summarize studies directly comparing monotherapy options (**Table 2**) and combinations of different classes of medications (**Table 3**). Although the focus of this review is pharmacotherapy of pediatric bipolar disorder, psychosocial interventions are important and should not be discounted.

## ACUTE MONOTHERAPY OF MANIC AND MIXED STATES
### Lithium and Anticonvulsants

Lithium has been the gold standard for treatment of bipolar disorder in adults. It is also the first medication approved by the FDA for pharmacotherapy of bipolar disorder in children 12 years and older. At the time of its approval, all recommendations regarding dosing, safety, and efficacy were adapted from adult data. In efforts to bridge this gap, the Collaborative Lithium Trials (CoLT) examined dosing strategies, pharmacokinetics, safety, and short-term and long-term efficacy of lithium in youth aged 7 to 17.[7] In an open-label trial, lithium was found to be reasonably effective in reducing symptoms of a manic or mixed episode. Interestingly, only initial responders to lithium during the first 8 weeks maintained mood stabilization over the next 16 weeks.[8] The efficacy of lithium as a treatment for bipolar disorder has been further documented in a double-blind placebo-controlled trial[9] (**Table 4**). Lithium was superior to placebo in reducing symptoms during manic or mixed episode as well as increasing Clinical Global Impression-Improvement scores.

The Treatment of Early Age Mania Study (TEAM) describes a direct comparison of lithium, divalproex, and risperidone. In this randomized clinical trial, more youngsters with bipolar disorder responded to risperidone than to lithium or divalproex.[10,11] However, the risperidone group had higher rates of metabolic side effects.

Based on a randomized placebo-controlled trial and open-label studies discussed previously, lithium has been shown to be effective for acute treatment of manic and mixed states of pediatric bipolar disorder. However, acutely, it is less effective when compared with antipsychotics. In addition, lithium requires careful monitoring due to a narrow therapeutic window, which limits its use in some patients.

**Table 1**
**Medications approved by the Food and Drug Administration for the treatment of pediatric bipolar disorder**

| Medication | Phase of Bipolar Disorder | Age, y | Daily Dose Range, mg/d |
|---|---|---|---|
| Lithium | Mixed/manic | 12–17 | 300–2400 |
| Risperidone | Mixed/manic | 10–17 | 0.25–2.5 |
| Olanzapine | Mixed/manic | 13–17 | 2.5–20 |
| Aripiprazole | Mixed/manic | 10–17 | 2–30 |
| Quetiapine | Mixed/manic | 10–17 | 50–600 |
| Olanzapine/fluoxetine combination | Depressive episode | 10–17 | 3/25–12/50 |

**Table 2**
Select comparison studies

| Medications | Dose/Serum Level | Study Design | Age, y | Number of Subjects | Results | Common Side Effects |
|---|---|---|---|---|---|---|
| Lithium[11] Divalproex Risperidone | Lithium max 1.1–1.3 mEq/L; Divalproex 111–25 µg/mL; Risperidone 4–6 mg/d | Controlled, randomized | 6–15 | 279 | Mean CGI-BP-IM for Risperidone (68.5), lithium (35.6), divalproex (24.0) | Weight gain, increase in prolactin level and thyrotropin with risperidone. |
| Divalproex[12] Quetiapine | Divalproex 80–120 µg/mL; Quetiapine 400–600 mg/c | Double-blind, randomized | 12–18 | 50 | No significant difference in YMRS scores between groups; more rapid improvement in quetiapine group | No difference in rates of side effects between groups. |
| Lithium[19] Divalproex Carbamazepine | Maximum serum concentrations: lithium 0.8–1.2 mEq/L; divalproex 85–110 µg/mL; carbamazepine 7–10 µg/L | Open-label | 6–18 | 42 | Mean reduction in YMRS scores was 14.53 for divalproex, 9.46 for lithium, 9.00 for carbamazepine | Nausea was the most common side effect across all groups. Other side effects in lithium group included increased appetite, polyuria and diarrhea; in divalproex group, sedation; and in carbamazepine group, sedation, rash and dizziness. |
| Risperidone[32] Divalproex | Risperidone 0.5–2 mg/d Divalproex 60–120 µg/mL | Double-blind, randomized | 8–18 | 66 | YMRS score decreased from 30.59 to 7.58 with risperidone; and from 25.09 to 9.0 with divalproex | Increased appetite, stomach discomfort, sleepiness and fatigue was reported among both groups. Increased irritability was reported with divalproex. |

*Abbreviations:* CGI-BP-IM, clinical global impressions for bipolar illness improvement-mania; YMRS, Young Mania Rating Scale.

**Table 3**
Select medications for combination therapy

| Medications | Dose | Study Design | Phase of Bipolar Disorder | Age, y | Number of Subjects | Results | Common Side Effects |
|---|---|---|---|---|---|---|---|
| Divalproex[62] Quetiapine | Divalproex 20 mg/kg Quetiapine 450 mg/d | Randomized, double-blind, placebo-controlled | Acute manic/ mixed episode | 12–18 | 30 | Combination treatment resulted in greater reduction in YMRS scores compared with divalproex + placebo | Sedation was more common with combination treatment. Nausea, headache, gastrointestinal distress occurred in both groups. |
| Lithium[63] Divalproex | Serum levels: Lithium 0.6–1.2 mEq/L Divalproex 50–100 µg/mL | Open-label | Acute manic/ hypomanic episode within 3 mo | 5–17 | 90 | Significant reduction in YMRS (from 21.8 to 5.7), CDRS (from 31.7 to 21.0) and CGAS (from 50.1 to 68.1) | Emesis, enuresis, stomach pain, tremor, increased thirst, headache, nausea, sedation, increased appetite, diarrhea. |
| Lithium+ Risperidone[65] Divalproex+ Risperidone | Risperidone: up to 3 mg/d; Lithium serum level: 0.6–1.0 mEq/L; Divalproex serum level: 50–120 µg/mL | Prospective open-label | Acute mixed/ manic episode | 5–18 | 37 | Mean reduction in YMRS scores was 23.53 for lithium + risperidone; and 22.0 for divalproex + risperidone | Weight gain, sedation, nausea, increased appetite, stomach pain, tremors occurred in both groups. |
| Olanzapine[47] Fluoxetine | 6/25 12/50 | Randomized, placebo-controlled | Depressive episode | 10–17 | 255 | Mean change in CDRS-R score was greater in active treatment group (−28.4) vs placebo (−23.4) | Weight gain, increased appetite, somnolence, hyperlipidemia, increases in hepatic analytes, prolactin, QTc. |

Abbreviations: CDRS, children's depression rating scale; CDRS-R, children's depression rating scale, revised; CGAS, children's global assessment scale; YMRS, Young Mania Rating Scale.

**Table 4**
Select acute randomized placebo-controlled trials for monotherapy in manic/mixed states of pediatric bipolar disorder

| Medication | Dose | Age, y | Number of Subjects | Results | Common Side Effects |
|---|---|---|---|---|---|
| Lithium[9] | Serum level up to 1.4 mEq/L | 7–17 | 81 | Mean change in YMRS scores greater for lithium (−14) vs placebo (−7) | Vomiting, nausea, headache, fatigue, increase in TSH |
| Divalproex[16] | Serum level of 80–125 μg/mL | 10–17 | 150 | No significant difference in YMRS scores for divalproex (−8.8) vs placebo (−7.9) | No difference between groups |
| Risperidone[31] | 0.5–2.5 mg/d; 3–6 mg/d | 10–17 | 169 | Mean change in YMRS scores greater for high dose of risperidone (−16.5) and low dose of risperidone (−18.5) vs placebo (−9.1) | Somnolence, headache, fatigue |
| Olanzapine[33] | 2.5–20 mg | 13–17 | 161 | Mean change in YMRS scores greater for olanzapine (−17.65) vs placebo (−9.99) | Olanzapine group had more weight gain, higher levels of hepatic enzymes, prolactin, fasting glucose, fasting total cholesterol, and uric acid |
| Quetiapine[34] | 400 mg 600 mg | 10–17 | 277 | Mean change in YMRS scores greater for lower dose of quetiapine (−14.25) and higher dose of quetiapine (−15.60) vs placebo (−9.04) | Sedation, dizziness, heacache, and average weight gain of 1.7 kg; notable increases in total cholesterol and triglycerides |
| Aripiprazole[36] | 10 mg 30 mg | 10–17 | 296 | Mean change in YMRS scores greater for lower (−14.2) and higher (−16.5) doses of aripiprazole vs placebo (−8.2) | EPS and somnolence |
| Ziprasidone[37] | 40–160 mg/d | 10–17 | 237 | Mean change in YMRS greater for ziprasidone (−13.83) vs placebo (−8.61) | Sedation, headache, fatigue, nausea |
| Asenapine[39] | 5 mg/d 10 mg/d 20 mg/d | 10–17 | 403 | Mean change in YMRS scores greater for asenapine 5 mg/d (−12.8), asenapine 10 mg/d (−14.9) and asenapine 20 mg/d (−15.8) vs placebo (−9.6) | Somnolence, sedation, oral hypoesthesia and paresthesia, increased appetite, weight gain, increase in fasting lipids and glucose |

*Abbreviations:* EPS, extrapyramidal symptoms; TSH, thyroid stimulating hormone; YMRS, Young Mania Rating Scale.

Anticonvulsants have been found to have mood-stabilizing properties in adults, but available evidence is weaker in children. Divalproex is approved by the FDA for the treatment of manic and/or mixed episodes in adults, but not in youth. There are several positive open-label studies and a chart review suggesting the benefit of divalproex in the treatment of manic/mixed states.[12–14] A double-blind study compared divalproex with quetiapine in treating acute mania and showed higher response with quetiapine.[12] A randomized placebo-controlled study comparing lithium, divalproex, and placebo demonstrated effectiveness of divalproex over placebo.[15] However, a randomized placebo-controlled, industry-sponsored trial of divalproex for the treatment of acute mania failed to show separation from placebo during the first 4 weeks of treatment.[16] The discrepancy observed in the results of the 2 clinical trials was possibly due to the use of different formulations of the medication. In addition, the number of sites was larger in the negative study but so was the statistical power.

Although there is some evidence suggesting effectiveness of divalproex in the management of acute manic episodes, the available data are quite limited. In addition, divalproex may be toxic at higher doses, requires serum drug level monitoring, and has a potential for multiple drug interactions and teratogenic effects. Therefore, we believe it should not be used as a first-line agent for the treatment of acute mania in pediatric bipolar disorder.

Carbamazepine is currently approved by the FDA for the treatment of manic and mixed episodes of bipolar disorder in adults but not in children. Although there are no randomized, placebo-controlled clinical trials available to this date, several open-label studies suggest variable benefit of carbamazepine in a pediatric population. In a 26-week study of youth suffering from an acute manic or mixed episode, there was a significant decrease of a Young Mania Rating Scale (YMRS) score.[17] However, in another open-label study, many patients remained symptomatic despite treatment.[18] Carbamazepine was directly compared with divalproex and lithium in a small open-label study of youth with bipolar disorder I or II.[19] This study reported large effect sizes for divalproex (1.63), lithium (1.06), and carbamazepine (1.00).

Given the lack of randomized placebo-controlled trials evaluating the effectiveness, safety and pharmacokinetics of carbamazepine in the treatment of pediatric bipolar disorder, it would be prudent to consider other mood stabilizers when treating manic or mixed episode in children.

Lamotrigine is not approved by the FDA for the management of bipolar disorder in children, but it has an indication for maintenance treatment in adults. At this time, there are no randomized placebo-controlled trials of lamotrigine in the pediatric population, in spite of several positive open-label studies.[20] Currently, there is insufficient evidence to recommend its use for the treatment of acute manic or mixed episode of pediatric bipolar disorder.

Topiramate is currently not approved by the FDA for the treatment of bipolar disorder in children or adults. There are 2 chart reviews of adjunctive therapy with topiramate suggesting improvement in youth with manic/mixed episode.[21,22] In a study investigating the effect of topiramate on weight gain related to second-generation antipsychotics, the use of topiramate was associated with lower YMRS scores.[23] Adjunctive use of topiramate with olanzapine did not help reduce YMRS scores, but it did lead to reduced weight gain compared with olanzapine alone.[24] The only double-blind, placebo-controlled trial was stopped before completion in pediatric patients due to failure to separate from placebo in adult studies. Yet, despite the low power, analysis of the data provided some evidence for possible effectiveness.[25] Further studies are needed to establish effectiveness of topiramate in the treatment of manic episodes of bipolar disorder in children.

Although case reports suggested efficacy of oxcarbazepine in the treatment of pediatric manic/mixed states,[26] in a 7-week randomized controlled trial of 116 patients, it failed to separate from placebo.[27] Therefore, its use is not recommended in children with bipolar disorder.

It has been our experience that gabapentin is sometimes prescribed by clinicians for the treatment of bipolar disorder; nonetheless, there are only 2 case reports showing some improvement in youth.[28] To this date, there are no clinical trials examining the effect of gabapentin in children. However, studies in an adult population did not support its use for bipolar disorder.[29] Given the lack of evidence, gabapentin is not recommended for treatment of bipolar disorder.

### Antipsychotics

Meta-analysis of pharmacologic treatments of bipolar disorder revealed that second-generation antipsychotics are generally more effective than mood stabilizers, but have greater burden of side effects (weight gain and metabolic changes).[30] In addition, risperidone, quetiapine, aripiprazole, and asenapine carry FDA approval for the treatment of acute mixed and manic episodes of bipolar disorder in children based on randomized placebo-controlled trials.

Haas and colleagues[31] reported significant improvement in manic symptoms with low (0.5–2.5 mg/d) and high (3–6 mg/d) doses of risperidone in a randomized placebo-controlled trial. In a direct comparison with divalproex, the risperidone group improved earlier and with a greater response and remission rates.[32] In addition, the discontinuation rate was lower in the risperidone group. As described earlier, the response rate in the risperidone group was significantly higher than in divalproex and lithium groups.[11]

Olanzapine is currently approved by the FDA for the treatment of acute manic/mixed episodes in adolescents 13 to 17 years of age based on a 3-week double-blind study, in which more patients on medication met response and remission criteria when compared with placebo.[33] However, there was a significant increase in weight in the olanzapine group compared with placebo (3.7 kg vs 0.3 kg).

A randomized placebo-controlled trial of quetiapine demonstrated high response rates with either 400 mg or 600 mg quetiapine compared with placebo.[34] In a double-blind, randomized study comparing divalproex and quetiapine in adolescents 12 to 18 years of age, the response and remission rates were greater in the quetiapine group.[12] In addition, youth receiving quetiapine improved faster compared with divalproex

An open-label, dose-escalation study of 20 mg, 25 mg, and 30 mg per day of aripiprazole showed safety and efficacy of aripiprazole in the treatment of youth with bipolar disorder and schizophrenia.[35] Two doses of aripiprazole (10 mg and 30 mg) were given to youth ages 10 to 17 in a 4-week double-blind, placebo-controlled trial, which showed significant reduction in manic symptoms when compared with placebo.[36]

Ziprasidone is approved by the FDA for the treatment of mania in adult but not pediatric bipolar disorder. A randomized placebo-controlled trial, in which 237 subjects 10 to 17 years of age received flexible doses of ziprasidone or placebo, showed significant changes in YMRS scores in the active medication group.[37] Although electrocardiogram changes were minimal in this study, a different trial reported a notable prolongation of QTc interval in youth.[38]

A randomized placebo-controlled study of 3 doses of asenapine (2.5 mg twice a day, 5 mg twice a day, 10 mg twice a day) was conducted with 403 patients aged 10 to 17 years. During the course of the study, all groups showed significant improvement in YMRS scores compared with placebo.[39]

To date, there are no randomized placebo-controlled trials of clozapine for the treatment of podiatric bipolar disorder, but retrospective chart reviews suggested potential benefit.[40,41] Due to the severity of the side-effect profile and the lack of randomized controlled trials, the use of clozapine in children with bipolar disorder is not recommended.

There is only one prospective open-label study of paliperidone in the treatment of pediatric bipolar disorder. Adolescents 16 to 17 years of age received monotherapy with paliperidone for 8 weeks and had a significant improvement in YMRS scores.[42]

To date, there are no published clinical studies on the use of lurasidone and iloperidone for the treatment of mania in youth. A search of the clinical trials Web site (www.clinicaltrials.gov) revealed an ongoing open-label study of lurasidone as a treatment for mania in youth 6 to 17 years of age.

## ACUTE TREATMENT OF DEPRESSIVE EPISODES

Depressive episodes are less common than manic or mixed states in the pediatric population[43] and fewer treatment studies are available to date. Although selective serotonin reuptake inhibitors improve depressive symptoms in youth with bipolar disorder, they increase the risk of switching to a manic state.[44,45] Antidepressants are recommended only in addition to a mood stabilizer for the treatment of a depressive episode.[45,46] The only medication that is currently approved by the FDA for the treatment of bipolar depression in youth of 10 to 17 years of age is olanzapine/fluoxetine combination, which was superior to placebo in an 8-week randomized trial.[47]

There are no other trials of antidepressants in pediatric bipolar depression available to date. However, a pilot study of youth with a genetic risk for bipolar disorder presenting with depressive symptoms was conducted.[48] Children were randomized to receive paroxetine or paroxetine/divalproex combination. Both treatment options were not effective and more than 50% of patients had manic symptoms or suicidality, which led to the early termination of the study.

Two randomized placebo-controlled studies of quetiapine for the treatment of bipolar depression in children have been reported. In both studies, the response rates did not demonstrate a significant separation from placebo.[49,50] However, in one of the trials, the response rate in the placebo group was high and could have contributed to the lack of statistical significance.[49]

Open label trials with lithium and lamotrigine demonstrated effectiveness for the treatment of pediatric bipolar depression.[51,52] Although these studies show some promise, they should be interpreted with caution given the open-label design and high YMRS scores before treatment. In addition, more randomized trials are needed to establish efficacy and safety of antidepressants and other mood stabilizers for the treatment of bipolar depression.

## MAINTENANCE THERAPY

Bipolar disorder is a chronic and life-long illness, requiring not only treatment of acute episodes, but also maintenance therapy to prevent relapse.[5] There is a paucity of randomized data available on maintenance treatment of youth with bipolar disorder. Trials that exist focus mostly on open-label extension after acute treatment.[8,37,53–57]

Two randomized, double-blind, placebo-controlled trials of aripiprazole for maintenance treatment of pediatric bipolar disorder have been performed. In a 30-week trial, youth 10 to 17 years of age were first assigned to acute treatment for 4 weeks with 10 mg or 30 mg of aripiprazole or placebo, followed by 26 weeks of double-blind extension.[58] Both doses of medication resulted in a significant reduction of YMRS scores. In another trial, children 4 to 9 years of age were randomized to receive pla-cebo or aripiprazole for 72 weeks after the initial acute stabilization.[59] The time to discontinuation was longer in the active treatment group.

Two trials evaluated the efficacy of lamotrigine in maintenance treatment of pediat-ric bipolar disorder. In an open-label trial, 46 pediatric patients, 8 to 18 years of age, with manic/mixed or hypomanic episode received lamotrigine for 14 weeks with high response and remission rates.[60] Findling and colleagues[61] conducted a discontinua-tion study in which lamotrigine was investigated as an add-on to conventional treat-ment in youth 10 to 17 years of age. Patients receiving a stable dose of lamotrigine for 2 weeks were randomized to continue lamotrigine treatment or placebo for an addi-tional 36 weeks. The overall time to occurrence of a bipolar event did not differ be-tween groups, but was significantly longer in the subset of patients aged 13 to 17 years of age.

In summary, lithium, divalproex, aripiprazole, ziprasidone, asenapine, and lamotri-gine have shown promising results in maintenance treatment of pediatric bipolar dis-order. However, more randomized placebo-controlled studies are needed to evaluate long-term safety and effectiveness of these pharmacologic interventions.

## COMBINATION TREATMENT

Although many studies have reported significant symptom reduction during acute manic episode with monotherapy, many children continue to be symptomatic despite being treated. Several studies explored the possibility of combination therapy for treatment-resistant youth.

A randomized placebo-controlled study of combination treatment with divalproex and quetiapine showed greater symptom reduction when compared with divalproex alone and placebo.[62] Combination therapy of lithium and divalproex was effective in an open-label trial of 90 youth presenting with manic or hypomanic episode within 3 months before the study.[63,64]

A significant reduction in YMRS scores was achieved in an open-label trial of com-bination treatment with risperidone and either divalproex or lithium, respectively.[65] Risperidone augmentation was also explored in a 12-month prospective open-label trial.[66] In this study, children with preschool onset of bipolar disorder, who did not respond to lithium monotherapy or relapsed, showed decrease in manic symptoms with addition of risperidone.

In general, the augmentation with an antipsychotic may improve manic symptoms when monotherapy with an anticonvulsant or lithium has not been sufficient. However, more studies are needed to evaluate the effectiveness of other antipsychotics in com-bination treatments, as well as to assess the initial response to monotherapy versus combination therapy.

## SUMMARY

Despite an increasing interest in pharmacotherapy of pediatric bipolar disorder and more clinical trials of second-generation antipsychotics published over the past several years, there still remains a paucity of data to inform clinicians on the appro-priate medication management. Based on the available data, initial monotherapy is preferable when treating an acute mixed or manic state. Generally, atypical antipsy-chotics have shown higher response rates when compared with lithium or anticon-vulsants. However, higher efficacy is usually accompanied by metabolic side effects. Lithium is effective and generally well tolerated. Results for divalproex in the treatment of pediatric mania are mixed, but overall show some promise. Studies of carbamazepine and topiramate show potential in children with bipolar disorder, but randomized placebo-controlled trials are needed to establish efficacy. The use of oxcarbazepine is not recommended.

Even fewer data are available on the treatment of bipolar depression. The olanzapine/fluoxetine combination was approved by the FDA after it was shown to be effective in a randomized placebo-controlled trial. Quetiapine failed to show efficacy in 2 randomized placebo-controlled trials.

There is only a modest amount of research available on maintenance treatment of bipolar disorder in youth. Randomized placebo-controlled clinical trials were conducted with aripiprazole, which showed positive results. Lithium and divalproex are promising medications, but further studies are needed to evaluate the long-term efficacy. Lamotrigine may be more effective in adolescents but not in younger children.

Despite the advances in pharmacotherapy of pediatric bipolar disorder over the past 15 years, more research is needed to bridge the gap between clinical practice and available data. Head-to-head comparison trials, as well as long-term studies, can help guide medical decision making. Studies of combination treatment are promising and further research should focus on combining medications for more effective management of bipolar disorder.

## REFERENCES

1. Lish JD, Dime-Meenan S, Whybrow PC, et al. The National Depressive and Manic-depressive Association (DMDA) survey of bipolar members. J Affect Disord 1994;31(4):281–94.
2. Perlis RH, Miyahara S, Marangell LB, et al. Long-term implications of early onset in bipolar disorder: data from the first 1000 participants in the systematic treatment enhancement program for bipolar disorder (STEP-BD). Biol Psychiatry 2004;55(9):875–81.
3. Goldstein BI, Birmaher B. Prevalence, clinical presentation and differential diagnosis of pediatric bipolar disorder. Isr J Psychiatry Relat Sci 2012;49(1):3–14.
4. Gore FM, Bloem PJ, Patton GC, et al. Global burden of disease in young people aged 10-24 years: a systematic analysis. Lancet 2011;377(9783):2093–102.
5. McClellan J, Kowatch R, Findling RL, Work Group on Quality Issues. Practice parameter for the assessment and treatment of children and adolescents with bipolar disorder. J Am Acad Child Adolesc Psychiatry 2007;46(1):107–25.
6. Wiznitzer M, Findling RL. Why do psychiatric drug research in children? Lancet 2003;361(9364):1147–8.
7. Findling RL, Frazier JA, Kafantaris V, et al. The Collaborative Lithium Trials (CoLT): specific aims, methods, and implementation. Child Adolesc Psychiatry Ment Health 2008;2(1):21.
8. Findling RL, Kafantaris V, Pavuluri M, et al. Post-acute effectiveness of lithium in pediatric bipolar I disorder. J Child Adolesc Psychopharmacol 2013;23(2):80–90.
9. Findling RL, Robb A, McNamara NK, et al. Lithium in the acute treatment of bipolar I disorder: a double-blind, placebo-controlled study. Pediatrics 2015;136(5): 885–94.
10. Vitiello B, Riddle MA, Yenokyan G, et al. Treatment moderators and predictors of outcome in the Treatment of Early Age Mania (TEAM) study. J Am Acad Child Adolesc Psychiatry 2012;51(9):867–78.
11. Geller B, Luby JL, Joshi P, et al. A randomized controlled trial of risperidone, lithium, or divalproex sodium for initial treatment of bipolar I disorder, manic or

mixed phase, in children and adolescents. Arch Gen Psychiatry 2012;69(5): 515–28.

12. DelBello MP, Kowatch RA, Adler CM, et al. A double-blind randomized pilot study comparing quetiapine and divalproex for adolescent mania. J Am Acad Child Adolesc Psychiatry 2006;45(3):305–13.

13. Wagner KD, Weller EB, Carlson GA, et al. An open-label trial of divalproex in children and adolescents with bipolar disorder. J Am Acad Child Adolesc Psychiatry 2002;41(10):1224–30.

14. Papatheodorou G, Kutcher SP, Katic M, et al. The efficacy and safety of divalproex sodium in the treatment of acute mania in adolescents and young adults: an open clinical trial. J Clin Psychopharmacol 1995;15(2):110–6.

15. Kowatch R, Findling R, Scheffer R, et al. Pediatric bipolar collaborative mood stabilizer trial. Paper presented at: Annual Meeting of the American Academy of Child and Adolescent Psychiatry; Boston, MA; October 23–28, 2007.

16. Wagner KD, Redden L, Kowatch RA, et al. A double-blind, randomized, placebo-controlled trial of divalproex extended-release in the treatment of bipolar disorder in children and adolescents. J Am Acad Child Adolesc Psychiatry 2009;48(5): 519–32.

17. Findling RL, Ginsberg LD. The safety and effectiveness of open-label extended-release carbamazepine in the treatment of children and adolescents with bipolar I disorder suffering from a manic or mixed episode. Neuropsychiatr Dis Treat 2014; 10:1589–97.

18. Joshi G, Wozniak J, Mick E, et al. A prospective open-label trial of extended-release carbamazepine monotherapy in children with bipolar disorder. J Child Adolesc Psychopharmacol 2010;20(1):7–14.

19. Kowatch RA, Suppes T, Carmody TJ, et al. Effect size of lithium, divalproex sodium, and carbamazepine in children and adolescents with bipolar disorder. J Am Acad Child Adolesc Psychiatry 2000;39(6):713–20.

20. Biederman J, Joshi G, Mick E, et al. A prospective open-label trial of lamotrigine monotherapy in children and adolescents with bipolar disorder. CNS Neurosci Ther 2010;16(2):91–102.

21. Barzman DH, DelBello MP, Kowatch RA, et al. Adjunctive topiramate in hospitalized children and adolescents with bipolar disorders. J Child Adolesc Psychopharmacol 2005;15(6):931–7.

22. DelBello MP, Kowatch RA, Warner J, et al. Adjunctive topiramate treatment for pediatric bipolar disorder: a retrospective chart review. J Child Adolesc Psychopharmacol 2002;12(4):323–30.

23. Tramontina S, Zeni CP, Pheula G, et al. Topiramate in adolescents with juvenile bipolar disorder presenting weight gain due to atypical antipsychotics or mood stabilizers: an open clinical trial. J Child Adolesc Psychopharmacol 2007;17(1): 129–34.

24. Wozniak J, Mick E, Waxmonsky J, et al. Comparison of open label, 8 week trials of olanzapine monotherapy and topiramate augmentation of olanzapine for the treatment of pediatric bipolar disorder. J Child Adolesc Psychopharmacol 2009;19(5):539–45.

25. Delbello MP, Findling RL, Kushner S, et al. A pilot controlled trial of topiramate for mania in children and adolescents with bipolar disorder. J Am Acad Child Adolesc Psychiatry 2005;44(6):539–47.

26. Davanzo P, Nikore V, Yehya N, et al. Oxcarbazepine treatment of juvenile-onset bipolar disorder. J Child Adolesc Psychopharmacol 2004;14(3):344–5.

27. Wagner KD, Kowatch RA, Emslie GJ, et al. A double-blind, randomized, placebo-controlled trial of oxcarbazepine in the treatment of bipolar disorder in children and adolescents. Am J Psychiatry 2006;163(7):1179–86.

28. Soutullo CA, Casuto LS, Keck PE. Gabapentin in the treatment of adolescent mania: a case report. J Child Adolesc Psychopharmacol 1998;8(1):81–5.

29. Pande AC, Crockatt JG, Janney CA, et al. Gabapentin in bipolar disorder: a placebo-controlled trial of adjunctive therapy. Gabapentin Bipolar Disorder Study Group. Bipolar Disord 2000;2(3 Pt 2):249–55.

30. Liu HY, Potter MP, Woodworth KY, et al. Pharmacologic treatments for pediatric bipolar disorder: a review and meta-analysis. J Am Acad Child Adolesc Psychiatry 2011;50(8):749–62.e9.

31. Haas M, Delbello MP, Pandina G, et al. Risperidone for the treatment of acute mania in children and adolescents with bipolar disorder: a randomized, double-blind, placebo-controlled study. Bipolar Disord 2009;11(7):687–700.

32. Pavuluri MN, Henry DB, Findling RL, et al. Double-blind randomized trial of risperidone versus divalproex in pediatric bipolar disorder. Bipolar Disord 2010;12(6):593–605.

33. Tohen M, Kryzhanovskaya L, Carlson G, et al. Olanzapine versus placebo in the treatment of adolescents with bipolar mania. Am J Psychiatry 2007;164(10):1547–56.

34. Pathak S, Findling RL, Earley WR, et al. Efficacy and safety of quetiapine in children and adolescents with mania associated with bipolar I disorder: a 3-week, double-blind, placebo-controlled trial. J Clin Psychiatry 2013;74(1):e100–9.

35. Findling RL, Kauffman RE, Sallee FR, et al. Tolerability and pharmacokinetics of aripiprazole in children and adolescents with psychiatric disorders: an open-label, dose-escalation study. J Clin Psychopharmacol 2008;28(4):441–6.

36. Findling RL, Nyilas M, Forbes RA, et al. Acute treatment of pediatric bipolar I disorder, manic or mixed episode, with aripiprazole: a randomized, double-blind, placebo-controlled study. J Clin Psychiatry 2009;70(10):1441–51.

37. Findling RL, Cavuş I, Pappadopulos E, et al. Efficacy, long-term safety, and tolerability of ziprasidone in children and adolescents with bipolar disorder. J Child Adolesc Psychopharmacol 2013;23(8):545–57.

38. Blair J, Scahill L, State M, et al. Electrocardiographic changes in children and adolescents treated with ziprasidone: a prospective study. J Am Acad Child Adolesc Psychiatry 2005;44(1):73–9.

39. Findling RL, Landbloom RL, Szegedi A, et al. Asenapine for the acute treatment of pediatric manic or mixed episode of bipolar I disorder. J Am Acad Child Adolesc Psychiatry 2015;54(12):1032–41.

40. Kant R, Chalansani R, Chengappa KN, et al. The off-label use of clozapine in adolescents with bipolar disorder, intermittent explosive disorder, or posttraumatic stress disorder. J Child Adolesc Psychopharmacol 2004;14(1):57–63.

41. Masi G, Mucci M, Millepiedi S. Clozapine in adolescent inpatients with acute mania. J Child Adolesc Psychopharmacol 2002;12(2):93–9.

42. Joshi G, Petty C, Wozniak J, et al. A prospective open-label trial of paliperidone monotherapy for the treatment of bipolar spectrum disorders in children and adolescents. Psychopharmacology (Berl) 2013;227(3):449–58.

43. Chang K. Challenges in the diagnosis and treatment of pediatric bipolar depression. Dialogues Clin Neurosci 2009;11(1):73–80.

44. Biederman J, Mick E, Spencer TJ, et al. Therapeutic dilemmas in the pharmacotherapy of bipolar depression in the young. J Child Adolesc Psychopharmacol 2000;10(3):185–92.

45. Pacchiarotti I, Bond DJ, Baldessarini RJ, et al. The International Society for Bipolar Disorders (ISBD) task force report on antidepressant use in bipolar disorders. Am J Psychiatry 2013;170(11):1249–62.

46. Kowatch RA, Fristad M, Birmaher B, et al. Treatment guidelines for children and adolescents with bipolar disorder. J Am Acad Child Adolesc Psychiatry 2005; 44(3):213–35.

47. Detke HC, DelBello MP, Landry J, et al. Olanzapine/Fluoxetine combination in children and adolescents with bipolar I depression: a randomized, double-blind, placebo-controlled trial. J Am Acad Child Adolesc Psychiatry 2015;54(3): 217–24.

48. Findling RL, Lingler J, Rowles BM, et al. A pilot pharmacotherapy trial for depressed youths at high genetic risk for bipolarity. J Child Adolesc Psychopharmacol 2008;18(6):615–21.

49. DelBello MP, Chang K, Welge JA, et al. A double-blind, placebo-controlled pilot study of quetiapine for depressed adolescents with bipolar disorder. Bipolar Disord 2009;11(5):483–93.

50. Findling RL, Pathak S, Earley WR, et al. Efficacy and safety of extended-release quetiapine fumarate in youth with bipolar depression: an 8 week, double-blind, placebo-controlled trial. J Child Adolesc Psychopharmacol 2014;24(6):325–35.

51. Patel NC, DelBello MP, Bryan HS, et al. Open-label lithium for the treatment of adolescents with bipolar depression. J Am Acad Child Adolesc Psychiatry 2006; 45(3):289–97.

52. Chang K, Saxena K, Howe M. An open-label study of lamotrigine adjunct or monotherapy for the treatment of adolescents with bipolar depression. J Am Acad Child Adolesc Psychiatry 2006;45(3):298–304.

53. Findling RL, McNamara NK, Youngstrom EA, et al. Double-blind 18-month trial of lithium versus divalproex maintenance treatment in pediatric bipolar disorder. J Am Acad Child Adolesc Psychiatry 2005;44(5):409–17.

54. Kafantaris V, Coletti DJ, Dicker R, et al. Lithium treatment of acute mania in adolescents: a placebo-controlled discontinuation study. J Am Acad Child Adolesc Psychiatry 2004;43(8):984–93.

55. Redden L, DelBello M, Wagner KD, et al. Long-term safety of divalproex sodium extended-release in children and adolescents with bipolar I disorder. J Child Adolesc Psychopharmacol 2009;19(1):83–9.

56. Boarati MA, Wang YP, Ferreira-Maia AP, et al. Six-month open-label follow-up of risperidone long-acting injection use in pediatric bipolar disorder. Prim Care Companion CNS Disord 2013;15(3) [pii:PCC.12m01368].

57. DelBello MP, Versavel M, Ice K, et al. Tolerability of oral ziprasidone in children and adolescents with bipolar mania, schizophrenia, or schizoaffective disorder. J Child Adolesc Psychopharmacol 2008;18(5):491–9.

58. Findling RL, Correll CU, Nyilas M, et al. Aripiprazole for the treatment of pediatric bipolar I disorder: a 30-week, randomized, placebo-controlled study. Bipolar Disord 2013;15(2):138–49.

59. Findling RL, Youngstrom EA, McNamara NK, et al. Double-blind, randomized, placebo-controlled long-term maintenance study of aripiprazole in children with bipolar disorder. J Clin Psychiatry 2012;73(1):57–63.

60. Pavuluri MN, Henry DB, Moss M, et al. Effectiveness of lamotrigine in maintaining symptom control in pediatric bipolar disorder. J Child Adolesc Psychopharmacol 2009;19(1):75–82.

61. Findling RL, Chang K, Robb A, et al. Adjunctive maintenance lamotrigine for pediatric bipolar I disorder: a placebo-controlled, randomized withdrawal study. J Am Acad Child Adolesc Psychiatry 2015;54(12):1020–31.e3.

62. Delbello MP, Schwiers ML, Rosenberg HL, et al. A double-blind, randomized, placebo-controlled study of quetiapine as adjunctive treatment for adolescent mania. J Am Acad Child Adolesc Psychiatry 2002;41(10):1216–23.

63. Findling RL, McNamara NK, Gracious BL, et al. Combination lithium and divalproex sodium in pediatric bipolarity. J Am Acad Child Adolesc Psychiatry 2003;42(8):895–901.

64. Findling RL, McNamara NK, Stansbrey R, et al. Combination lithium and divalproex sodium in pediatric bipolar symptom re-stabilization. J Am Acad Child Adolesc Psychiatry 2006;45(2):142–8.

65. Pavuluri MN, Henry DB, Carbray JA, et al. Open-label prospective trial of risperidone in combination with lithium or divalproex sodium in pediatric mania. J Affect Disord 2004;82(Suppl 1):S103–11.

66. Pavuluri MN, Henry DB, Carbray JA, et al. A one-year open-label trial of risperidone augmentation in lithium nonresponder youth with preschool-onset bipolar disorder. J Child Adolesc Psychopharmacol 2006;16(3):336–50.

# New Psychoactive Substances in Pediatric Patients

 CrossMark

Brandon J. Warrick, MD[a],*, Anita Paula Tataru, MSc (Pharm), PharmD[b],
Roy Gerona, PhD[c]

## KEYWORDS

- Designer drug • Cathinone • Cannabinoid • Synthetic opioid • Fentanyl analogue
- Illicit drug analogue • Pediatric • Adolescent

## KEY POINTS

- New psychoactive substances (NPS) have grown in popularity over the last decade resulting in thousands of deaths and even more hospitalizations.
- NPS are bought over the Internet, in headshops, or on the streets as counterfeit pills mimicking prescription medications; they may also be contaminants in illicit drugs.
- There are little to no pharmacologic or toxicologic data for most NPS.
- Commonly available urine drug tests are of minimal utility because of numerous false positives and false negatives. Laboratory testing using nontargeted analysis allows identification of previously unreported NPS.
- Treatment is primarily supportive with benzodiazepines for agitation and seizures, and naloxone for opioid toxidrome reversal.

## INTRODUCTION

New psychoactive substances (NPS) are psychoactive substances not approved for therapeutic use and not yet listed under the 1971 United Nations Convention on Psychotropic Substances. They are typically analogues of controlled substances, designed to produce effects similar to the controlled substances they mimic. By 2015, 560 NPS have been reported to the European Monitoring Center for Drugs and Drug Addiction (EMCDDA) with most (380) only detected in the last 5 years.[1] A

Disclosure Statement: The authors have nothing to disclose.
[a] University of New Mexico, NMPDIC MSC07 4390, 1 University of New Mexico, Albuquerque, NM 87107-0001, USA; [b] Faculty of Pharmaceutical Sciences, University of British Columbia, British Columbia, Canada; [c] Clinical Toxicology and Environmental Biomonitoring Lab, University of California, San Francisco, 513 Parnassus Avenue, Medical Sciences Building S864, San Francisco, CA 94143, USA
* Corresponding author.
E-mail address: brandon_warrick@hotmail.com

http://dx.doi.org/10.1016/j.pcl.2017.08.003
0031-3955/17/© 2017 Elsevier Inc. All rights reserved.
pediatric.theclinics.com

wide variety of NPS are rapidly spreading worldwide, and various classification systems published in the literature have made navigating this drug landscape confusing.[2–5] Such inconsistency often creates challenges in facilitating the accurate documentation of their pharmacologic, clinical, and toxicologic effects, which can derail establishing effective regimens that can be administered to specifically address intoxications for each class of NPS. A more chemistry-based approach adopted by the EMCDDA classifies NPS into 13 categories that are largely based on their characteristic functional moiety (**Table 1**).[6] EMCDDA classification scheme defines clear boundaries between classes of NPS, and their familiarization by medical practitioners can facilitate accurate documentation of their toxicologic profiles in patients.

The prevalence of NPS use in the United States may be greater than elsewhere. The United Nations World Drug Report noted the problem of NPS is twice as widespread in the United States as it is in Europe.[7] This trend is reflected in the number of calls received by the American Association of Poison Control Centers (PCC) on exposures to just a single class of NPS: synthetic cannabinoids. Since the sudden increase in calls noted in 2010, the number of exposures reported annually continues to increase.[8]

NPS are also easily accessible over the Internet or in headshops in a wide variety of formulations, including bulk powders, tablets, pills, capsules, liquids, blotter papers, and herbal preparations. To skirt drug laws, they are often deceptively packaged as "food supplement," "plant food," "bath salts," "incense," or "research chemical" and almost always labeled with the disclaimer "not for human consumption."[9]

| Table 1 Classification of new psychoactive substances according to chemical class proposed by the European Monitoring Centre for Drugs and Drug Addiction | |
|---|---|
| **Class** | **Examples** |
| Synthetic cannabinoid receptor agonists | JWH-018, AM-2201, XLR 11, PB-22, AB-CHMINACA, AMB-FUBINACA (Common Drug of Abuse: THC) |
| Synthetic cathinones | Mephedrone, Methylone, MDPV, alpha-PVP (Common Drug of Abuse: Cathinone) |
| Phenethylamines | 2C-B, 2C-I-NBOMe |
| Tryptamines | DiPT, 5-MeO-DALT (Common Drugs of Abuse: DMT, Psilocybin) |
| Aminoindanes | 2-AI, MDAI |
| Arylalkylamines | Ethylamphetamine, MDE, DOC (Common Drugs of Abuse: Methamphetamine, MDMA) |
| Arylcyclohexyamines | 4-methoxy-PCP, Methoxetamine (Common Drugs of Abuse: Ketamine, Phencyclidine) |
| Benzodiazepines | Etizolam, Flubromazolam, Flubromazepam (Common Drugs of Abuse: Diazepam, Alprazolam) |
| Opioids | AH-7921, U-4770, W-18, Carfentanil (Common Drugs of Abuse: Heroin, Morphine, Fentanyl) |
| Piperidines and pyrrolidines | Ethylphenidate, Desoxypipradrol Common Drug of Abuse: Methylphenidate) |
| Piperazines | m-CPP, TFMPP |
| Plants and extracts | Kratom |
| Others | Allocaine, 4'-Fluorococaine |

Recently, opioids have been detected in counterfeit prescription pills more frequently.[10]

Most NPS have limited or no pharmacologic and toxicologic data in humans, outside of personal experiences found on drug forums. Because their structures are often different enough from common illicit drugs, they are often not detected on commonly used drug screens. This presents a challenge in recognizing and treating emergency cases with NPS cause; pediatricians face an even greater challenge because the presentation may be different in younger patients from the limited cases of adult intoxications reported in the literature. This review focuses on the three most prevalent classes of NPS used in the United States: synthetic cannabinoids receptor agonists (SCRA), synthetic cathinones (SCs), and opioids, and provides pediatricians with the most recent information on their pharmacology, clinical presentations, and management strategies. Although several compounds have been grouped into categories for ease of comparison, it cannot be overstated that each compound has unique pharmacology, and significant variations between groups within each category exist.

## SYNTHETIC CANNABINOIDS

The first synthetic cannabinoid receptor agonists (SCRAs) were research chemicals developed in the 1980s intended to mimic the effects of tetrahydrocannabinol (THC). They appeared on the European market in 2004, and their first seizure in the United States dates back to 2008. SCRAs are frequently found mixed with dried plant material. More recently, SCRAs were found in cannabis resin mimics, in e-cigarette fluid, and as adulterants in other illicit drugs such as ecstasy.

### Epidemiology

Use of SCRAs varies worldwide. Although the use is increasing in some parts such as Spain, Latvia, and Germany,[11] it still remains fairly low in the general population at 1.7% in France in 2014, 0.5% in Spain in 2013, and 0.5% in the United Kingdom in 2014/2015.[12] In the United States, a survey[13] found that, aside from alcohol and tobacco, SCRAs are the third most popular drug among 10th and 12th graders after marijuana and amphetamines, and the fourth most popular among 8th graders after marijuana, inhalants, and amphetamines. Overall, past year, prevalence of SCRAs self-reported use among adolescents aged 13 to 19 years decreased between 2012 and 2016.[13,14] Past year use of SCRAs dropped from 11.3% in 2012 to 7.9% in 2013, 5.8% in 2014, 5.2% in 2015, and 3.5% in 2016 among 12th grade students in 2012.[13]

Paradoxically, with the decrease in self-reported use of SCRAs, the number of calls to PCC and emergency departments (EDs) has increased. PCC SCRA-related calls have increased from 2668 in 2013 and 3682 in 2014, to 7794 in 2015.[15] Fifty percent (5493) of SCRA calls between 2009 and 2012 involved patients aged 19 or less, with 48.8% being aged 13 to 19 years.[16] The number of ED visits related to SCRAs increased from 11,406 in 2010[17] to 28,531 in 2011.[18] More specifically, ED visits involving teenagers aged 12 to 17 years have doubled (3780 visits in 2010, 7584 in 2011) and for patients aged 18 to 20 years have tripled (1881 in 2010, 8212 in 2011) within 1 year.[17] These age groups also represented 27% and 29%, respectively, of total ED admissions related to SCRAs in 2011. Although SCRAs are advertised as legal alternatives to cannabis, their users have a 30-fold (95% CI 17.5–51.2) increased relative risk of requiring emergency medical care compared with cannabis users.[11] It is hypothesized that newer generations of SCRAs are more toxic than the previous ones.

## Pharmacology

No prior pharmacological and toxicological characterization have been done on most of the newer synthetic cannabinoid products available in the recreational drug market. Moreover, it is difficult to extrapolate data from one SCRA to another because this class of compounds is quite heterogeneous. Their shared properties are as follows[19,20]:

- Cannabinoid receptor agonists
- Highly lipophilic and nonpolar
- Able to undergo extensive metabolism
- Significantly excreted metabolites in the urine

There are two main cannabinoid receptors: the CB1 subtype is found mostly in the central nervous system and is associated with psychoactive effects, whereas the CB2 subtype is found peripherally, especially in the immune system.[19] Each SCRA has different relative selectivity for these receptors. Moreover, they also have different affinities to CB1: when compared with THC, ADB-FUBINACA has 143 times higher affinity; AMB-FUBINACA has 85 times higher affinity; and MDMB-CHMICA has 17 times higher affinity.[21,22] When compared with JWH-018, one of the first synthetic cannabinoids, ADB-FUBINACA, AMB-FUBINACA, and MDMB-CMICA have 15 times, 9 times, and almost twice more affinity to CB1, respectively.[20,21,23] Interestingly, all three compounds have been involved in outbreaks of mass poisonings.[12,23]

SCRAs and their metabolites may have additional pharmacologic targets that have not been explored and could explain the different clinical presentation from marijuana. For example, compounds possessing an indole group resembling serotonin may interact with serotonin receptors.[24] Some SCRAs, such as WIN 55,212-2, also possess monoamine oxidase inhibitory activity that could explain serotonin syndrome features in those intoxicated.[25]

## Clinical Presentation and Toxicology

Clinical presentation of SCRA intoxication is highly variable, ranging from severe agitation to unresponsiveness. The difficulty predicting signs and symptoms is likely multifactorial but may include varying amounts and purities of the products, route of administration, presence of coingestants or contaminants, lack of analytical confirmation of SCRA exposure in reported cases, and individual risk factors and genetic predispositions to specific adverse events.

The most common adverse effects reported by the Texas PCCs were tachycardia (37.3%), agitation (18.5%), drowsiness (18.5%), vomiting (15.7%), hallucinations (10.8%), nausea (9.9%), hypertension (9.7%), confusion (9.1%), dizziness (8.6%), and chest pain (6.7%) in 464 patients, of which 190 (41%) were aged 19 years or less.[26] Metabolic findings include hyperglycemia,[27] hypokalemia,[27,28] and acidosis.[27] In addition, Tait and colleagues[28] found pediatric reports of confusion, bizarre behavior, agitation, psychosis, hallucinations, delusions, syncope, mydriasis, hypokalemia, and hyperreflexia.

Severe adverse events reported in children include seizure,[29] hypothermia,[30] acute respiratory failure,[29,31] and aggression[29] following analytically confirmed exposure to MAB-CHMINACA and AB-PINACA, junctional bradycardia with JWH-018 and JWH-073,[32] and death from hypothermia with JWH-210.[33] Myocardial infarction,[27,28] catatonia, and severe agitation[28] were also reported in children without analytically confirmed exposures. Additional severe adverse events reported in adults include subarachnoid hemorrhage, ischemic stroke, cannabinoid hyperemesis, liver failure, hematuria, acute kidney failure, rhabdomyolysis, sudden cardiac death, and indirect death (accidents, suicide, self-injury).[27,28]

## SYNTHETIC CATHINONES

SCs are derivatives of cathinone, a psychoactive substance found in the khat plant *Catha edulis*.[34] They are marketed as legal substitutes to stimulants like methamphetamine and 3,4-methylenedioxymethamphetamine (MDMA) and sold as plant food, bath salts, or jewelry cleaner. They are also sold as ecstasy or "molly" to unsuspecting users.

SCs are related to amphetamine, and subtle structural variations distinguish them from methamphetamine and MDMA.[35] Structurally, SCs are beta-ketoamphetamines, that is, a ketone group is present two carbons away from the amino group in the alkyl chain. SCs are more hydrophilic than their amphetamine counterparts and are less able to cross the blood-brain barrier.[34] Methcathinone, the first popular SC, was developed in 1928 and gained popularity only in the 1990s.[36]

### Epidemiology

Mephedrone was introduced in 2009 in United Kingdom and Holland, with its popularity increasing in the nightlife scene reportedly because of the poor quality or difficulty in finding cocaine and MDMA.[24,37] SCs enjoyed similar popularity in the United States until 2011 when a temporary ban was placed by the Drug Enforcement Administration. Calls to PCCs initially increased from 304 in 2010 to a peak of 6137 in 2011, followed by a decrease to 2691 in 2012, 996 in 2013,[18] 587 in 2014, and 522 in 2015.[38] There were 22,904 ED visits involving "bath salts" in the United States in 2011 during its peak popularity.[39] Annual self-reported use by US adolescents has remained fairly constant since 2012 at around 1% of 8th, 10th, and 12th graders.[13] One caveat of self-reported prevalence use is it does not capture the unintended use of cathinones that are found as adulterants or misleadingly sold as MDMA to unaware users.[40]

### Pharmacology

SCs are central nervous system stimulants,[41] increasing postsynaptic neurotransmission: they inhibit the reuptake of serotonin, dopamine, and norepinephrine, and, to a lesser extent, increase presynaptic release of these monoamines by reversing the flux of their transport from inside to outside the neuron.

- Methylenedioxypyrovalerone (MDPV) is a pure monoamine reuptake inhibitor, with an affinity for dopamine and norepinephrine transporters 10 and 50 times stronger than cocaine, respectively, but 10 times less strong for serotonin.[42]
- Alpha-PVP is also a pure reuptake inhibitor, with an affinity for dopamine and norepinephrine transporters 15 and 20 times stronger, respectively, than cocaine and almost no serotonin activity.[43]
- Mephedrone, methylone, ethylone, and butylone are reuptake inhibitors of the 3 catecholamines, and similarly to MDMA, also serotonin releasers.[42]
- Ephedrone and flephedrone are selective dopamine and norepinephrine reuptake inhibitors, and similar to amphetamines, dopamine releasers as well.[42]

The increase in norepinephrine in the synaptic cleft is linked to sympathomimetic effects, dopamine to psychostimulant and addictive features, and serotonin to paranoia and hallucinations.[42]

SCs are typically ingested orally, but can also be smoked, insufflated, and injected intravenously.[44,45] There are reports of rectal, intramuscular, and other routes of administration. Typical mephedrone and methylone oral doses range from 100 to 200 mg, with the onset of psychostimulant effects starting 30 to 45 minutes later, and the duration of action being 2 to 5 hours.[35] When insufflated, a dose of mephedrone ranging from 20 to 75 mg has a quick onset and lasts less than 2 hours, whereas an intravenous dose has a quicker onset, with a "high" lasting 10 to 15 minutes, and psychoactive effects lasting less than 30 minutes.[42] On the other hand, the MDPV oral dose is about 10 to 15 mg, has a quicker onset at 15 to 30 minutes, and a duration of 2 to 7 hours.[35] MDPV is more lipophilic than other SCs and efficiently crosses the blood-brain barrier.[42] Jolliff and colleagues[46] have also suggested MDPV crosses the placenta because it was found in the blood, urine, and cord blood of a newborn.

SCs are thought to undergo hepatic phase I and II metabolism, where they could be affected by drug interactions. For mephedrone, cytochrome CYP2D6 is mainly involved in its phase I metabolism,[42] whereas for methylone, it is CYP2C19, 2D6, and 1A2.[35] Methylone, butylone, and ethylone were found to be metabolized by catechol O-methyltransferase.[42]

### Clinical Presentation and Toxicology

Like amphetamines, intoxications with SCs present with sympathomimetic and neuropsychiatric symptoms.[34] The Texas PCC retrospectively looked at 51 pediatric patients aged 12 to 19 years between 2010 and 2011 and found the main features at presentation following analytically unconfirmed exposures to SCs were agitation (43%), tachycardia (37.3%), drowsiness (13.7%), hallucinations (9.8%), fever (9.8%), vomiting (9.8%), and hypertension (7.8%).[47] Similarly, the American Association of PCCs found that among 1328 analytically unconfirmed pediatric exposures, the most common signs were tachycardia (48.8%), hallucinations and/or delusions (21.6%), hypertension (16%), seizures (5.5%), fever (5.3%), and acidosis (2.4%).[48] There are also pediatric cases of analytically confirmed intoxications with MDPV, mephedrone, and methylone, whereby the patients presented with paranoia, insomnia, diaphoresis, mydriasis, tremor,[49] catatonia,[50] transudative ascites and hepatosplenomegaly,[51] death,[52] and sexual assault facilitated by intoxication.[53]

Clinical presentation following exposure to SCs varies widely for the same reasons as with SCRAs.[34] Generally speaking, more severe adverse reactions are reported after insufflation and intravenous use, compared with other routes of administration. Moreover, the most commonly found SC in the blood and urine of patients self-reporting taking "bath salts" after presenting to the ED is MDPV, which implies that MDPV is more toxic than other SCs.[54]

"Comedown" or aftereffects can also be experienced with higher doses of SCs, redosing, or use of potent SCs like MDPV[42]; this could be linked to monoamine dopamine and serotonin receptor downregulation. It includes, but is not limited to, anxiety, depression, irritability, insomnia, anhedonia, muscle cramping, and fatigue.

## OPIOIDS

AH-7921, U-47700, MT-45, and fentanyl analogues (eg, carfentanil) are emerging synthetic opioids that were originally patented in the 1970s but introduced on the recreational drug market only in the early 2010s. Designer opioids are illicitly manufactured and either sold in place of another illicitly produced drug, unknowingly to the customer, or used to "cut" another illicit drug. Their use is thought to have fueled the increase in the opioid overdose epidemic in the last 2 years.[55]

## Epidemiology

Opioid misuse is a rapidly growing epidemic in North America. There were 28,647 deaths related to opioid poisonings in the United States in 2014 alone[56] and 33,091 in 2015.[57] Deaths from synthetic opioids other than methadone have increased by 72.2% from 2014 to 2015, with 9580 deaths in 2015.[58] Currently, little is known about the prevalence of use of designer opioids. Their use is difficult to capture because most intoxications result from unintentional exposure,[59] where they pose a public health risk for being used as adulterants to "cut" other illicitly manufactured drugs and as counterfeit pills. At risk of such exposure are the 0.3% of 8th, 10th, and 12th grade students in the United States who self-reported heroin use at least once in 2016, and 4.8% of 12th graders that took "narcotics" other than heroin.[13] It is thought that fentanyl and analogues are popularly used to intensify the euphoric state induced by other drugs such as heroin;[60] they are also quite inexpensive to manufacture.

## Pharmacology

Designer opioids are opioid receptor agonists found in pill, powder, liquid, and nasal spray[61] and can be used orally, sublingually, parenterally, rectally,[62] by nasal insufflation or spray, or by heating the drug and inhaling the vapor.

AH-7921 is a compound structurally related to fentanyl and phencyclidine.[63] It is an agonist of mu- and kappa-opioid receptors with a moderate selectivity toward mu-opioid receptors; it has a potency similar or slightly lower than morphine for analgesia in animal models,[62,63] but is 1.7 times more potent for respiratory inhibition.[63] Its activity at other pharmacologic targets has not been studied. Usual oral doses range from 40 to 150 mg.

U-47700 is an isomer of AH-7921, but is thought to have an affinity 7.5 times stronger than morphine for the mu-opioid receptor and a much higher selectivity for the mu than the kappa-opioid receptor.[59] U-47700 is popularly known as "Pink" among its users.

MT-45, also called I-C6, is a piperazine derivative analgesic that is an agonist of mu-, delta-, and kappa-opioid receptors[62] and possibly other receptors.[64] Each enantiomer has a different potency and affinity at the receptors, with the (S) enantiomer being more potent than morphine in some rodent models and more selective toward the delta and kappa receptors, and the (R) enantiomer being less potent than morphine and less selective.[64] An experimental pain model in mice showed a smaller difference in therapeutic and toxic doses than for morphine, suggesting a higher risk of overdose.[65] Usual oral doses reported on the Internet is 25-75 mg and insufflation is 15-30 mg.[65] The onset of action is 15 minutes after insufflation or up to 60 minutes after oral intake and lasts for up to 2 hours.[65]

Fentanyl analogues are lipophilic compounds, selective agonists of mu-opioid receptor. Some examples include the following:

- Acryloylfentanyl,[66] or acrylfentanyl, is particularly challenging to detect analytically because its structure is closely related to fentanyl. Compared with fentanyl, its potency was found to be similar in a rat brain model, but its duration of action prolonged, still maintaining analgesic effects two hours after intraperitoneal administration in mice.
- Acetylfentanyl[67] is structurally similar to fentanyl, with an extra methyl group. It was found to be 15 times more potent than morphine and 3 times less potent than fentanyl for analgesia in an animal model, but also 6 times more toxic than fentanyl in a dose-finding animal model, meaning that acetylfentanyl has a narrow therapeutic index compared with fentanyl.

- Carfentanil is currently used in veterinary medicine for general anesthesia of large animals and as a radioligand for PET imaging in humans.[68] It is 10,000 times more potent than morphine and 100 times more potent than fentanyl,[69] making it one of the most potent opioids known and the strongest commercially available. A veterinarian developed drowsiness within 2 minutes following accidental ocular and oral mucous membrane exposure despite immediate decontamination,[69] suggesting this compound is readily bioavailable after mucous membrane exposure and has a quick onset of action. Half-life in humans was also found to be around 40 minutes.[68]
- Little is known about other fentanyl analogues. Butyrfentanyl is reported to be several times more potent than morphine but retains approximately one-sixth of the potency of fentanyl,[70] and ocfentanil is reported to be 90 times more potent than morphine and twice as potent as fentanyl.[71]

### Clinical Presentation and Toxicology

Opioids induce euphoria, relaxation, and a state of well-being. MT-45 is reported by some users to induce sedation without euphoria.[64] Self-limited adverse events include itching, sedation, somnolence, dizziness, and nausea. Typical opioid overdose presentation such as deep sedation, respiratory depression, cyanosis, miosis, tachycardia, hypertension, and hypothermia are also observed in intoxications involving various fentanyl analogs.[61,62] Seizures were also reported in patients intoxicated with AH-7921[72] and MT-45.[64]

MT-45 was linked to transient tinnitus and hearing loss, and neurologic effects (paresthesia, blurred vision, and seizures).[62] Another particularity is that its (S) isomer is linked to excitation, whereas the (R) isomer is linked to sedation.[64]

A literature search identified only two published pediatric case reports involving designer opioids: Coopam and colleagues[71] describe the forensic aspects of a lethal intoxication with ocfentanil in a 17-year-old male adolescent, and Cole and colleagues[70] describe the clinical management of an 18-year-old male adolescent that presented with hemoptysis, acute lung injury, and diffuse alveolar hemorrhage after insufflating butyrfentanyl.

## LABORATORY TESTING OF NEW PSYCHOACTIVE SUBSTANCES

Clinical testing of common illicit drugs is routinely done in two stages: urine drug screening (UDS) that typically uses immunoassays, followed by a confirmatory assay that is either performed using gas chromatography-mass spectrometry (GC-MS) or liquid chromatography-mass spectrometry (LC-MS).[72–75] These assays are targeted, that is, they are developed with a predefined set of drugs as analytes. The rapid turnover of NPS drug composition does not lend itself tractable to this type of drug testing. Hence, identifying and confirming NPS in emergency cases pose a unique and almost insurmountable challenge to clinical laboratories.

Evasion of detection by UDS is one of the major appeals of NPS to its users. Although NPS are derivatives or analogues of common illicit drugs, their structures may differ enough to evade cross-reaction with immunoassays used to screen for common drugs of abuse. Several studies have evaluated the cross-reactivity of several classes of NPS to commonly used immunoassays in clinical and forensic laboratories (**Table 2**).[76–81]

As what has been the common experience in most clinical laboratories, these studies demonstrate that NPS do not cross-react with UDS for common drugs of abuse. Likewise, the reliability of immunoassays developed for specific classes of NPS like SCRAs and SCs is dismal even in detecting newer compounds within their class.

**Table 2**
**Selected studies on the cross-reactivity of cathinones and cannabinoids to commercially available immunoassays**

| Reference | Study | Findings |
|---|---|---|
| Beck et al,[76] 2014 | Tested the detectability of 45 different NPS including 14 cathinones spiked in urine in 3 commonly used immunoassay platforms (CEDIA, EMIT, and KIMS) | Of the 17 immunoassays tested, 11 did not show cross-reactivity to any of the 45 NPS tested<br>Seven of the 14 cathinones cross-reacted with the EMIT or CEDIA amphetamine assay but at concentrations $\geq$10 µg/mL<br>Few cathinones like $\alpha$-PPP and MPPP were observed to give false positive results in the CEDIA cocaine assay albeit at low cross-reactivity rate of 5.4% and 1.2%, respectively |
| Swortwood et al,[77] 2014 | Tested the cross-reactivity of 30 NPS, including 8 cathinones spiked in serum in 16 different enzyme-linked immunosorbent assay (ELISA) reagents | All but one have cross-reactivities of <4% to the ELISA reagents<br>Most have no cross-reactivity and only mephedrone at 40 ng/mL showed 25% cross-reactivity in the Orasure methamphetamine assay |
| Ellefsen et al,[78] 2014 | Validated a commercially available immunoassay for SCs (Randox) | When applied to urine specimens, the validated immunoassays for mephedrone/methcathinone (Randox BSI) and MDPV/MDPBP (Randox BSII) showed only 4 of the 97 (4.1%) presumptive positive specimens from the 2 assays confirmed for one or more SCs at the manufacturer's prescribed cutoff concentration for a positive response<br>Few cathinones cross-reacted with the immunoassays (eg, methedrone and butylone for BS I and MDPPP, pentedrone and butylone for BS II) but most of the other cathinones did not cross-react with the immunoassays |
| Franz et al,[79] 2017 | Evaluated the diagnostic efficiency of immunoassay screening of synthetic cannabinoids in urine using the "JWH-018" kit (Immunalysis SC1) and "UR-144" kit (Immunalysis SC II) | In applying the immunoassays to a study with confirmed 8% prevalence of SC use (n = 549), none of the samples tested positive in the immunoassays<br>In a second study (n = 200), the 2 assays showed a combined sensitivity of 2% and diagnostic efficiency of 51%<br>Samples with confirmed metabolites of AB-CHMINACA, AB-FUBINACA, ADB-CHMINACA, AM-2201, MDMB-CHMICA, or 5F-PB-22 were not detected as positive by both assays |

(continued on next page)

**Table 2**
*(continued)*

| Reference | Study | Findings |
|-----------|-------|----------|
| Spinelli et al,[80] 2015 | Evaluated the performance of an SPICE ELISA kit that targets JWH-018 N-pentanoic acid (Neogen) | Applying the assay to 2469 urine specimens, the assay exhibited 79.9% sensitivity, 99.4% specificity, and 97.6% efficiency at a cutoff of 5 ng/mL when the results were confirmed by LC-MS/MS<br>Only 18 of 73 other synthetic cannabinoid markers evaluated exhibited >10% cross-reactivity to the assay at concentrations of 10–100 ng/mL |
| Barnes et al,[81] 2015 | Validated an ELISA synthetic cannabinoids urine assay that targets the JWH-018 N-(5-hyrdroxypentyl) metabolite (NMS) | Applying the assay to 2492 urine specimens, the assay exhibited 83.4% sensitivity, 99.7% specificity, and 97.4% efficiency at a cutoff of 5 ng/mL when the results were confirmed by LC-MS/MS<br>Only 19 of 73 other synthetic cannabinoid markers evaluated exhibited >10% cross-reactivity to the assay at concentrations of 10–100 ng/mL |

*Abbreviations:* α- PPP- α-Pyrrolidinopropiophenone, CEDIA, Cloned Enzyme Donor Immunoassay; EMIT, Enzyme Multiplied Immunoassay Technique; MDPBP, 3′4′-Methylenedioxy-α-pyrrolidinobutiophenone; MDPPP- 3′4′-Methylenedioxy-α-pyrrolidinopropiophenone; MPPP, 4′-Methyl-α-pyrrolidinopropiophenone.

A large number of confirmatory testing for NPS by targeted GC-MS or liquid chromatography-tandem mass spectrometry assay (LC-MS/MS) has been published in the last five years. For SCRAs, SCs and opioid analogues alone, more than a hundred publications on GC-MS and LC-MS methods have been reported since 2012. A few reviews that comprehensively summarize these methods and the specific NPS they cover are good sources of information on the extent of targeted NPS testing currently available.[82–87] Although targeted assays using GC-MS and LC-MS/MS are currently the gold standard for quantitative analysis, they are not adequate for NPS testing. Even comprehensive targeted NPS assays are limited to a few hundred analytes and are not able to detect previously unidentified NPS, which are now appearing at a rapidly accelerating turnover rate as more aggressive scheduling of identified NPS is being pursued.

Recently, more advanced laboratories have used high-resolution mass spectrometry (HRMS) for the comprehensive analysis of NPS. HRMS platforms like the Orbitrap and quadrupole time-of-flight mass spectrometer have the capacity to perform nontargeted data acquisition, that is, no predefined list of analytes is used to acquire data from a sample.[82] Instead, all accurate masses in a sample are acquired, and the sum of all acquired masses (total ion chromatogram) is later queried using a database of suspect compounds. If a reference standard of a compound in the database is available, the process is no different from targeted analysis. However, if the compound in the database has no available reference standard, a tentative identification of a possible compound is done through a process called suspect screening. The suspect compound is later confirmed by acquiring its reference standard. Suspect screening enables the detection of previously unidentified NPS, a capability that is compatible with the fast turnover rate of chemical composition of most NPS products. More recently, published HRMS methods for analyzing NPS in urine and serum are reviewed by Meyer and Maurer.[87]

It is worth remembering that most NPS are not detected by common UDS assays. Even the newer immunoassays developed for specific classes of NPS do not cross-react with all compounds in its class. Hence, in interpreting the results of immunoassays for SCRAs, SCs, and opioid analogues, it is important to ask for the specific compounds for which the immunoassay has been developed and tested to avoid making a diagnosis from false negative results. The same applies for interpreting targeted NPS assays. A positive result confirms the presence of specific NPS, but a negative result does not exclude the possibility that a new NPS not covered by the targeted assay may be in the sample. By far, suspect screening using HRMS provides the more comprehensive and reliable method for NPS testing in the clinical laboratory.

Although urine is the most commonly used sample for drug testing, the clinician should also consider sending serum or plasma for NPS testing to laboratories that have such capabilities using HRMS especially if an NPS cause is being considered for a case. Urine is a suitable matrix to assess exposure to a drug, but because some drugs may persist in urine beyond 72 hours after they were taken, results of a urine drug assay may not always be associated with a patient's symptoms. In cases whereby urine is the only available matrix, however, it is important to note that some NPS are rapidly metabolized, such as most SCRAs. Hence, in assessing whether a test covers a specific NPS, one should also consider whether the assay also detects its metabolites. When drug testing is needed in neonates to identify what they were exposed to in utero, hair and meconium samples are suitable matrices to test. Because hair is subject to external contamination, it is best to obtain hair sample as close to the neonate's time of delivery as possible.

### Assessment and Treatment

Assessment of suspected NPS toxicity is complicated by multiple factors, including limited or misleading case information, polydrug ingestion, and severe limitations of testing in the acute setting. Therefore, a good physical assessment is critical. Because a true antidote only exists for opioids, most management is supportive. Because there are no controlled trials for the treatment of NPS, experts generally extrapolate from other pharmacologically similar agents and rely on observational data.

The following principles are not intended to be complete, but a starting point. An early discussion with the medical toxicologist or the PCC especially for ill patients should be considered. In addition, most medical toxicologists and PCC are involved in NPS from a public health standpoint. In the United States, the local PCC can be reached at all times at 1-800-222-1222.

### Loss of airway reflexes/respiratory failure

The loss of airway reflexes or respiratory failure is a medical emergency and should be managed consistently with the Pediatric Advanced Life Support guidelines. Naloxone, a mu-opioid receptor antagonist, is used to reverse opioid toxidrome, with the goal being the restoration of adequate breathing and airway reflexes, as opposed to complete reversal to full consciousness that may precipitate withdrawal.[88] The effective dose of naloxone depends on the patient's weight, amount of opioid to be reversed, and binding affinities at the mu receptor for naloxone compared with the opioid. For children, the initial dose is 0.1 mg/kg. For adolescents, following adult dosing may be beneficial especially if opioid dependency is considered. Boyer[88] recommends an initial adult dose of naloxone of 0.04 mg, which may be lower than the initial pediatric dose. The dose is then escalated every 2 minutes until ventilation is preserved or until 15 mg of naloxone has been given. If the patient does not respond to 15 mg of naloxone, it is unlikely they will respond to higher doses. Naloxone can be given by parenteral, intranasal, or endotracheal routes. Because it has a short duration of action, patients should be observed closely, especially 45 to 90 minutes because additional naloxone may be needed. There is scarce information on human and animal naloxone reversal of ultrapotent opioids, that is, carfentanil, and higher than usual doses may be necessary.[69]

### Chest pain

With chest pain, shortness of breath, or severe intoxications, an electrocardiogram and serial troponins are helpful in evaluating for acute myocardial damage.[89] In patients with myocardial infarction or unstable angina following drug intoxication, the best data available are for cocaine. The American Heart Association recommends intravenous fluids, benzodiazepines, and nitroglycerine as the primary treatments, while avoiding beta-blockers because they increase the risk of exacerbating coronary spasms.[89] In a case of a 16-year-old male adolescent with unconfirmed SCRA exposure presenting with chest pain and ST-elevation myocardial infarction, sublingual nitroglycerin spray and acetylsalicylic acid by mouth were used initially, followed by a nitroglycerin infusion titrated to pain relief. Cardiac catheterization later suggested vasospasm.[90]

### Hypertension

Hypertension needs to be addressed in the setting of hypertensive emergency or signs of end-organ damage. As for chest pain, hypertension in the setting of cocaine intoxication provides most of the literature for guidance. Treatment with benzodiazepines and avoidance of beta-blockers are the cornerstone, whereas nitroglycerin and phentolamine may be useful in cases refractory to benzodiazepines.[89]

### Dysrhythmia

Tachycardia is treated primarily with fluids, benzodiazepines, and supportive care.[44,45] In addition to tachycardia, QRS prolongation and QT prolongation may exist. QRS prolongations are generally mediated through sodium channel blockade and are seen, for example, with intoxications to bupropion, an SC,[91] or lidocaine that has been found as contaminant in NPS.[92] Treatment of QRS prolongation is sodium bicarbonate intravenously until QRS is less than 100 ms, or serum pH 7.45 to 7.55 and sodium of 145 to 150 meq/L.[91] Treatment of QT prolongation begins with optimizing electrolytes, especially potassium, calcium, and magnesium. In addition to cardioversion, overdrive pacing can be used. In refractory, life-threatening dysrhythmias, intravenous 20% lipid emulsion dosed at 1.5 mL/kg can be considered.[93]

### Seizures

Seizures require immediate attention with escalating doses of a benzodiazepine every 5 to 10 minutes and dosing that may exceed the package insert. The data for the best second-line agent are unclear. Second-line agents include barbiturates, propofol, and levetiracetam. Phenytoin and fosphenytoin have failed to show benefit for terminating active toxin-induced seizures and should be avoided.[94] Once seizure control is obtained, imaging should be performed.

### Fever

Fever is a medical emergency in intoxicated patients. In contrast to an infectious cause, the fever is from extreme motor neuromotor excitation. Consequently, antipyretics are generally unhelpful and not recommended. In addition to intravenous fluids and cooling measures, benzodiazepines should be given to get the patient calm and cooperative. In cases of very high fevers, that is, greater than 40°C, chemically induced coma may be beneficial with or without a paralytic. When using paralytics, ensuring proper sedation is critical. If available, continuous electroencephalogrammonitoring is helpful in identifying seizures.

### Agitation and hallucinations

Benzodiazepines are the most common first-line agents.[44,45,95] Benzodiazepines are GABA agonists that hyperpolarize membranes and suppress neuroexcitation. In severe intoxication, higher doses than the package insert may be needed.[44,45,95] Because all benzodiazepines share the same mechanism of action, there is little benefit switching agents if the desired effect is not achieved. Instead, consider escalating the dose every 10 to 15 minutes until the patient is calm. In controlled trials of undifferentiated delirium and agitation, midazolam was the fastest among benzodiazepines and antipsychotics. Antipsychotics are used in less than 20% of cases[44,45,95] because, although they are sedatives, they do not offer protection from seizures, cause QT prolongation, and may interfere with the body's ability to cool itself. Typically, an antipsychotic is given with a benzodiazepine and doses do not exceed the package insert.[44,95] Ketamine may be an additional option as a second-line agent.[96] Physical restraints are a recognized primary risk factor in sudden death in acutely delirious patients.[97,98] Restraints should only be used as a last resort, applied simultaneously with chemical restraint, removed as soon as possible, and used only if patients can be supervised closely.[99,100]

### Rhabdomyolysis

To prevent kidney damage, treatment is aggressive fluids with close monitoring of urine output, electrolytes, and renal function.[44,45,95]

### SUMMARY

NPS have been evolving rapidly in the past decade with dozens of new compounds emerging every year. Recently, NPS have also been found in counterfeit pills such as Norco and OxyContin. Clinicians should consider an NPS cause when someone presents with physical signs and symptoms that may be similar to a drug intoxication after taking an unknown substance, a product obtained from the Internet or headshops, a "prescription pill" obtained from the black or gray market, or a product with the warning "not for human consumption." A thorough history and physical examination should be performed and the identified signs and symptoms treated supportively in the absence of an antidote. Typical immunoassays may not capture the new drug taken, and additional testing either by comprehensive NPS targeted testing or by suspect screening should be considered.

### REFERENCES

1. EMCDDA and Europol, 2016 EU Drug Markets Report: In-Depth Analysis. 2016. Available at: http://www.emcdda.europa.eu/publications/joint-publications/eu-drug-markets-2016-in-depth-analysis. Accessed May 5, 2017.

2. Drugwise. New psychoactive substances. 2016. Available at: http://www.drugwise.org.uk/new-psychoactive-substances. Accessed May 5, 2017.

3. United Nations Office on Drugs and Crime. The challenge of new psychoactive substances: a report from the Global SMART Programme. 2013. Available at: https://www.unodc.org/documents/scientific/NPS_2013_SMART.pdf. Accessed May 5, 2017.

4. Martinotti G, Lupi M, Carlucci L, et al. Novel psychoactive substances: use and knowlodge among adolescents and young adults in urban and rural areas. Hum Psychopharmacol 2015;30(4):295–301.

5. Schifano F, Orsolini L, Duccio Papanti G, et al. Novel psychoactive substances of interest for psychiatry. World Psychiatry 2015;14(1):15–26.

6. Wood DM, Dargan PI. The toxicity of the novel psychoactive substances. In: Gall JAM, Payne-James JJ, editors. Current practice in forensic medicine. West Sussex (United Kingdom): John Wiley and Sons, Ltd; 2016. p. 35–46.

7. UNODC, World Drug Report 2013. 2013. Available at: https://www.unodc.org/unodc/secured/wdr/wdr2013/World_Drug_Report_2013.pdf. Accessed May 5, 2017.

8. American Association of Poison Control Centers. AAPCC issues statement on the synthetic drug abuse prevention act. 2012. Available at: http://www.aapcc.org/press/2/. Accessed May 5, 2017.

9. Musselman ME, Hampton JP. "Not for human consumption": a review of emerging designer drugs. Pharmacotherapy 2014;34(7):745–57.

10. Drug Enforcement Agency Strategic Intelligence Section. Counterfeit prescription pills containing fentanyls: a global threat. 2016. Available at: https://www.dea.gov/docs/Counterfeit%20Prescription%20Pills.pdf. Accessed May 5, 2017.

11. Loeffler G, Delaney E, Hann M. International trends in spice use: prevalence, motivation for use, relationship to other substances, and perception of use and safety for synthetic cannabinoids. Brain Res Bull 2016;126(Pt 1):8–28.

12. European Monitoring Center for Drugs and Drug Addiction. Synthetic cannabinoids in Europe (Perspectives on drugs). 2016. Available at: http://www.emcdda.europa.eu/system/files/publications/2753/att_212361_EN_EMCDDA_POD_2013_Synthetic%20cannabinoids.pdf. Accessed April 30, 2017.

13. Johnston LD, Miech RA, O'Malley PM, et al. Teen use of any illicit drug other than marijuana at new low, same true for alcohol. Table 2: trends in annual prevalence of use of various drugs in grades 8, 10, and 12. University of Michigan news service. 2016. Available at: http://www.monitoringthefuture.org/data/16data/16drtbl2.pdf. Accessed April 30, 2017.

14. Keyes KM, Rutherford C, Hamilton A, et al. Age, period, and cohort effects in synthetic cannabinoid use among US adolescents, 2011-2015. Drug Alcohol Depend 2016;166:159–67.

15. American Association of Poison Control Centers. Synthetic cannabinolds. 2017. Available at: http://www.aapcc.org/alerts/synthetic-cannabinoids/. Accessed April 30, 2017.

16. Wood KE. Exposure to bath salts and synthetic tetrahydrocannabinol from 2009 to 2012 in the United States. J Pediatr 2013;163(1):213–6.

17. Substance Abuse and Mental Health Services Administration, Center for Behavioral Health Statistics and Quality. The DAWN report: drug-related emergency department visits involving synthetic cannabinoids. 2012. Available at: https://www.samhsa.gov/data/sites/default/files/DAWN105/DAWN105/SR105-synthetic-marijuana.pdf. Accessed April 30, 2017.

18. Bush DM, Woodwell DA, on behalf of the Substance Abuse and Mental Health Services Administration. Center for Behavioral Health Statistics and Quality. The CBHSQ report – Update: drug-related emergency department visits involving synthetic cannabinoids. 2014. Available at: https://www.samhsa.gov/data/sites/default/files/SR-1378/SR-1378.pdf. Accessed April 30, 2017.

19. European Monitoring Center for Drugs and Drug Addiction. Understanding the 'Spice' phenomenon. 2009. Available at: http://www.emcdda.europa.eu/system/

files/publications/537/Spice-Thematic-paper-final-version.pdf. Accessed April 30, 2017.

20. European Monitoring Center for Drugs and Drug Addiction. EMCDDA-Europol joint report on MDMB-CHMICA. 2016. Available at: http://www.emcdda. europa.eu/system/files/publications/2873/2016.4528_WEB.pdf. Accessed April 28, 2017.

21. Banister SD, Moir M, Stuart J, et al. Pharmacology of indole and indazole synthetic cannabinoid designer drugs AB-FUBINACA, ADB-FUBINACA, AB-PINACA, ADB-PINACA, 5F-AB-PINACA, 5F-ADB-PINACA, ADBICA, and 5F-ADBICA. ACS Chem Neurosci 2015;6(9):1546–59.

22. Banister SD, Longworth M, Kevin R, et al. Pharmacology of valinate and tert-leucinate synthetic cannabinoids 5F-AMBICA, 5F-AMB, 5F-ADB, AMB-FUBINACA, MDMB-FUBINACA, MDMB-CHMICA, and their analogues. ACS Chem Neurosci 2016;7(9):1241–54.

23. Adams AJ, Banister SD, Irizarry L, et al. "Zombie" outbreak caused by the synthetic cannabinoid AMB-FUBINACA in New York. N Engl J Med 2017;376(3): 235–42.

24. Abdulrahim D, Bowden-Jones O, on behalf of the NEPTUNE Expert Group. Guidance on the clinical management of acute and chronic harms of club drugs and novel psychoactive substances. 2015. Available at: http://neptune-clinical-guidance.co.uk/wp-content/uploads/2015/03/NEPTUNE-Guidance-March-2015. pdf. Accessed April 30, 2017.

25. Fisar Z. Inhibition of monoamine oxidase activity by cannabinoids. Naunyn Schmiedebergs Arch Pharmacol 2010;381(6):563–72.

26. Forrester MB, Kleinschmidt K, Schwarz E, et al. Synthetic cannabinoid exposures reported to Texas poison centers. J Addict Dis 2011;30(4):351–8.

27. Castellanos D, Gralnik LM. Synthetic cannabinoids 2015: an update for pediatricians in clinical practice. World J Clin Pediatr 2016;5(1):16–24.

28. Tait RJ, Caldicott D, Mountain D, et al. A systematic review of adverse events arising from the use of synthetic cannabinoids and their associated treatment. Clin Toxicol (Phila) 2016;54(1):1–13.

29. Adamowicz P, Gieroń J. Acute intoxication of four individuals following use of the synthetic cannabinoid MAB-CHMINACA. Clin Toxicol (Phila) 2016;54(8):650–4.

30. Hawkins JA, Ryan ML, Arnold TC. Severe toxicity after synthetic cannabinoid exposure in an infant [67]. Clin Toxicol (Phila) 2015;53(7):670.

31. Thornton SL, Akpunonu P, Glauner K, et al. Unintentional pediatric exposure to a synthetic cannabinoid (AB-PINACA) resulting in coma and intubation. Ann Emerg Med 2015;66(3):343–4.

32. Young AC, Schwarz E, Medina G, et al. Cardiotoxicity associated with the synthetic cannabinoid, K9, with laboratory confirmation. Am J Emerg Med 2012; 30(7):1320.e5-7.

33. Kronstrand R, Roman M, Andersson M, et al. Toxicological findings of synthetic cannabinoids in recreational users. J Anal Toxicol 2013;37(8):534–41.

34. European Monitoring Center for Drugs and Drug Addiction. Synthetic cathinones drug profile. 2015. Available at: http://www.emcdda.europa.eu/publications/ drug-profiles/synthetic-cathinones. Accessed April 18, 2017.

35. Rosenbaum CD, Carreiro SP, Babu KM. Here today, gone tomorrow...and back again? A review of herbal marijuana alternatives (K2, Spice), synthetic cathinones (bath salts), kratom, Salvia divinorum, methoxetamine, and piperazines. J Med Toxicol 2012;8(1):15–32.

36. Benzer TI, Nejad SH, Flood JG. Case records of the Massachusetts General Hospital. Case 40-2013. A 36-year-old man with agitation and paranoia. N Engl J Med 2013;369(26):2536–45.

37. European Monitoring Center for Drugs and Drug Addiction, Europol. EU drug markets report: in-depth analysis. 2016. Available at: http://www.emcdda. europa.eu/system/files/publications/2373/TD0216072ENN.PDF. Accessed April 28, 2017.

38. Drug Policy Alliance. Fact sheet: synthetic cathinones. 2016. Available at: http:// www.drugpolicy.org/sites/default/files/DPA_Fact_Sheet_Synthetic_Cathinones_% 28June%202016%29.pdf. Accessed April 28, 2017.

39. Substance Abuse and Mental Health Services Administration. The DAWN report: "bath salts" were involved in over 20,000 drug-related emergency department visits in 2011. 2013. Available at: https://www.samhsa.gov/data/sites/default/ files/spot117-bath-salts-2013/spot117-bath-salts-2013.pdf. Accessed April 28, 2017.

40. Palamar JJ, Salomone A, Vincenti M, et al. Detection of "bath salts" and other novel psychoactive substances in hair samples of ecstasy/MDMA/"Molly" users. Drug Alcohol Depend 2016;161:200–5.

41. Rech MA, Donahey E, Cappiello Dziedzic JM, et al. New drugs of abuse. Pharmacotherapy 2015;35(2):189–97.

42. Valente MJ, Guedes de Pinho P, de Lourdes Bastos M, et al. Khat and synthetic cathinones: a review. Arch Toxicol 2014;88(1):15–45.

43. European Monitoring Center for Drugs and Drug Addiction. EMCDDA-Europol joint report on a new psychoactive substance: 1-phenyl-2-(1-pyrrolidinyl)-1-pentanone (α-PVP). 2015. Available at: http://www.emcdda.europa.eu/system/files/ publications/1814/TDAS15001ENN.pdf. Accessed April 28, 2017.

44. Warrick BJ, Hill M, Hekman K, et al. A 9-state analysis of designer stimulant, "bath salt," hospital visits reported to poison control centers. Ann Emerg Med 2013;62(3):244–51.

45. Froberg BA, Levine M, Beuhler MC, et al. Acute methylenedioxypyrovalerone toxicity. J Med Toxicol 2015;11(2):185–94.

46. Jolliff HA, Keyes JS, Magers JA, et al. "Bath salts" toxicity and withdrawal in a newborn [229]. Clin Toxicol (Phila) 2013;51(7):679.

47. Forrester MB. Adolescent synthetic cathinone exposures reported to Texas poison centers. Pediatr Emerg Care 2013;29(2):151–5.

48. Tekulve K, Alexander A, Tormoehlen L. Seizures associated with synthetic cathinone exposures in the pediatric population. Pediatr Neurol 2014;51(1):67–70.

49. Osterhoudt KC, Cook MD. Clean but not sober: a 16-year-old with restlessness. Pediatr Emerg Care 2011;27(9):892–4.

50. Antunes J, Urbano N, Estrada J, et al. Catatonia in a teenager after use of mephedrone as a recreational drug. Sci Med 2013;23(3):175–9.

51. Stanisz J, Terry J, Zeidler J, et al. Unexplained ascites in an adolescent female: possible association with excessive ingestion of methylone [A189]. Can J Gastroenterol Hepatol 2016;2016:4792898.

52. Kovacs K, Toht AR, Kereszty EM. A new designer drug: methylone related death. Orv Hetil 2012;153(7):271–6.

53. Hagan KS, Reidy L. Detection of synthetic cathinones in victims of sexual assault. Forensic Sci Int 2015;257:71–5.

54. National Institute on Drug Abuse. Synthetic cathinones ("Bath salts"). 2016. Available at: https://www.drugabuse.gov/publications/drugfacts/synthetic-cathinones-bath-salts. Accessed April 30, 2017.

55. Drug Enforcement Administration. DEA report: counterfeit pills fueling U.S. fentanyl and opioid crisis. Problems resulting from abuse opioid drugs continue to grow. 2016. Available at: https://www.dea.gov/divisions/hq/2016/hq072216.shtml. Accessed April 30, 2017.

56. Lucyk SN, Nelson LS. Novel synthetic opioids: an opioid epidemic within an opioid epidemic. Ann Emerg Med 2017 Jan;69(1):91–3.

57. Centers for Disease Control and Prevention. Drug overdose death data. 2016. Available at: https://www.cdc.gov/drugoverdose/data/statedeaths.html. Accessed April 30, 2017.

58. Centers for Disease Control and Prevention. Synthetic opioid data. 2016. Available at: https://www.cdc.gov/drugoverdose/data/fentanyl.html. Accessed April 30, 2017.

59. Armenian P, Olson A, Anaya A, et al. Fentanyl and a novel synthetic opioid U-47700 masquerading as street "Norco" in central California: a case report. Ann Emerg Med 2017;69(1):87–90.

60. Centers for Disease Control and Prevention. Opioid data analysis. 2017. https://www.cdc.gov/drugoverdose/data/analysis.html. Accessed April 30, 2017.

61. Helander A, Bäckberg M, Signell P, et al. Intoxications involving acrylfentanyl and other novel designer fentanyls - results from the Swedish STRIDA project. Clin Toxicol (Phila) 2017. http://dx.doi.org/10.1080/15563650.2017.1303141.

62. Zawilska JB, Andrzejczak D. Next generation of novel psychoactive substances on the horizon - a complex problem to face. Drug Alcohol Depend 2015 Dec 1; 157:1–17.

63. European Monitoring Center for Drugs and Drug Addiction. EMCDDA-Europol joint report on a new psychoactive substance: AH-7921. 2014. Available at: http://www.emcdda.europa.eu/system/files/publications/816/AH-7921_465209.pdf. Accessed April 28, 2017.

64. European Monitoring Center for Drugs and Drug Addiction. EMCDDA-Europol joint report on a new psychoactive substance: 1-cyclohexyl-4-(1,2-diphenylethyl)piperazine ('MT-45'). 2014. http://www.emcdda.europa.eu/system/files/publications/810/TDAS14007ENN_477731.pdf. Accessed April 28, 2017.

65. European Monitoring Center for Drugs and Drug Addiction. Report on the risk assessment of MT-45 in the framework of the Council Decision on new psychoactive substances. 2015. Available at: http://www.emcdda.europa.eu/system/files/publications/1865/TDAK14006ENN.pdf. Accessed April 28, 2017.

66. European Monitoring Center for Drugs and Drug Addiction. EMCDDA-Europol joint report on a new psychoactive substance: N-(1-phenethylpiperidin-4-yl)-N-phenylacrylamide (acryloylfentanyl). 2017. Available at: http://www.emcdda.europa.eu/system/files/publications/3873/TI_PUBPDF_TDAS17001ENN_PDFWEB_20170221105322.pdf. Accessed April 28, 2017.

67. European Monitoring Center for Drugs and Drug Addiction. EMCDDA-Europol joint report on acetylfentanyl. 2016. Available at: http://www.emcdda.europa.eu/system/files/publications/2693/TDAS16001ENN.PDF. Accessed April 28, 2017.

68. Minkowski CP, Epstein D, Frost JJ, et al. Differential response to IV carfentanil in chronic cocaine users and healthy controls. Addict Biol 2012;17(1):149–55.

69. George AV, Lu JJ, Pisano MV, et al. Carfentanil—an ultra potent opioid. Am J Emerg Med 2010;28(4):530–2.

70. Cole JB, Dunbar JF, McIntire SA, et al. Butyrfentanyl overdose resulting in diffuse alveolar hemorrhage. Pediatrics 2015;135(3):e740–3.

71. Coopam V, Cordonnier J, De Leeuw M, et al. Ocfentanil overdose fatality in the recreational drug scene. Forensic Sci Int 2016;266:469–73.

72. European Monitoring Center for Drugs and Drug Addiction. Report on the risk assessment of 3,4-dichloro-N-{[1-(dimethylamino)cyclohexyl]methyl}benzamide (AH-7921) in the framework of the Council Decision on new psychoactive substances. 2014. Available at: http://www.emcdda.europa.eu/system/files/publications/774/TDAK14002ENN_480892.pdf. Accessed April 28, 2017.

73. Markway EC, Baker SN. A review of the methods, interpretation, and limitations of the urine drug screen. Orthopedics 2011;34(11):877–81.

74. Eldridge DL, Holstege CP. Utilizing the laboratory in the poisoned patient. Clin Lab Med 2006;26(1):13–30, vii.

75. Erickson TB, Thompson TM, Lu JJ. The approach to the patient with an unknown overdose. Emerg Med Clin North Am 2007;25(2):249–81 [abstract: vii].

76. Beck O, Rausberg L, Al-Saffar Y, et al. Detectability of new psychoactive substances, 'legal highs', in CEDIA, EMIT, and KIMS immunochemical screening assays for drugs of abuse. Drug Test Anal 2014;6(5):492–9.

77. Swortwood MJ, Hearn WL, DeCaprio AP. Cross-reactivity of designer drugs, including cathinone derivatives, in commercial enzyme-linked immunosorbent assays. Drug Test Anal 2014;6(7–8):716–27.

78. Ellefsen KN, Anizan S, Castaneto MS, et al. Validation of the only commercially available immunoassay for synthetic cathinones in urine: Randox Drugs of Abuse V Biochip Array Technology. Drug Test Anal 2014;6(7–8):728–38.

79. Franz F, Angerer V, Jechle H, et al. Immunoassay screening in urine for synthetic cannabinoids - an evaluation of the diagnostic efficiency. Clin Chem Lab Med 2017;55:1375–84.

80. Spinelli E, Barnes AJ, Young S, et al. Performance characteristics of an ELISA screening assay for urinary synthetic cannabinoids. Drug Test Anal 2015;7(6):467–74.

81. Barnes AJ, Young S, Spinelli E, et al. Evaluation of a homogenous enzyme immunoassay for the detection of synthetic cannabinoids in urine. Forensic Sci Int 2014;241:27–34.

82. Wu AH, Gerona R, Armenian P, et al. Role of liquid chromatography-high-resolution mass spectrometry (LC-HR/MS) in clinical toxicology. Clin Toxicol (Phila) 2012;50(8):733–42.

83. Peters FT. Recent developments in urinalysis of metabolites of new psychoactive substances using LC-MS. Bioanalysis 2014;6(15):2083–107.

84. Znaleziona J, Ginterova P, Petr J, et al. Determination and identification of synthetic cannabinoids and their metabolites in different matrices by modern analytical techniques – a review. Anal Chim Acta 2015;874:11–25.

85. Castaneto MS, Wohlfarth A, Desrosiers NA, et al. Synthetic cannabinoids pharmacokinetics and detection methods in biological matrices. Drug Metab Rev 2015;47(2):124–74.

86. Namera A, Kawamura M, Nakamoto A, et al. Comprehensive review of the detection methods for synthetic cannabinoids and cathinones. Forensic Toxicol 2015;33(2):175–94.

87. Meyer MR, Maurer HH. Review: LC coupled to low- and high-resolution mass spectrometry for new psychoactive substance screening in biological matrices - where do we stand today? Anal Chim Acta 2016;927:13–20.

88. Boyer EW. Management of opioid analgesic overdose. N Engl J Med 2012;367(2):146–55.

89. McCord J, Jneid H, Hollander JE, et al. Management of cocaine-associated chest pain and myocardial infarction: a scientific statement from the American

Heart Association Acute Cardiac Care Committee of the Council on Clinical Cardiology. Circulation 2008;117(14):1897–907.

90. McKeever RG, Vearrier D, Jacobs D, et al. K2—not the spice of life; synthetic cannabinoids and ST elevation myocardial infarction: a case report. J Med Toxicol 2015;11(1):129–31.

91. Curry SC, Kashani JS, LoVecchio F, et al. Intraventricular conduction delay after bupropion overdose. J Emerg Med 2005;29(3):299–305.

92. Schneir A, Ly BT, Casagrande K, et al. Comprehensive analysis of "bath salts" purchased from California stores and the internet. Clin Toxicol (Phila) 2014; 52(7):651–8.

93. Levine M, Hoffman RS, Lavergne V, et al. Systematic review of the effect of intravenous lipid emulsion therapy for non-local anesthetics toxicity. Clin Toxicol (Phila) 2016;54(3):194–221.

94. Choosing Wisely Work Group. The American College of Medical Toxicology and the American Academy of Clinical Toxicology—Ten things physicians and patients should question. 2015. Available at: http://www.choosingwisely.org/wp-content/uploads/2015/02/ACMT-AACT-Choosing-Wisely-List.pdf. Accessed April 14, 2017.

95. Benzie F, Hekman K, Cameron L, et al. Emergency department visits after use of a drug sold as "bath salts" –- Michigan, November 13, 2010–March 31, 2011. MMWR Morb Mortal Wkly Rep 2011;60:624–7.

96. Nazarin DJ, Broder JS, Thiessen MEW, et al. Clinical policy: critical issues in the diagnosis and management of the adult psychiatric patient in the Emergency Department. Ann Emerg Med 2017;69:480–90.

97. Stratton SJ, Rogers C, Brickett K, et al. Factors associated with sudden death of individuals requiring restraint for excited delirium. Am J Emerg Med 2001;19(3): 187–91.

98. Mash DC. Excited delirium and sudden death: a syndromal disorder at the extreme end of the neuropsychiatric continuum. Front Physiol 2016;7:435, eCollection 2016.

99. Crisis Prevention Institute. Joint commission standards on restraint and seclusion/ Nonviolent Crisis Intervention® training program. 2009. Available at: https://www. crisisprevention.com/CPI/media/Media/Resources/alignments/Joint-Commission-Restraint-Seclusion-Alignment-2011.pdf. Accessed April 4, 2017.

100. American College of Emergency Physicians Board of Directors. Use of patient restraints. ACEP, 2014. Available at: https://www.acep.org/Clinical—Practice-Management/Use-of-Patient-Restraints/. Accessed September 6, 2017.

# Dietary Supplements in Children

Susan C. Smolinske, PharmD, DABAT

## KEYWORDS

- Dietary supplements • Children • Homeopathy

## KEY POINTS

- High-quality systematic reviews of use of herbal or homeopathic remedies in children often suffer from design flaws, such as not following PRISMA guidelines, inconsistent outcome measurements, and paucity of high-quality studies.
- Homeopathic remedies demonstrate lack of efficacy for pediatric patients and are associated with risk of serious adverse reactions, particularly with teething products.
- High-risk supplements used in adolescents include energy drinks, which are associated with adverse behaviors and medical complaints. Children should not consume more than 2.5 mg/kg or 100 mg of caffeine daily.
- With an increase in obesity in children, the use of weight-loss supplements is concerning. These supplements have a high rate of adulteration with unlabeled stimulants that are associated with serious adverse effects.

## INTRODUCTION

Dietary supplements are a form of complementary and alternative medicine (CAM) that include amino acids, biological/animal extracts, herbals, minerals, and vitamins. Homeopathic remedies are not included in the US regulation of dietary supplements (DS). They are included in this review because of widespread use in infants and concern about safety. This review considers only published systematic reviews or meta-analyses that include children. One notable review of pediatric CAM reviews found that PRISMA guidelines are often not followed for CAM therapy reviews, which creates inconsistency in effectiveness interpretation. The investigators also found only 3 acceptable reviews related to DSs: ivy leaf extract for asthma, *Echinacea* for common cold, and chamomile tea for colic symptoms. Finally, many reviews only contained 1 or 2 studies, highlighting a paucity of evidence.[1]

---

Disclosure Statement: The author has nothing to disclose.
New Mexico Poison and Drug Information Center, Pharmacy Practice and Administration, University of New Mexico, MSC 07 4390, 1 University of New Mexico, Albuquerque, NM 87131-0001, USA
*E-mail address:* SSmolinske@salud.unm.edu

Pediatr Clin N Am 64 (2017) 1243–1255
https://doi.org/10.1016/j.pcl.2017.09.001
0031-3955/17/© 2017 Elsevier Inc. All rights reserved.

**pediatric.theclinics.com**

## PREVALENCE OF DIETARY SUPPLEMENT USE IN PEDIATRICS

The 2007 National Health Interview Survey conducted by the Centers for Disease Control and Prevention found that 11.8% of children had used a CAM. The most common form of CAM was nonvitamin, nonmineral, natural products (3.9%). Children whose parent used CAMs were more than twice as likely as all children to have used a natural product (9.2%). Of the natural products, the most commonly used in 2007 were *Echinacea* (37.2%); fish oil, omega-3 fatty acids, or docosahexaenoic acid (DHA) (30.5%); combination products (17.9%); and flaxseed oil (16.7%).[2] An update of this survey in 2012 showed so significant change in prevalence, but fish oil became the most commonly used, followed by probiotics. Use of melatonin increased.[3]

Homeopathy was used in 1.3% of children in the 2007 National Health Interview Survey[2] and in 1.8% of children in the 2012 survey.[3] In a later systematic review, prevalence rates were 0.8% to 39.0% lifetime use, and up to 30.0% in the prior year.[4] The Australian National Health and Medical Research Council summarized 57 systematic reviews on effectiveness of homeopathy. They found no reliable evidence that homeopathy was effective for any condition. There were no high-quality, well-designed studies with sufficient sample size to compare homeopathy with placebo or active treatments (**Table 1**).[5–9]

## ATTENTION-DEFICIT/HYPERACTIVITY DISORDER

It has been estimated that 12% to 68% of parents use CAM to treat children with attention-deficit/hyperactivity disorder (ADHD).[1] A few studies have shown positive benefits on attention and memory with normal doses of multivitamins, omega-3 fatty acids, and *Bacopa monnieri*, whereas other supplements have shown no greater efficacy than stimulants or do not significantly improve symptoms (**Table 2**).[10–13]

## ASTHMA

A literature search to categorize prevalence of use of CAM in patients with asthma found 17 studies that were of poor or moderate quality. Ten surveys focused on pediatric patients and found prevalence ranging from 33% to 89%. When isolated to more

**Table 1**
**Homeopathy remedy systematic reviews in children**

| Author, Year | DS Type | Condition | No. RCTs | Result | Comment |
|---|---|---|---|---|---|
| Mathie et al,[6] 2015 | Oscillococcinum | Influenza | 6 | No difference between placebo RR 0.48 (CI 0.17–1.34) | Overall quality poor |
| Simonart et al,[7] 2011 | Various | Dermatologic conditions | 12 | 9/12 trials no positive effect | Positive trials were low quality |
| Ernst,[8] 2012 | Not specified | Eczema | 3 | No efficacy | All trials had weak methodology |
| Altunç et al,[9] 2007 | Various | Pediatric ailments | 16 | No efficacy other than mixed results for ADHD and acute diarrhea | Single trials were available for 4/9 conditions |

*Abbreviations:* ADHD, attention-deficit/hyperactivity disorder; CI, confidence interval; DS, dietary supplement; RCT, randomized controlled trial; RR, relative risk.

**Table 2**
Dietary supplement (DS) systematic reviews in children with ADHD

| Author, Year | DS Type | Condition | No. RCTs | Result | Comment |
|---|---|---|---|---|---|
| Hurt et al,[10] 2011 | Multivitamins, minerals at RDA | ADHD | 2 | Improved nonverbal IQ, concentration, attention, motor behavior | May benefit children with poor nutrition |
| Hurt et al,[10] 2011 | Essential fatty acids (marine oils) | ADHD | 13 | Medium benefit for attention at 1 g/d of omega-3 after 3 mo, DHA alone ineffective | Children with polymorphism of FADS2 gene have lower ability to make EFAs |
| Anheyer et al,[11] 2017 | GLA (evening primrose oil 3 g/d) | ADHD | 2 | No significant improvement | Present in human but not cow's milk. One child had severe diarrhea |
| Hurt et al,[10] 2011 | L-Carnitine | ADHD | 3 | Equivocal results; may improve attention | Low adverse effects |
| Hurt et al,[10] 2011 | DMAE (deanol) | ADHD | — | Equivocal results, less effective than stimulant medication | Trials are from 1960-1976 |
| Anheyer et al,[11] 2017 | Valerian root | ADHD | 1 | Improvement in most subscales rated by parents and teachers | Pilot study, methodology issues |
| Anheyer et al,[11] 2017 | Ginkgo biloba 80–120 mg/d | ADHD | 2 | No significant improvement | Mild to moderate side effects |
| Anheyer et al,[11] 2017 | Pine bark extract 1 mg/kg/d (Pycnogenol) | ADHD | 1 | No significant improvement | Study funded by manufacturer; GI distress in 2/61 |
| Anheyer et al,[11] 2017 | St. John's wort 300 mg 3X/d | ADHD | 1 | No significant improvement | Low risk of bias |
| Wong et al,[12] 2012 | Traditional oriental medicine | ADHD | 12 | Some formulas have comparable efficacy to methylphenidate | Adverse effects less than methylphenidate; formulations varied or were not disclosed |
| Kean et al,[13] 2016 | Bacopa monnieri | ADHD/cognitive impairment | 5 | Consistent improvement in language behavior, cognition, and memory span | Adverse effects in 2.3% (gastrointestinal) |

*Abbreviations:* ADHD, attention-deficit/hyperactivity disorder; DHA, docosahexaenoic acid; EFA, essential fatty acid; GI, gastrointestinal; RCT, randomized controlled trial; RDA, recommended dietary allowance.

rigorous studies, the prevalence was 50% to 60%.[14] Of the herbal supplements stud ied, pycnogenol was the only herb that appeared to reduce use of albuterol and improve pulmonary function, whereas eucalyptol, *Tylophora indica*, and propolis showed potential benefit (**Table 3**).[15–17]

## CANCER

Herbal remedies may be used in children with cancer to reduce nausea and vomiting from chemotherapy or as part of cancer therapy. Prevalence of use of herbal remedies in children with cancer ranged from 2% to 47% and use of homeopathy in 1% to 17% of children.[18] Efficacy data are largely lacking or have shown negative outcomes (**Table 4**).[19]

## COMMON COLD

Studies with zinc lozenges, vitamin C, and *Echinacea* to prevent or treat common cold in children have shown no efficacy in treatment once a cold occurs and modest, likely clinically insignificant reductions in cold duration that may not warrant the risk of chronic therapy. Both vitamin C and zinc showed a dose-relationship, with only higher doses being effective (**Table 5**).[20–22]

## INFANTILE COLIC

Several reviews examined nonhomeopathic herbal remedies for treatment of infantile colic. All studies had positive results for fennel-containing products. However, adverse

**Table 3**
**Dietary supplement (DS) systematic reviews in children with asthma**

| Author, Year | DS Type | Condition | No. RCTs | Result | Comment |
|---|---|---|---|---|---|
| Clark et al,[15] 2010 | 20 herbal preparations | Chronic asthma | 6 | Pycnogenol was the only herb studied in children with positive effect; use of albuterol decreased | Only modest absolute change in lung volume; inadequate blinding and randomization was frequent |
| Song et al,[16] 2016 | Chinese herbal medicine | Childhood cough variant asthma | 20 | 19 trials had effective rate with OR 3.52; CI 2.57–4.82 | All studies were in Chinese; only 4 trials measured lung function |
| Arnold et al,[17] 2008 | 21 herbal preparations | Chronic asthma | 27 | Eucalyptol was steroid-sparing, *Tylophora indica* showed some benefit but side effects were significant; Propolis, pycnogenol may improve pulmonary function | Cochrane review |

*Abbreviations:* CI, confidence interval; OR, odds ratio; RCT, randomized controlled trial.

**Table 4**
**Dietary supplement (DS) systematic reviews in children with cancer**

| Author, Year | DS Type | Condition | No. RCTs | Result | Comment |
|---|---|---|---|---|---|
| Momani & Berry,[19] 2017 | Bergamot oil inhalation aromatherapy | Nausea in cancer | 1 | Higher anxiety and nausea with aromatherapy | — |

*Abbreviation:* RCT, randomized controlled trial.

effects did occur in most studies and the volume of liquid needed may not be practical (**Table 6**).[23,24]

## NEUROLOGIC DISORDERS

CAMs are used more frequently in children with neurologic conditions, such as headache, migraine, or seizures, than in healthy children. In one Canadian survey, the most commonly used products were multivitamins (86%), vitamin C (25%), herbal medicine (18%), fish oil (19%), and homeopathic and colic teething remedies (12%).[25] A systematic review found studies were either of poor quality, lacking primary outcomes to determine reduction in seizure frequency, or of insufficient duration (**Table 7**).[26,27]

## ADVERSE REACTIONS TO DIETARY SUPPLEMENTS

In a systematic review of serious adverse reactions to DSs, reactions to non-adulterated DS included allergies or coma from eucalyptus (149 cases), Ghee-related tetanus (102 cases), hemolysis from *Acalypha* (4 cases), and liver failure from pennyroyal (3 cases) and pyrrolizidine alkaloids (22 cases). The investigator also related many cases of indirect risk of herbal remedies in children, due to discontinuation of conventional therapy, many resulting in death.[28] A systematic review of

**Table 5**
**Dietary supplement (DS) systematic reviews in children with cancer**

| | | | | | |
|---|---|---|---|---|---|
| Karsch-Völk et al,[20] 2014 | Echinacea | Common cold prevention or treatment | 24 | No efficacy for treatment; pooling of results showed possible RR reduction of 10%–20% as prevention | Wide difference in formulations used |
| Hemilä,[21] 2011 | Zinc lozenges | Dose relationship to cold treatment | 13 | Total daily doses of <75 mg had no effect; higher doses reduced duration 20%–42% | Only one study involved children, Cochrane Review |
| Hemilä & Chalker,[22] 2013 | Vitamin C, daily use | Common cold prevention | 29 | No decrease in incidence; 14 trials included children | Cochrane Review |
| Hemilä & Chalker[22] 2013 | Vitamin C, daily use | Common cold duration | 31 | Duration decreased by 14% (7%–21%); ingestion of 1–2 g/d shortened duration by 18% | Cochrane Review |

**Table 6**
**Dietary supplement (DS) systematic reviews in children with infantile colic**

| Author, Year | DS Type | Condition | No. RCTs | Result | Comment |
|---|---|---|---|---|---|
| Garrison & Christakis,[23] 2000 | Chamomile/ vervain/ licorice/fennel/ Melissa tea | Infantile colic | 1 | Decreased symptoms but not number of night awakenings (RR = 0.57; CI 0.37–0.89) | Volume of tea needed (32 mL/kg/d) could impact milk consumption |
| Perry et al,[24] 2011 | Chamomile/ fennel/ Melissa tea | Infantile colic | 1 | Crying reduced 50% in 85.4% vs 48.9% in placebo | Adverse reactions vomiting, sleepiness, restlessness, rash, constipation |
| Perry et al,[24] 2011 | Fennel seed oil 0.1% in water, 5–20 mL 4X/d up to 12 mL/kg/d | Infantile colic | 1 | Significant improvement; no colic in 65% vs 23.7% in control; reduced crying hours 8.8 h/wk vs 12.3 h/wk | No adverse effects; less volume consumed in intervention group |

*Abbreviations:* CI, confidence interval; RCT, randomized controlled trial; RR, relative risk.

published case reports of adverse events to herbal products in children found 96 articles representing 128 cases. Of those, 37% were in children younger than 2 years, 38% in children 2 to 8 years old, and 23% in children 9 to 18 years old. Intentional ingestion represented 29%, unintentional ingestion 36%, topical exposure 17%, and prenatal exposure 8%. The most common herbal products mentioned were eucalyptus,[12] camphor,[10] fennel,[6] jin bu huan (known to be adulterated with tetrahydropalmitine),[6] svanuri Marili,[6] kharchos suneli,[6] tea tree,[5] lavender,[4] blue cohosh,[3] buckthorn,[3] licorice,[3] and garlic.[3,29]

**Table 7**
**Dietary supplement (DS) systematic reviews in children with epilepsy**

| Author, Year | DS Type | Condition | No. RCTs | Result | Comment |
|---|---|---|---|---|---|
| Sarmento Vasconcelos et al,[26] 2016 | EPA/DHA | Refractory epilepsy | 3 | Seizure freedom relative effect only for children RR 20 (CI 2.84–141); 50% reduction in seizures RR 33 (CI 4.77–228) | Study had high risk of bias |
| Brigo et al,[27] 2016 | Melatonin 5 mg or 10 mg | Add-on therapy for epilepsy | 6 | One trial showed decrease in diurnal seizures (7.75 for placebo and 4.6 with melatonin) | Insufficient data to show reduction in seizure frequency |

*Abbreviations:* DHA, docosahexaenoic acid; EFA, essential fatty acid; RCT, randomized controlled trial.

An observational study of emergency department (ED) visits and hospital admissions due to DS adverse events in the United States over 10 years estimated that 23,005 ED visits per year are related to DSs, with 21% of those representing unintentional ingestions by children and 25% of the remainder related to weight-loss supplements.[30] A retrospective analysis of the National Poison Data System for 13 years found an average of 21,154 exposures annually. Most exposures were to children younger than 6 years and were unintentional. Serious medical outcomes occurred in 4.5% of exposures, most of them in older children and adults. Supplements associated with greater severity were energy products, botanicals (with yohimbe the greatest), and cultural medicines. Homeopathic products accounted for 35% of exposures, with 93% in younger children, resulting in 0.5% serious outcomes and 3 deaths.[31]

Energy drinks are a form of CAM that has been associated with a high prevalence of use and adverse reaction in adolescents, and is generally not included with other reviews of natural products. These supplements contain caffeine derived from plants as well as added pure caffeine, with total amount often unlabeled, and ranging from 80 to more than 500 mg per can when measured.[32] Energy supplements, primarily beverages, are widely used, with one prospective survey finding that 33% of survey respondents were frequent energy drink consumers. These adolescents were more likely than infrequent energy drink consumers to report headache, anger, increased urination, and medical evaluation for difficulty breathing or headache in the prior 6 months.[33] A broader study of 916 adolescent students found a higher prevalence with increased age, 17.8% of sixth graders and 56.2% of eighth graders.[34]

Several studies have shown that adolescent energy drink consumption is associated with high-risk and negative behaviors, such as alcohol, tobacco and drug abuse, negative school experiences (fighting, bullying, poor achievement, truancy), and frequent health complaints.[34,35] Trends in ED visits captured by the Drug Abuse Warning Network involving energy drink toxicity increased from 10,068 visits in 2007 to 20,783 visits in 2011; however adolescent visits increased only slightly and did not reach significance.[32] A review of 46 publications found that boys were more likely to report energy drink use than girls, and in higher quantities. Those who consumed alcohol mixed with energy drinks had higher odds of driving violations and accidents.

**Table 8**
**Specific dietary supplement (DS) systematic reviews in children with adverse reactions**

| Author, Year | DS Type | Condition | No Studies | Result | Comment |
|---|---|---|---|---|---|
| Huntley et al,[39] 2006 | Echinacea | Whooping cough or tuberculosis | 36 | All pediatric studies were with injectables (fever, pain, headache, vomiting) | Serious allergic reactions are reported in adults, including anaphylaxis |
| Stub et al,[40] 2016 | Homeopathy | various | 41 | 68% of trials reported ADE, mostly GI, headache/dizziness, or dermatitis; 66% were minor and 33% moderate or severe | Rate of adverse effects were not different from placebo |

*Abbreviations:* ADE, adverse dry effect; GI, gastrointestinal; RCT, randomized controlled trial.

**Table 9**
Adulterants found in weight-loss/performance-enhancing supplements

| Author | Adulterant | Adulterant Class | Botanic Ingredient | Adverse Reactions | Comments |
|---|---|---|---|---|---|
| Pawar & Grundel,[41] 2017 | DMAA | Stimulant | Geranium | • 80 reports<br>• Cerebral hemorrhage, cardiac arrest, cardiac failure, heat stroke, death | Geranium does not contain this purported constituent |
| Cohen et al,[42] 2017 | DMBA | Stimulant | Pouchong tea (Camellia sinensis) | None | Not found naturally in this plant |
| Pawar & Grundel,[41] 2017 | N-methyl PEA, N-methyltyramine | Stimulant | Acacia rigidula | None | Up to 800 mg/d could be supplied; supplements contain higher amounts than present in plant material |
| Pawar & Grundel,[41] 2017 | Hordenine (N-dimethyl tyramine) | Stimulant, nootropic | Hordeum vulgare (barley) | — | — |
| Pawar & Grundel,[41] 2017 | Meta-synephrine | Stimulant | Citrus aurantium | — | Only para-synephrine is found naturally; meta is more active |
| Pawar & Grundel,[41] 2017 | Aegeline | Hepatotoxin | Aegle marmelos | Cluster of liver toxicity in 2013 | — |
| Pawar & Grundel,[41] 2017 | B-MePEA | Stimulant | Acacia rigidula | Hemorrhagic stroke | Not found naturally in this plant; 52.4% of supplements contained this |
| Pawar & Grundel,[41] 2017 | N,N-DMPPA | Stimulant | Acacia rigidula | Found in urine of athletes | Not found naturally in this plant |
| Cohen et al,[42] 2017 | Methylsynephrine (oxilofrine) | Stimulant | Citrus aurantium | Cardiac arrest, heart palpitations, chest pain; 26 cases | Not found naturally in this plant |

| Reference | Name | Category | Source | Adverse effects | Notes |
|---|---|---|---|---|---|
| Pawar & Grundel,[41] 2017 | N-Isopropyloctopamine | Stimulant | — | — | Not found naturally |
| Pawar & Grundel,[41] 2017 | Alpha-Ethyl Phenethylamine (NADEP) | Stimulant | Dendrobium stem | — | Not found naturally in this plant |
| Pawar & Grundel,[41] 2017 | Clenbuterol | Anabolic Beta-2 agonist | — | — | — |
| Pawar & Grundel,[41] 2017 | Fenfluramine | Stimulant | Traditional Chinese Medicine | Heart valve disease, coma | — |
| Pawar & Grundel,[41] 2017 | Dexfenfluramine | Stimulant | Traditional Chinese Medicine | — | — |
| Pawar & Grundel,[41] 2017 | Sibutramine and analogs | Stimulant | Weight-loss products | Increased risk of heart attack, stroke, and cardiovascular death, psychosis | Very high frequency of adulteration, often with phenolphthalein |
| Pawar & Grundel,[41] 2017 | Lorcaserin | Serotonin agonist | Weight-loss products | Hallucinations, euphoria | Drug Enforcement Administration Schedule IV drug |
| Pawar & Grundel,[41] 2017 | Nitroso-fenfluramine | Stimulant | Traditional Chinese Medicine | More than 800 cases of liver damage | — |

Four health symptoms were highly associated with daily use: headache, sleeping disorders, irritation, and fatique.[36] Poison center studies have relayed serious adverse events, including seizures, rhabdomyolysis, hypertension, tachycardia, heart failure, palpitations, myocardial infarction, and death. The lowest caffeine dose was 1 mg/kg in a 13-year-old with jitteriness, and the highest was 35.5 mg/kg in a 14-year-old. It is recommended that children and adolescents should not consume more than 2.5 mg/kg or 100 mg of caffeine daily.[37]

Although homeopathic remedies have a low incidence of adverse effects cited in clinical trials, the US Food and Drug Administration (FDA) found more than 400 Medwatch adverse events in infants and children associated with homeopathic teething products. These included tremors, seizures, fever, shortness of breath, lethargy, vomiting, agitation, and irritability, with 10 deaths. After a report of status epilepticus in an infant, the FDA issued a warning to consumers to stop using these products. This was followed by voluntary recalls of many homeopathic teething products, some after FDA investigation showed inconsistent amounts of belladonna in several products that far exceeded the labeled amount. The FDA has issued more than 40 warning letters regarding homeopathic products, such as a zinc nasal inhaler that was associated with more than 100 cases of loss of smell, penicillin found in products for cold or yeast infection, and asthma products that lack evidence for efficacy (**Table 8**).[38]

## ADULTERATION OF DIETARY SUPPLEMENTS

Adulteration of DSs has occurred with heavy metals, such as lead and mercury, corticosteroids, and pharmaceuticals. A systematic review of pediatric adverse reactions to DSs found 21 reports related to lead, 2 to mercury, and 2 to corticosteroids.[28] The FDA has estimated that more than 700 DS products were adulterated with pharmaceuticals, pharmaceutical analogs such as novel stimulants or novel anabolic steroids, banned weight-loss drugs, and sildenafil analogs. Two broad classifications of DSs used in children and adolescents have high rates of adulteration, weight-loss products, and performance-enhancing supplements. Often the manufacturer lists a botanic name ingredient that claims to contain the stimulant compound. Analysis of these plants has always failed to confirm the natural occurrence, thus these are considered to be adulterants. Examples of adulterants are listed in **Table 9**.[41]

## SUMMARY

High-quality studies and systematic reviews of use of herbal or homeopathic remedies in children often suffer from design flaws, such as not following PRISMA guidelines, inconsistent outcome measurements, insufficient duration, and paucity of original high-quality studies. In this review, conditions in children with ADHD, asthma, common cold, cancer, infantile colic, and epilepsy found limited or modest efficacy with most remedies where sufficient methodology was followed. There are also many concerns regarding use of homeopathic remedies. Aside from overall agreement of lack of efficacy, there is evidence of serious adverse reactions to these products in children, so much that a large number of homeopathic teething products have been withdrawn from the market. Homeopathy and herbal medicine also carry the indirect risk of replacing effective traditional therapies, resulting in poor disease control or death.

Although well-designed clinical studies and systematic reviews of adverse effects of herbal remedies in children are limited, there is growing evidence of harm to adolescents from energy drink consumption. There is also concern that many weight-loss and performance-enhancing supplements used by adolescents contain unlabeled adulterant stimulants that are associated with life-threatening toxicity. Pediatricians are encouraged to discuss use of supplements with parents in an open and honest manner. Medication histories should always include DS use. Future research should focus on randomized controlled trials with high-quality designs and methodology.

## REFERENCES

1. Hunt K, Ernst E. The evidence-base for complementary medicine in children: a critical overview of systematic reviews. Arch Dis Child 2011;96(8):769–76.
2. Barnes PM, Bloom B, Nahin RL. Complementary and alternative medicine use among adults and children: United States, 2007. Natl Health Stat Rep 2008;(12):1–23.
3. Black LI, Clarke TC, Barnes PM, et al. Use of complementary health approaches among children aged 4-17 years in the United States: National Health Interview Survey, 2007-2012. Natl Health Stat Rep 2015;(78):1–19.
4. Italia S, Wolfenstetter SB, Teuner CM. Patterns of complementary and alternative medicine (CAM) use in children: a systematic review. Eur J Pediatr 2014;173(11): 1413–28.
5. National Health and Medical Research Council. NHMRC information paper: evidence on the effectiveness of homeopathy for treating health conditions. Canberra (Australia): National Health and Medical Research Council; 2015.
6. Mathie RT, Frye J, Fisher P. Homeopathic Oscillococcinum® for preventing and treating influenza and influenza-like illness. Cochrane Database Syst Rev 2015;(1):CD001957.
7. Simonart T, Kabagabo C, De Maertelaer V. Homoeopathic remedies in dermatology: a systematic review of controlled clinical trials. Br J Dermatol 2011; 165(4):897–905.
8. Ernst E. Homeopathy for eczema: a systematic review of controlled clinical trials. Br J Dermatol 2012;166(6):1170–2.
9. Altunç U, Pittler MH, Ernst E. Homeopathy for childhood and adolescence ailments: systematic review of randomized clinical trials. Mayo Clin Proc 2007; 82(1):69–75.
10. Hurt EA, Arnold LE, Lofthouse N. Dietary and nutritional treatments for attention-deficit/hyperactivity disorder: current research support and recommendations for practitioners. Curr Psychiatry Rep 2011;13(5):323–32.
11. Anheyer D, Lauche R, Schumann D, et al. Herbal medicines in children with attention deficit hyperactivity disorder (ADHD): a systematic review. Complement Ther Med 2017;30:14–23.
12. Wong YW, Kim DG, Lee JY. Traditional oriental herbal medicine for children and adolescents with ADHD: a systematic review. Evid Based Complement Alternat Med 2012;2012:520198.
13. Kean JD, Downey LA, Stough C. A systematic review of the Ayurvedic medicinal herb Bacopa monnieri in child and adolescent populations. Complement Ther Med 2016;29:56–62.
14. Slader CA, Reddel HK, Jenkins CR, et al. Complementary and alternative medicine use in asthma: who is using what? Respirology 2006;11(4):373–87.
15. Clark CE, Arnold E, Lasserson TJ, et al. Herbal interventions for chronic asthma in adults and children: a systematic review and meta-analysis. Prim Care Respir J 2010;19(4):307–14.
16. Song P, Zeng L, Liang Z, et al. Clinical efficacy and safety of Chinese herbal medicine auxiliary therapy for childhood cough variant asthma: a systematic review

and meta-analysis of 20 randomized controlled trials. Intern Med 2016;55(18): 2135–43.

17. Arnold E, Clark CE, Lasserson TJ, et al. Herbal interventions for chronic asthma in adults and children. Cochrane Database Syst Rev 2008;(1):CD005989.

18. Bishop FL, Prescott P, Chan YK, et al. Prevalence of complementary medicine use in pediatric cancer: a systematic review. Pediatrics 2010;125(4):768–76.

19. Momani TG, Berry DL. Integrative therapeutic approaches for the management and control of nausea in children undergoing cancer treatment: a systematic review of literature. J Pediatr Oncol Nurs 2017;34(3):173–84.

20. Karsch-Völk M, Barrett B, Kiefer D, et al. *Echinacea* for preventing and treating the common cold. Cochrane Database Syst Rev 2014;(2):CD000530.

21. Hemilä H. Zinc lozenges may shorten the duration of colds: a systematic review. Open Respir Med J 2011;5:51–8.

22. Hemilä H, Chalker E. Vitamin C for preventing and treating the common cold. Cochrane Database Syst Rev 2013;(1):CD000980.

23. Garrison MM, Christakis DA. A systematic review of treatments for infant colic. Pediatrics 2000;106(1 Pt 2):184–90.

24. Perry R, Hunt K, Ernst E. Nutritional supplements and other complementary medicines for infantile colic: a systematic review. Pediatrics 2011;127(4):720–33.

25. Galicia-Connolly E, Adams D, Bateman J, et al. CAM use in pediatric neurology; an exploration of concurrent use with conventional medicine. PLOS ONE 2014; 9(4):e94078.

26. Sarmento Vasconcelos V, Macedo CR, de Souza Pedrosa A, et al. Polyunsaturated fatty acid supplementation for drug-resistant epilepsy. Cochrane Database Syst Rev 2016;(8):CD011014.

27. Brigo F, Igwe SC, Del Felice A. Melatonin as add-on treatment for epilepsy. Cochrane Database Syst Rev 2016;(8):CD006967.

28. Ernst E. Serious adverse effects of unconventional therapies for children and adolescents: a systematic review of recent evidence. Eur J Pediatr 2003;162(2): 72–80.

29. Gardiner P, Adams D, Filippelli AC, et al. A systematic review of the reporting of adverse events associated with medical herb use among children. Glob Adv Health Med 2013;2(2):46–55.

30. Cohen PA. Emergency department visits and hospitalisations for adverse events related to dietary supplements are common. Evid Based Med 2016;21(2):79.

31. Rao N, Spiller HA, Hodges NL, et al. An increase in dietary supplement exposures reported to US poison control centers. J Med Toxicol 2017. [Epub ahead of print].

32. Mattson ME. Update on emergency department visits involving energy drinks: a continuing public health concern. The CBHSQ report. Rockville (MD): Substance Abuse and Mental Health Services Administration (US); 2013.

33. Bashir D, Reed-Schrader E, Olympia RP, et al. Clinical symptoms and adverse effects associated with energy drink consumption in adolescents. Pediatr Emerg Care 2016;32(11):751–5.

34. Gallimberti L, Buja A, Chindamo S, et al. Energy drink consumption in children and early adolescents. Eur J Pediatr 2013;172(10):1335–40.

35. Holubcikova J, Kolarcik P, Madarasova Geckova A, et al. Regular energy drink consumption is associated with the risk of health and behavioural problems in adolescents. Eur J Pediatr 2017;176(5):599–605.

36. Visram S, Cheetham M, Riby DM, et al. Consumption of energy drinks by children and young people: a rapid review examining evidence of physical effects and consumer attitudes. BMJ Open 2016;6(10):e010380.
37. Seifert SM, Schaechter JL, Hershorin ER, et al. Health effects of energy drinks on children, adolescents, and young adults. Pediatrics 2011;127(3):511–28.
38. Abbasi J. Amid reports of infant deaths, FTC cracks down on homeopathy while FDA investigates. JAMA 2017;317(8):793–5.
39. Huntley AL, Thompson Coon J, Ernst E. The safety of herbal medicinal products derived from *Echinacea* species: a systematic review. Drug Saf 2005;28(5): 387–400.
40. Stub T, Musial F, Kristoffersen AA, et al. Adverse effects of homeopathy, what do we know? A systematic review and meta-analysis of randomized controlled trials. Complement Ther Med 2016;26:146–63.
41. Pawar RS, Grundel E. Overview of regulation of dietary supplements in the USA and issues of adulteration with phenethylamines (PEAs). Drug Test Anal 2017; 9(3):500–17.
42. Cohen PA, Avula B, Venhuis B, et al. Pharmaceutical doses of the banned stimulant oxilofrine found in dietary supplements sold in the USA. Drug Test Anal 2017;9(1):135–42.

# Anticoagulation Therapies in Children

Guy Young, MD

## KEYWORDS

- Anticoagulation • Children • Heparin • Low-molecular-weight heparin • Warfarin
- Argatroban • Bivalirudin • Fondaparinux

## KEY POINTS

- The coagulation system in the youngest children (<1 year of age) has not fully matured, which affects the way anticoagulants exert their effect in this age group.
- The properties of anticoagulant drugs that are prescribed in children are varied and the clinician should be familiar with the pros and cons of the standard anticoagulants.
- Clinicians should understand when nonstandard anticoagulants should be considered for use in children.
- Anticoagulation in children will undergo a dramatic shift and the standard agents will largely be replaced by direct oral anticoagulants currently being evaluated.

## INTRODUCTION

The incidence of venous thromboembolism (VTE) in children has been increasing steadily over the past 20 years.[1–3] This increase is attributed primarily to the increasing use of central venous access devices and the significant advances made in the management of children with chronic and/or serious medical conditions.[3] The increase in the prevalence of VTE has resulted in a corresponding increase in the use of anticoagulants.[1] Although the rationale for prescribing anticoagulation to children in many situations in mirrors the use in adults (VTE, extracorporeal circulation, heart disease), anticoagulating children results in problems specific to this population. First, the coagulation system in the youngest children (<1 year of age) has not fully matured, such that the very coagulation proteins that anticoagulants exert their effect on have much lower physiologic levels in children in this age group. Somewhat paradoxically, higher weight-based doses of anticoagulants are, nevertheless, required for these children owing to the pharmacokinetic differences in drug metabolism. Second, there exist significant issues with the seemingly simple act of administering medications to children. Whereas adults can swallow tablets and tolerate subcutaneous injections

Hemostasis and Thrombosis Center, Children's Hospital Los Angeles, Department of Pediatrics, Division of Pediatric Hematology/Oncology, University of Southern California Keck School of Medicine, 4650 Sunset Blvd, Los Angeles, CA 90027, USA
E-mail address: gyoung@chla.usc.edu

Pediatr Clin N Am 64 (2017) 1257–1269
http://dx.doi.org/10.1016/j.pcl.2017.08.004
0031-3955/17/© 2017 Elsevier Inc. All rights reserved.

with relative ease, children, especially younger ones, may have difficulty swallowing tablets (the only available formulation for vitamin K antagonists [VKA]) and will not likely not be cooperative with injectable drugs. This consideration is in addition to the fact that It puts parents In the uncomfortable and awkward position of inducing pain in their children. Furthermore, children who require anticoagulation often have serious medical conditions that could potentially exacerbate the risk for serious bleeding or result in serious adverse drug interactions, making the use of VKA even more challenging. Last, in comparison with adults, there are relatively few data from prospective clinical trials of anticoagulation in children, rendering decision making that much more difficult.

Regardless, there remains a need to treat children with anticoagulant medications for several indications. The clinical conditions and their corresponding duration of therapy are highly variable ranging from hours to days for the prevention of thrombosis in children on extracorporeal circulation (cardiac bypass and extracorporeal membrane oxygenation) to lifelong anticoagulation for children with recurrent deep vein thrombosis and cardiac valve replacement. In addition to therapeutic anticoagulation, there is a movement to bring the ubiquitous practice of prophylactic anticoagulation in adult patients with the proper indications to pediatric practice. Although few scenarios in pediatrics exist where there is consensus regarding the use of prophylactic anticoagulation,[4,5] current studies evaluating newer anticoagulants, specifically, the direct oral anticoagulants (DOACs) are exploring prophylactic indications. Although there is widespread use of anticoagulation, especially in hospitalized patients, there is precious little high-level evidence on which to base decisions such as choice of anticoagulant, intensity of treatment, and duration of treatment. There are published treatment guidelines, albeit with low levels of evidence, providing recommendations for the management of thrombosis for children in general[4] and more specifically for children with heart disease.[6] Thus, this review focuses more specifically on the properties of the anticoagulants themselves and review the pros and cons of the standard anticoagulants (heparin, low-molecular-weight heparin [LMWH], and VKA), followed by a discussion on the alternative anticoagulants, which are not widely used in clinical practice (argatroban, bivalirudin, and fondaparinux). Finally, there will be a brief mention of the potential for treatment with DOACs[7] in children for a variety of indications by examining the properties of these agents and presenting the very limited published data. For a historical context on the anticoagulation in children, the reader is referred to **Table 1**.

## THE FUTURE LANDSCAPE OF ANTICOAGULATION IN CHILDREN

The standard anticoagulants currently in widespread use in children include unfractionated heparin, LMWH (of which there are several available), and VKA, primarily warfarin.

**Table 1**
**Historical context of new anticoagulants in children**

| Anticoagulant | Discovery | First Clinical Use in Adults | First Use in Children | First Prospective Study in Children |
|---|---|---|---|---|
| Heparin | 1916 | 1934 | 1954 | 1994 |
| Warfarin | 1929 | 1954 | 1976 | 1994 |
| Low-molecular-weight heparin | 1970s | 1980s | 1991 | 1996 |
| Direct thrombin inhibitors | 1884 | 1997 | 1999 | 2007 |
| Fondaparinux | 1985 | 2001 | 2004 | 2010 |
| Direct oral anticoagulants | 2005 | 2010 | 2013 | 2015 |

These agents could also be called multitargeted agents, as they were in a prior review, because they exert their anticoagulant effect on multiple coagulation proteins.[8] Although these agents have been used for decades in children, and despite the lack of published prospective studies, they have nevertheless gained the confidence of pediatric treaters. The experience physicians have developed with these agents combined with the relative lack of alternatives has led to a level of comfort such that they are the most frequently (by far) prescribed anticoagulants. Moving forward, however, the landscape of anticoagulation will undergo a dramatic shift and the standard agents will largely be replaced by the alternative agents and, a bit further into the future, by the DOACs that are currently being evaluated in a number of clinical trials worldwide.

## STANDARD ANTICOAGULANTS
### Unfractionated Heparin

Unfractionated heparin is so called to distinguish it from the LMWHs; however, in general parlance it is simply referred to as heparin. It is a polysaccharide compound derived from porcine intestine and exerts its anticoagulant effect by potentiating the inhibitory effects of antithrombin on thrombin and factor Xa. It has a short half-life and is, therefore, administered as a continuous infusion. As such, heparin is generally only used in the setting of hospitalized children and usually only in patients in critical care units. The major advantages of heparin include its short half-life (an advantage in the intensive care unit and cardiac catheterization laboratory) and the presence of an available antidote (protamine), allowing for rapid reversal should bleeding occur. Heparin, however, has several significant limitations. One of the most important issues involves the laboratory monitoring of heparin, which is challenging on a number of levels.[9] First, there are different assays used for therapeutic drug monitoring (the activated partial thromboplastin time [aPTT], the anti-factor Xa level, and the activated clotting time), all of which have their own limitations. Second, the degree to which these assays accurately reflect the degree of anticoagulation is not entirely clear.[10] Furthermore, several studies have demonstrated discrepancies between the aPTT and the anti-Xa assay, and it is not entirely clear which laboratory test reflects reality.[11,12] Aside from these issues, it is well-known that there is a high degree of interpatient and even intrapatient variability in the pharmacokinetics of heparin further complicating management.[13] Moreover, heparin therapy can result in heparin-induced thrombocytopenia (HIT), a serious adverse effect that can go unrecognized in children owing to its rarity.[14,15] Last, heparin is a biologic compound and, therefore, subject to potential contamination, which has in the past led to severe complications.[16] Despite these limitations, heparin is widely used in children, and is still considered the first-line therapy for the prevention of thrombosis in patients undergoing cardiac catheterization and cardiopulmonary bypass surgery, and for anticoagulation of extracorporeal circuits. Of note, there are only 2 prospective studies of heparin in children with 65 and 38 patients treated both prophylactically and for prevention of thrombosis in patients with congenital heart disease.[17,18] Despite that fact, many pediatric specialists involved in the care of such children have an almost cavalier level of comfort with heparin despite the concerns outlined.

### Low-Molecular-Weight Heparin

The LMWHs are heparin-like molecules derived from unfractionated heparin, but are composed of shorter lengths of the polysaccharide chains, which confers them with somewhat different properties. The LMWHs exert a more profound effect on factor Xa than on thrombin, and have more stable pharmacokinetics resulting in a more predictable dose response and a longer half-life, making them useful in the outpatient setting.[19,20] In addition, and in contradistinction to VKA, these medications do not have drug or food interactions and, combined with their predictable pharmacokinetics, obviate the need for frequent therapeutic drug monitoring. These features have led to the widespread use of LMWH in pediatrics in the past 20 years and today they are considered the first-line anticoagulant for both the initial and long-term treatment of VTE.[1] Several different LMWH preparations are available use throughout the world, and a number of pharmacokinetic and dose-finding studies have been completed.[21–27] Although their longer half-life allows for outpatient use, the treatment of VTE requires twice daily dosing as demonstrated by these pharmacokinetic studies of enoxaparin.[22,23] The LMWH have some similar limitations to heparin, such as risk for contamination and HIT, although at lower rates than unfractionated heparin. More relevant perhaps is the effect of LMWH on bone metabolism and, although there are no studies in children addressing this issue, both in vitro and in vivo data indicate that they exert a negative effect on bone mineral metabolism.[28] Last, the antidote protamine is only partially effective at reversing the anticoagulant effect of LMWH.

### Vitamin K Antagonists

The major advantage of VKAs are their oral route of administration; however, these medications are best with a number of significant limitations, which have resulted in a decrease in their use.[29] The most important drawback is the narrow therapeutic index of VKAs, which lead to an increased risk for serious bleeding.[30] In addition, VKAs have numerous drug interactions and can be affected by the vitamin K content of the diet, further complicating the ability to maintain a therapeutic dose. This problem is especially acute in children for a number of reasons. First, most children who require warfarin have serious chronic medical conditions and are often receiving numerous other drugs, many of which interact with VKA. Second, children, and especially infants, many of whom take in large amounts of vitamin K with their formulas, have a rapidly changing diet, altering their vitamin K consumption. Third, even otherwise healthy children receive antibiotic medications, many of which can significantly affect the International Normalized Ratio. Finally, although the oral route of administration is clearly a significant advantage in adults, this is not always the case with children. For example, the use of VKA in infants is difficult owing to their inability to swallow whole tablets and the fact that warfarin cannot be safely compounded into a liquid formulation. Last, a well-designed study demonstrated that the target International Normalized Ratio is not met on a sufficiently consistent basis in children, especially infants.[31]

## ALTERNATIVE ANTICOAGULANTS

In previous reviews,[32,33] anticoagulants other than heparin, LMWH, and VKA were referred to as "novel" anticoagulants when describing their use in children; however, because these agents are no longer novel, they are referred to herein as alternative anticoagulants. There are a number of ways to classify these agents: mechanism of action, route of administration, and half-life (**Table 2**). One approach is to consider the route of administration and to compare the standard anticoagulants with the alternative agents that are administered the same way. Thus, heparin, a continuous infusion, agent could be compared with bivalirudin and argatroban, and fondaparinux could be compared with LMWH and VKA with DOACs. The following section describes the available data on these agents. A more detailed discussion of their pharmacokinetics and pharmacodynamics can be found elsewhere.[29]

**Table 2**
**Basic properties of anticoagulants used in children**

| Anticoagulant | Route of Administration | Administration Interval[a] | Half-Life | Antithrombin Dependence | Antidote/Reversal Agent |
|---|---|---|---|---|---|
| Heparin | IV | Bolus followed by continuous infusion | 30 min | Yes | Protamine |
| Warfarin | Oral | Once daily | 24 h | No | Vitamin K prothrombin complex concentrates |
| Enoxaparin | Subcutaneous | q12 h | 6 h | Yes | Protamine (partial) |
| Bivalirudin | IV continuous infusion | Bolus followed by continuous infusion | 25 min | No | None |
| Argatroban | IV continuous infusion | Continuous infusion | 40 min | No | None |
| Fondaparinux | Subcutaneous | Once daily | 17 h | Yes | None |

*Abbreviation:* IV, intravenous.
[a] These doses are for treatment not prophylaxis.

### Parenteral Direct Thrombin Inhibitors

There are 2 parenteral direct thrombin inhibitors (argatroban and bivalirudin) that are commercially available. In the past decade, prospective studies evaluating bivalirudin (3 studies) and argatroban (1 study) in children have been published. Two prospective studies with bivalirudin evaluated the treatment of VTE[34,35] and another study assessed its ability to prevent thrombosis in patients undergoing cardiac catheterization.[36,37] The VTE studies differed in only 2 ways. First, they enrolled different age groups (<6 months and 6 months to 18 years, respectively) and second, the study in the older group collected pharmacokinetic data in addition to the pharmacodynamic data. These studies led to the following key findings: (1) dosing for children has been established (**Table 3**), (2) this agent seemed to be very safe and there were no serious bleeding events, albeit in a small number of patients (n = 34), and (3) the studies evaluated early clot resolution (at 48–72 hours after drug initiation) owing to the unique property of this agent to inhibit clot-bound thrombin, and found that 15 of the 34 subjects had partial or complete resolution of their thrombus at this early time point, a finding that is not known to occur with heparin. Of note, another report from a retrospective study[36] demonstrated rapid clot resolution in all 10 patients such that, together with the prospective studies, early clot resolution occurred in 57% of patients. Although it would be important to confirm this finding in comparative studies with heparin, it is unlikely such a study will be done. Finally, an important contribution of this research to pediatric anticoagulation revolves around the issue of therapeutic drug monitoring. The second bivalirudin study measured both pharmacokinetics (bivalirudin levels) and pharmacodynamics (aPTT) in all subject samples (182 paired samples) and it was noted that the better predictor of bivalirudin drug concentration was the infusion rate rather than the aPTT. In fact, the aPTT often led to dose adjustments that were deemed unnecessary based on the pharmacokinetics.

The third prospective study assessed the efficacy of bivalirudin as a prophylactic agent in children undergoing cardiac catheterization.[36] This study was a single-arm, safety, efficacy, and dose-finding study in children from birth to 16 years of age divided into 4 age cohorts that enrolled 110 patients using dosing similar to that for the adult licensed indication of bivalirudin. The results demonstrated a high degree of safety with only 2 of 110 patients experiencing major bleeding events (as defined by the protocol), which were relatively minor wound hematomas. Eight patients experienced thrombotic events; however, only 2 were deemed serious enough to be treated. This rate of thrombosis in this high-risk procedure is considered excellent.

**Table 3**
**Suggested dosing and monitoring for alternative anticoagulants**

| Anticoagulation | Dose | Interval | Monitoring Test | Target Range |
|---|---|---|---|---|
| Bivalirudin[a] | 0.125 mg/kg/h<br>0.125 mg/kg/h | Bolus<br>Continuous infusion | PTT | 1.5–2.5 baseline PTT |
| Argatroban | 0.1 μg/kg/min | Continuous infusion | PTT | 1.5–2.5 baseline PTT |
| Fondaparinux[b] | 0.1 mg/kg | Once daily | Anti-Xa level[c] | 0.5–1 mg/L |

*Abbreviation*: PTT, partial thromboplastin time.
[a] Bivalirudin has only been prospectively evaluated in children less than 6 months of age.
[b] Fondaparinux dosing has not been evaluated in children less than 1 year of age.
[c] Fondaparinux-based anti-Xa assay with results expressed as mg/L.

The only other prospective study of a direct thrombin inhibitor in children evaluated the use of argatroban in patients requiring an alternative to heparin, most of whom had either documented or suspected HIT.[38] This study enrolled 18 patients and demonstrated safety and efficacy as well as establishing dosing guidelines, which are now included in the prescribing information in the United States (a first for any anticoagulant in pediatrics). A detailed pharmacokinetic analysis was undertaken, resulting in a separate publication[39] that supports the dosing schema (see **Table 3**) now approved by the US Food and Drug Administration.

### Fondaparinux

Fondaparinux is a synthetic, antithrombin-dependent inhibitor of factor Xa composed of the pentasaccharide portion of heparin that binds to antithrombin. Two pediatric studies have been completed—a prospective, single-arm, open-label, dose-finding, pharmacodynamic and safety study and a follow-up long-term continuation study in which the data were collected retrospectively.[40,41] The prospective study enrolled 24 patients between 1 and 18 years of age in 3 age cohorts (patients <1 year of age could not be enrolled owing to an Investigational New Drug restriction imposed by the US Food and Drug Administration). Both studies demonstrated an excellent safety profile with a bleeding rate of 0.5 events per 1000 patient-days noted in the continuation study. With respect to dosing, a detailed pharmacologic analysis conducted in the prospective study led to 2 important findings. First, at a dose of 0.1 mg/kg/d, the pharmacodynamic profile in children was the same that found in adults supporting the once-daily dosing regimen and, second, 22 of 24 patients were therapeutic after the first dose with the other 2 becoming therapeutic after 1 dose adjustment. Furthermore, the second study demonstrated that 71% of the patients never required a dose adjustment despite a long treatment duration of 371 days (median, 152; range, 2–1566) and regular monitoring. Last, although the first study was not designed to assess efficacy, the continuation study demonstrated complete clot resolution in 64% of patients and partial resolution in 27%. Thus, fondaparinux can be considered as an excellent alternative to LMWH given its once-daily dosing and similar safety and efficacy profiles.

### Agents in Clinical Development

Although DOACs have found their place in the anticoagulant armamentarium of adult patients with various conditions, their use in children is appropriately rare, considering that there are no phase III studies published as of yet. However, in the forthcoming several years, pediatricians will likely begin prescribing DOACs in the same manner as we have seen the transition occur in adult medicine. Clearly, this change is because these compounds have several distinct advantages.[42] Of greatest importance is that these agents have demonstrated a high degree of safety (less bleeding) and efficacy (clot resolution or prevention) in very large clinical trials in adults. Although this finding is currently being evaluated in clinical trials in children, there is no reason to think that such results will not be replicated in children. In addition, these agents are given as a fixed dose with no requirement for laboratory monitoring, although this may not end up being the case in children. Finally, and in contradistinction to LMWH, the most commonly used anticoagulant in children, these agents have specific, targeted antidotes that have either recently become commercially available or will be so in the near future.[43]

Aside from the actual potential beneficial effects of the drugs themselves, there is a major additional benefit of these new compounds as it relates to the field of pediatric thrombosis, and this relates to the regulatory requirements imposed by the European Medicines Agency and the US Food and Drug Administration. Essentially, these

**Table 4**
Clinical trial programs for direct oral anticoagulants in children

| Medication | Indications | Primary Outcome Measures | Anticipated Study Conclusion |
|---|---|---|---|
| Rivaroxaban | VTE treatment | Recurrent VTE<br>Major and clinically relevant minor bleeding | November, 2018 |
| Apixaban | Prevention of VTE in leukemia patients | Composite of non-fatal VTE/PE, CSVT, and VTE-related death | May, 2019 |
| | VTE treatment | Composite of symptomatic and asymptomatic recurrent VTE and VTE-related death | October, 2020 |
| Dabigatran | VTE treatment | Composite of complete thrombus resolution, recurrent VTE and VTE-related death<br>Major Bleeding | March, 2018 |
| | Secondary VTE prevention | Recurrent VTE<br>Major and minor bleeding<br>VTE-related mortality<br>Overall mortality | June, 2018 |
| Edoxaban | VTE treatment | Recurrent VTE<br>VTE-related death<br>No VTE extension | March, 2021 |

*Abbreviations*: CSVT, Cerebral Venous Sinus Thrombosis; PE, pulmonary embolism; VTE, venous thromboembolism.

regulations have led to the initiation of the largest and most robust prospective clinical trials ever undertaken in the field. These data, once published, will eclipse the clinical trial data that are currently available for all the previous anticoagulants published, thereby allowing (hopefully) for the use of evidence-based guidelines for the use of these anticoagulants in children. Furthermore, these agents will overcome the critical issue of drug administration described, which likely affects adherence to treatment. An additional benefit of the regulations will lead to the development of child-friendly oral formulations of these new agents. This advance will ease the suffering of many parents and children by greatly facilitating the administration and perhaps improving the adherence to anticoagulant medications.

With respect to currently available data, the data are limited to just a handful of early study results; none of which can justify the routine use of these agents[44,45]; however, as stated, robust clinical development programs are under way for all of the commercially available DOACs in children for a variety of indications (**Table 4**).[46] Thus, until such data are published, these agents should not be prescribed to children less than 18 years of age with rare exceptions and provided that there is clear rationale to make such an exception.

## SUMMARY AND RECOMMENDATIONS

The standard anticoagulants used in children, namely, heparin, LMWH, and VKA, all have significant limitations and will eventually be replaced by a wide variety of newer anticoagulants. Based on the results of these studies of bivalirudin, argatroban, and fondaparinux, several recommendations for the use of alternative anticoagulants can be made that can be implemented into clinical practice currently (**Table 5**). Based

**Table 5**
**Treatment with alternative anticoagulants in pediatric practice**

| | Medical Condition | Medication Options | Pros | Cons |
|---|---|---|---|---|
| Required | Heparin-induced thrombocytopenia | Argatroban Bivalirudin Fondaparinux | Pediatric and adult clinical trial data available | Limited familiarity No antidotes |
| Recommended | Extensive VTE | Bivalirudin | Rapid clot resolution No need for laboratory monitoring | Limited familiarity |
| | Typical VTE | Fondaparinux | Once-daily dosing No risk for heparin-induced thrombocytopenia No impact on bone mineralization | Limited familiarity No antidote |
| Suggested | Typical VTE in hospitalized patients | Bivalirudin | Rapid clot resolution No need for laboratory monitoring | Limited familiarity |
| Not recommended | All situations | Direct oral anticoagulants | N/A | No pediatric data on safety/efficacy |

*Abbreviations:* N/A, not applicable; VTE, venous thromboembolism.

on the available data, the only clear indication for the use of one of these anticoagulants is the presence or suspicion of HIT, which requires avoidance of heparin and
LMWH and for which VKA is not appropriate at least for acute management. The
only agent studied in children specifically for this indication is argatroban and it is
thus the agent of choice for children with HIT.

The next best scenario for use of an alternative anticoagulant would be for the use of
bivalirudin for the prevention of thrombosis in children undergoing cardiac catheterization based on the excellent results of the published clinical trial.

With respect to the management of acute VTE for hospitalized or critically ill patients
in whom a continuous infusion medication is indicated, there are 2 points of view. One
is to consider the alternative agents as second-line therapy for patients who have a
poor response to or are difficult to manage with heparin. A contrary point of view is
to consider these agents, particularly bivalirudin, as the ideal first option. To this
end, it should be noted that there are as much (if not more) quality, prospective study
data for bivalirudin as there is for heparin, but, more important, bivalirudin has been
shown to rapidly resolve (partially and completely) thrombi in nearly 60% of the children evaluated in the clinical trials and the retrospective study. This phenomenon
has not been tested in patients receiving heparin. As such, this author recommends
bivalirudin for critically ill and/or hospitalized children for the acute management of
VTE or at least for those with extensive thrombi in whom thrombolysis is considered
but not undertaken owing to the risk for bleeding.

With respect to long-term anticoagulation, the standard options of LMWH and VKA
both have the limitations discussed. In contrast with LMWH, fondaparinux allows for
once-daily dosing, does not interfere with bone metabolism, and has no risk for HIT
or contamination. In addition, the quantity and quality of prospective clinical trial
data are similar.

In conclusion, a new era is emerging with respect to pediatric anticoagulation. After
approximately 20 years since the initial use of LMWH in children began, several newer
anticoagulants are available now that have undergone prospective studies, establishing the dosing, safety, and efficacy, and can be prescribed in the circumstances as
described. Furthermore, a wide variety of newer oral agents are being studied in children currently, and will likely shift the paradigm of anticoagulation in children in the
coming 3 to 5 years.

## REFERENCES

1. Raffini L, Huang Y, Witmer C, et al. Dramatic increase in venous thromboembolism in children's hospitals in the United States from 2001-2007. Pediatrics
   2009;124:1001–8.
2. Setty BA, O'Brien SH, Kerlin BA. Pediatric venous thromboembolism in the United
   States: a tertiary care complication of chronic diseases. Pediatr Blood Cancer
   2012;59:258–64.
3. Kanin M, Young G. Incidence of thrombosis in children with tunneled central
   venous access devices versus peripherally inserted central catheters (PICCs).
   Thromb Res 2013;132:527–30.
4. Stem J, Christensen A, Davis D, et al. Safety of prophylactic anticoagulation at a
   pediatric hospital. J Pediatr Hematol Oncol 2013;35:e287–91.
5. Monagle P, Chan AK, Goldenberg NA, et al. Antithrombotic therapy in neonates
   and children: antithrombotic therapy and prevention of thrombosis, 9th ed: American College of Chest Physicians evidence-based clinical practice guidelines.
   Chest 2012;141(suppl2):e737S–801.

6. Giglia TM, Massicotte P, Tweddell JS, et al. Prevention and treatment of thrombosis in pediatric and congenital heart disease: a scientific statement from the American Heart Association. Circulation 2013;128:2622–703.

7. Yeh CH, Gross PL, Weitz JI. Evolving use of new oral anticoagulants for treatment of venous thromboembolism. Blood 2014;124:1020–8.

8. Young G. Anticoagulants in children and adolescents. Hematol Am Soc Hematol Educ Program 2015;2015:111–6.

9. Chan AK, Black L, Ing C, et al. Utility of a PTT in monitoring unfractionated heparin in children. Thromb Res 2008;122:135–6.

10. Ignatovic V, Summerhayes R, Gan A, et al. Monitoring unfractionated heparin (UFH) therapy: which anti factor Xa assay is appropriate? Thromb Res 2007; 120:347–51.

11. Schechter T, Finkelstein Y, Ali M, et al. Unfractionated heparin dosing in young infants: clinical outcomes in a cohort monitored with anti-factor Xa levels. J Thromb Haemost 2012;10:368–74.

12. Trucco M, Lehmann CU, Mollenkopf N, et al. Retrospective cohort study comparing activated partial thromboplastin time versus anti-factor Xa activity nomograms for therapeutic unfractionated heparin monitoring in pediatrics. J Thromb Haemost 2015;13:788–94.

13. Kuhle S, Eulmesekian P, Kavanagh B, et al. Lack of correlation between heparin dose and standard clinical monitoring tests in treatment with unfractionated heparin in critically ill children. Haematologica 2007;92:554–7.

14. Obeng EA, Harney KM, Moniz T, et al. Pediatric heparin-induced thrombocytopenia: prevalence, thrombotic risk, and application of the 4Ts scoring system. J Pediatr 2015;166:144–50.

15. Avila ML, Shah V, Brandao LR. Systematic review on heparin-induced thrombocytopenia in children: a call to action. J Thromb Haemost 2013;11:660–9.

16. Kishimoto TK, Viswanathan K, Ganguly T, et al. Contaminated heparin associated with adverse clinical events and activation of the contact system. N Engl J Med 2008;358:2457–67.

17. Andrew M, Marzinott V, Massicotte P, et al. Heparin therapy in pediatric patients: a prospective cohort study. Pediatr Res 1994;35:78–83.

18. Kuhle S, Eulmesekian P, Kavanagh B, et al. A clinically significant incidence of bleeding in critically ill children receiving therapeutic doses of unfractionated heparin: a prospective cohort study. Haematologica 2007;92:244–7.

19. Hirsh J, Levine MN. Low molecular weight heparin. Blood 1992;79:1–17.

20. Samama MM, Gerotziafas GT. Comparative pharmacokinetics of LMWHs. Semin Thromb Hemost 2000;6(Suppl):131–8.

21. Massicotte P, Adams M, Marzinotto V, et al. Low-molecular-weight heparin in pediatric patients with thrombotic disease: a dose finding study. J Pediatr 1996;128: 313–8.

22. O'Brion SH, Loo H, Ritohoy AK. Onoo daily onoxaparin in podiatrio thromboombolism: a dose finding and pharmacodynamics/pharmacokinetics study. J Thromb Haemost 2007;5:1985–7.

23. Trame MN, Mitchell L, Krumpel A, et al. Population pharmacokinetics of enoxaparin in infants, children, and adolescents during secondary thromboembolic prophylaxis: a cohort study. J Thromb Haemost 2010;8:195–8.

24. Massicotte P, Julian JA, Marzinotto V, et al. Dose-finding and pharmacokinetic profiles of prophylactic doses of a low molecular weight heparin (reviparin-sodium) in pediatric patients. Thromb Res 2003;109:93–9.

25. Nohe N, Flemmer A, Rumler R, et al. The low molecular weight heparin dalteparin for prophylaxis and therapy of thrombosis in childhood: a report on 48 cases. Eur J Pediatr 1999;158(Suppl 3):S134–9.

26. Kuhle S, Massicotte P, Dinyari M, et al. Dose-finding and pharmacokinetics of therapeutic doses of tinzaparin in pediatric patients with thromboembolic events. Thromb Haemost 2005;94:1164–71.

27. O'Brien SH, Kulkarni R, Wallace A, et al. Multicenter dose-finding and efficacy and safety outcomes in neonates and children treated with dalteparin for acute venous thrombosis. J Thromb Haemost 2014;12:1822–5.

28. Rajgopal R, Bear MK, Shaugnessy SG. The effects of heparin and low molecular weight heparin on bone. Thromb Res 2008;122:293–8.

29. Yee DL, O'Brien SH, Young G. Pharmacokinetics and pharmacodynamics of anticoagulants in paediatric patients. Clin Pharmacokinet 2013;52:967–80.

30. Moffett BS, Kim S, Bomgaars LR. Readmissions for warfarin-related bleeding in pediatric patients after hospital discharge. Pediatr Blood Cancer 2013;60:1503–6.

31. Streif W, Andrew M, Marzinotto V, et al. Analysis of warfarin therapy in pediatric patients: a prospective cohort study of 319 patients. Blood 1999;94:3007–14.

32. Young G. New anticoagulants in children. Hematol Am Soc Hematol Educ Program 2008;245–50.

33. Young G. New anticoagulants in children: a review of recent studies and a look to the future. Thromb Res 2011;127:70–4.

34. Young G, Tarantino MD, Wohrley J, et al. Pilot dose-finding and safety study of bivalirudin in infants<6 months of age with thrombosis. J Thromb Haemost 2007;5:1654–9.

35. O'Brien SH, Yee DL, Lira J, et al. UNBLOCK: an open-label, dose-finding, pharmacokinetic, and safety study of bivalirudin in children with deep vein thrombosis. J Thromb Haemost 2015;13:1615–22.

36. Forbes TJ, Hijazi Z, Young G. Bivalirudin as a procedural anticoagulant in the pediatric population undergoing intravascular procedures for congenital heart disease. Catheter Cardiovasc Interv 2011;77:671–9.

37. Rayapudi S, Torres A, Deshpande GG, et al. Bivalirudin for anticoagulation in children. Pediatr Blood Cancer 2008;51:798–801.

38. Young G, Boshkov LK, Sullivan JE, et al. Argtroban therapy in pediatric patients requiring nonheparin anticoagulation: an open-label, safety, efficacy, and pharmacokinetic study. Pediatr Blood Cancer 2011;56:1103–9.

39. Madabushi R, Cox DS, Hossain M, et al. Pharmacokinetic and pharmacodynamic basis for effective argatroban dosing in pediatrics. J Clin Pharmacol 2011;51:19–28.

40. Young G, Yee DL, O'Brien S, et al. FondaKIDS: a prospective dose-finding, pharmacokinetic, and safety study of fondaparinux in children between 1-18 years of age. Pediatr Blood Cancer 2011;57:1049–54.

41. Ko RH, Michieli C, Lira JL, et al. Long-term follow-up data of children receiving fondaparinux for treatment of venous thromboembolic events. Thromb Res 2014;134:643–7.

42. Van Es N, Coppens M, Schulman S, et al. Direct oral anticoagulants compared with vitamin K antagonists for acute venous thromboembolism: evidence from phase 3 trials. Blood 2014;124:1968–75.

43. Ansell JE. Reversal agents for direct anticoagulants. Hematol Oncol Clin North Am 2016;30:1085–98.

44. Young G, Kubitza D, Chan A, et al. Development of a rivaroxaban dosing regimen for treatment of VTE in children aged 12 to 18 years. J Thromb Haemost 2015; 13(suppl 2):AS133.

45. Halton JM, Lehr T, Cronin L, et al. Safety, tolerability, and clinical pharmacology of dabigatran etexilate in adolescents. An open-label phase IIa study. Thromb Haemost 2016;116:461–71.

46. von Vajna E, Alam R, So TY. Current clinical trials on the use of direct oral anticoagulants in the pediatric population. Cardiol Ther 2016;5:19–41.

# Probiotics in Newborns and Children

Mary W. Lenfestey, MD[a], Josef Neu, MD[b],*

## KEYWORDS

- Probiotics • Children • Microbiota • Intestine

## KEY POINTS

- The relationship between the gastrointestinal tract and the gut flora has been implicated in several different disease pathologies.
- Probiotics are microbe-containing supplements used to alter the gut flora, and there are claims that these can be used to alter the disease course for many different pathologies.
- Data to support or refute the efficacy of probiotic therapy are quite variable and depend on the underlying disease as well as the strain of probiotic used.
- This review serves to evaluate the relationship of probiotic therapy to several common pediatric ailments: necrotizing enterocolitis, inflammatory bowel disease, irritable bowel disease, diarrhea, constipation, and autism.

## INTRODUCTION

Interest in probiotics among the public as well as medical professionals has markedly increased over the past 3 decades. The probiotic industry is large and is often highly motivated to aggressively market these agents. Numerous studies of varying quality are available to support the use of probiotics in children. However, significant confusion exists as to which circumstances probiotics may be most efficacious and safe. This review provides some of the relevant literature pertaining to the use of probiotics in children and a better evidence basis for clinical practice guidelines. While reading this review, it is important to understand that there are numerous probiotics with strain-specific effects. Because of this, it is critical that one does not extrapolate benefits or harms caused by one agent to others.

Disclosure statement: none (M.W. Lenfestey). Medela, research grant and scientific advisory board; Infant Bacterial Therapeutics, research grant and scientific advisory board; Nutricia, scientific advisory board (J. Neu).
[a] Division of Pediatric Gastroenterology, University of Florida, PO Box 100296, Gainesville, FL 32610, USA; [b] Department of Pediatrics, University of Florida, 6516 Southwest 93rd Avenue, Gainesville, FL 32608, USA
* Corresponding author.
E-mail address: neuj@peds.ufl.edu

## DEFINITION OF PROBIOTIC

The international Scientific Association for Probiotics and Prebiotics define probiotics as "live microorganisms that, when administered in adequate amounts, confer health benefits on the host."[1] Of critical importance is that probiotic products can be regulated differently. Regulated as a dietary supplement or food ingredient, they are generally intended for the healthy population. Examples of health claims would include benefits to general well-being or enhancement of natural resistance. It is common to see advertisements in the popular media that suggest such benefits. On the other hand, when the probiotic product is restricted to a population of patients whereby there is a medical claim, such as for the prevention of necrotizing enterocolitis (NEC), treatment of diarrhea, or prevention of preterm delivery, then it should be treated as a drug. When a probiotic product marketed as a drug, it must meet much more rigorous requirements. These requirements are often similar to those required by the pharmaceutical industry for development and assurance of purity of the product and supported by well-designed studies of safety and efficacy. Categories of health and medical claim legislations for these agents differ depending on the country[1] (**Table 1**).

## MECHANISMS OF ACTION

Numerous mechanisms of action for probiotics are proposed. However, these should not be confused with the action of normal microbiota that is found in various niches of the body, such as the gastrointestinal tract. The commensal microbiota offer a well-tuned ecosystem during the healthy state that may be perturbed by diet, antibiotics, stress, and numerous other environmental factors. When these environmental factors are not overwhelming, the commensal microbiota exhibit plasticity and after a short period of adjustment generally return to the normal state.

Probiotic bacterial mechanisms of action include short chain fatty acid production, competitive exclusion of pathogens, colonization resistance, bile salt metabolism, enzyme activity, and immunologic effects.[2] It is beyond the scope of this review to discuss these mechanisms in detail. Rather, the authors provide evidence for the effects of individual probiotics that may play a role in health and disease in neonates, infants, and children.

## PROBIOTICS AND NEONATAL NECROTIZING ENTEROCOLITIS

NEC is a devastating disease seen primarily in preterm infants that is extremely difficult to treat.[3] Because of the severity of this disease and its insidious onset, and because

| Table 1<br>Definitions of agents | |
|---|---|
| Probiotic | A supplement or food containing a sufficient number of viable microorganisms to alter microflora and has the potential for health benefit |
| Prebiotic | A nondigestible food ingredient that selectively stimulates favorable growth and/or activity of 1 or more indigenous probiotic bacteria |
| Synbiotic | A product containing both probiotics and prebiotics; synergy of a specific probiotic for a probiotic in the product not essential; may be separate supplements or added to food |
| Postbiotic | A metabolic byproduct generated by a probiotic microorganism that influences biological functions |
| Functional food | Any modified food that provides a health benefit beyond that ascribed to any specific nutrients it contains |

of a lack of predictive biomarkers, preventative measures that are broad based over entire populations of preterm infants rather than targeted to high-risk individuals are being studied. A major problem with such an approach is that NEC represents a multifactorial pathophysiology and is likely more than one disease, similar to cancer and diabetes. Because of this, finding a magic bullet that is directed at NEC is likely to miss its target and a large number of babies could be exposed to an unnecessary agent that may eventually be found to be harmful if not adequately evaluated. Neonatology certainly has a history of such therapeutic misadventures and this need to be avoided.

It is beyond the scope of this review to discuss the development of the normal microbiota in preterm infants. However, it should be noted that there are numerous factors, such as feeding, diet composition, use of antibiotics, use of gastric acid blocking agents, and other environmental factors, that play a role in modulation of the microbial environment of premature infants' gastrointestinal tract. Furthermore, meconium is not a sterile medium as previously thought and has derived a set of microbes that accumulate in the fetal gastrointestinal tract that may have a significant effect on the gastrointestinal development and may play a role in future health and disease.[4–6] However, after birth, there are numerous factors, such as vaginal versus cesarean delivery, human milk versus formula feeding, and the other agents previously mentioned, that affect the trajectory of the development of the intestinal microbial milieu.[7] It is intuitive that exogenous placement of microbes that may not clearly be residents of the developing preterm infant gastrointestinal tract in high doses (as probiotics) may become early colonizers and prevent the normal development of the microbial ecology of the gastrointestinal tract in these infants. Long-term studies to evaluate this hypothesis are needed.

One of the first probiotic studies in neonates involved adding *Lactobacillus* to formula to evaluate the growth of intestinal microorganisms. No differences were found in the colonization patterns between the treated and control infants.[8] Numerous other studies have been completed over the past few decades. Most of these have been relatively small and poorly controlled trials of probiotics for the prevention of NEC in preterm infants. Of major importance is the fact that many of these studies evaluated different probiotic agents. Meta-analyses of these studies have been published; when taken as a group, it seemed that these probiotics had a beneficial effect in decreasing NEC. Major controversy was engendered when a meta-analysis published in 2010[9] suggested that probiotics were highly efficacious in the prevention of NEC. This finding led to the suggestion that it was no longer necessary to do further clinical trials on probiotics.[10] It is important to note that in the meta-analysis, 10 different forms of probiotics were used in the individual studies rather than a single agent. This point raises the question in terms of which probiotic might actually be the most beneficial, what would be an optimal dosage, and what should be the timing of their initiation. Furthermore, the studies in this meta-analysis as well as subsequent meta-analyses, including a Cochrane review,[11] did not include studies that were adequately powered with the prospective a priori hypothesis focused only on NEC. No apparent benefits were found in the meta-analyses for infants weighting less than 1000 g, which is the group that is the most susceptible to NEC. Adequate sample size for studies of this type with typical baseline rates of NEC is more than 1000 subjects to be able to adequately address this a priori hypothesis. Furthermore, it is important to note that studies done retrospectively over different time periods are unacceptable to change practice using these agents. Such studies are usually considered as hypothesis generating. Too many confounding variables occur during different time periods, which include changes in feeding practice (human milk vs formula), institution of new feeding protocols, and changes in antibiotic or histamine 2 blocker usage. All of these changes in practice are known to affect the microbial environment of the gastrointestinal tract and could thereby also affect the incidence of NEC, confounding the results of any such studies if incidence of NEC is compared between two different eras.

A more recent study done in the United Kingdom by Costeloe and colleagues[12] used one probiotic agent, had an a priori hypothesis based on NEC, and was adequately powered to evaluate whether this agent would decrease NEC. Comparison between probiotic versus placebo controls showed no difference in NEC, sepsis, death, or any other morbidity. Although it could be argued that the one probiotic agent used in this study was different than the ones used in previous studies that were evaluated in the meta-analyses, it is also clear from this study that probiotics should not be evaluated as a group. Rather, if a meta-analysis is to be done, it should be done on a single probiotic or discrete group of probiotics used in all of the individual studies that were used in a similar fashion in the studies being meta-analyzed.

In terms of the regulatory issues, probiotics have not been scrutinized with the same standards as those required for a pharmaceutical agent. Thus, concern should be raised about the quality and consistency of the probiotics being used for the prevention of NEC. This is especially concerning in that preterm infants are a highly vulnerable population with an immature immune system that could be detrimentally affected by inappropriate quantities of the probiotic agent or by poor quality-control measures. As an example, a preterm neonate, who died after receiving a probiotic preparation, was found to be infected with mucormycosis, possibly due to a tainted batch of product.[13]

Additional studies are being done in the United States and Europe that involve randomized controlled studies with regulatory agency approval for phase 2 studies. If safety is proven in the studies, and if the regulatory agencies allow, these studies are likely to continue with much more extensive phase 3 efficacy studies. These studies will provide important additional information on individual probiotic preparations that are studied using stringent methodologies.

It is currently clear that the use of probiotics for the prevention of NEC remains controversial, and future well-controlled randomized trials will provide us with the rigorous evidence to satisfy us for the nonuse or use of these agents in the preterm neonate population. It is concerning that neonatologists who insist on using probiotics without additional safety and efficacy studies are often times using probiotics that have not previously been evaluated for safety and efficacy in preterm infants. This is partially because the probiotics have all been lumped into one category. We need to be cognizant of the fact that these are different agents with different properties and different safety margins. The studies that are currently underway with collaboration of the regulatory agencies, such as the Food and Drug Administration, will be very important for clinical decisions in the future.

## INFLAMMATORY BOWEL DISEASE

Inflammatory bowel disease (IBD) is composed primarily of two main subsets of disease: ulcerative colitis (UC) and Crohn disease (CD). Both UC and CD have distinct clinical presentations and pathologic findings, with the main similarity of both processes being autoimmune in nature with resultant inflammation and disease of the gastrointestinal tract. CD can affect any portion of the gastrointestinal tract, from the oral cavity to the anus, and is characterized by transmural inflammation. UC is limited to the colon and results in only superficial mucosal inflammation.[14] Over the past several decades, there have been increasing incidences of pediatric inflammatory bowel disease, more notably in CD cases. However, despite increasing disease burden, the underlying cause of IBD is unclear. Possible contributing factors likely include diet,[15] genetics,[16] and early childhood antibiotic exposures[17–19]; there are many other factors under investigation, including vitamin D deficiency[20] and the role of the intestinal microbiome.[21,22] There is specific interest in the interactions between the enteric immune system and the microbiome, with some suggestion that interaction between the gut microbiome in genetically predisposed people may be a driving force in disease pathogenesis.[22] In UC, correlations in overall decreased biodiversity with increased abundance of Enterobacteriaceae has been noted.[23,24] In CD, there is a similar phenotype, with overall reduction in microbial diversity but an increased overall population of bacteria within the gut, specifically more pathogenic strains, such as *Bacteroides* and *Proteobacteria*.[25–30]

There are many therapeutic options for the treatment of IBD, including immunosuppressants (antitumor necrosis factor alpha agents, methotrexate, thiopurines), antiinflammatory medications (aminosalicylates), and adjuvant therapy with antimicrobial medications (specifically with metronidazole and ciprofloxacin). Based on the alterations in the microbiome found in patients with IBD compared with healthy controls, there has also been discussion as to whether probiotics could be a useful adjuvant therapy.

In CD, there is currently no consensus of data to support any benefit to using probiotics. A Cochrane review was completed in 2006 that evaluated the utility of probiotics in CD for maintenance of remission, which found no evidence to suggest that probiotics were beneficial in maintaining remission.[31] However, one limitation of this review was that, of the 7 randomized controlled trials (RCTs), there were different dosing and strains of probiotics used; in addition, many of the studies had small numbers of patients, which lacked statistical power. In fact, 2 of the studies included in the review had participants who withdrew from the respective studies because of gastrointestinal side effects (nausea, abdominal pain, vomiting, and/or diarrhea).[32,33] A second Cochrane review was completed in 2008 evaluating the use of probiotics for induction of remission in CD. This review found a lack of RCTs on the topic and insufficient data to make any conclusions on the efficacy of probiotics inducing remission.[34] Another review by Doherty and colleagues[35] evaluated the role of probiotics in the prevention of postoperative recurrence of CD, which did not show efficacy as a postoperative prophylactic measure. In summation, for CD there are not adequate data to support the use of probiotics, with mixed data in the studies that have been published. Lack of consistent selection in probiotic type and dose, in conjunction with small study sizes, limit what data are currently available.

There are more data in UC that show a favorable response to probiotic treatments. A study by Guslandi and colleagues[36] found that 68% of adults with active mild to moderate UC entered remission after 4 weeks of treatment with *Saccharomyces boulardii*. In a separate pilot study by Huynh and colleagues,[37] 61% of children with mild to moderately active UC went into remission after taking VSL#3, a commercially available proprietary mix of probiotic bacteria. A randomized control trial of 29 pediatric patients with newly diagnosed UC by Miele and colleagues[38] found that VSL#3 used in combination with standard therapy for systemic steroids and mesalamine resulted in higher rates of remission when compared with the placebo group (93% compared with 36%) and had lower rates of disease relapse over a 1-year time frame (21.4% vs 73.3%). There are studies involving other strains of probiotics as well, including *Escherichia coli* 1917 Nissle. However, although many studies do show benefit in probiotic therapy in patients with UC, it is not without risk. As patients with IBD are typically immunosuppressed, there is a risk of systemic infection. A case report by Vahabnezhad and colleagues[39] described a pediatric patient with UC managed with steroids and infliximab infusions who was taking *Lactobacillus rhamnosus* GG probiotics, who developed *Lactobacillus bacteremia*.

The North American Society of Pediatric Gastroenterology, Hepatology, and Nutrition's (NASPGHAN) Nutrition Report Committee published clinical practice guidelines based on a review of the available data. Their summary of the recommendations was that there is no clear efficacy for the use of probiotics in CD at this time (based primarily on *Lactobacillus* GG data) but that there is a role in UC management, as probiotic therapy has been found equivalent to the Aminosalicylates mode of therapy.[40]

## CONSTIPATION

Constipation is a very common complaint among the pediatric population and has been found to affect up to 30% of children.[41] Functional constipation, or constipation in which there is no underlying disease but rather is due to dietary and/or behavioral factors, is the source of more than 95% of constipation cases in healthy children.[42] There are many known organic causes of constipation, including anatomic anomalies (imperforate anus or anal stenosis), nervous issues (hypotonia, Hirschsprung disease, spinal dysraphisms), hormone abnormalities (hypothyroidism), electrolyte derangements, and a variety of other underlying disease processes (celiac disease), all of which should be considered in a constipated child and if found have unique management strategies. As functional constipation is the most common type of childhood constipation, this section focuses on the utility of probiotics in the management of functional constipation.

A study by Zoppi and colleagues[43] found a difference in the underlying microbiome in a set of pediatric patients with constipation, as compared with controls. The constipated children were noted to have higher clostridia and bifidobacteria species in their stool, indicating differences in their underlying microbiome. It is clear that diet also plays a role in constipation; it is unclear as to whether these differences in microbiome are due to the constipation process itself or a result of possible dietary differences. There have been studies that indicated that administration of *Bifidobacterium* or *Lactobacillus* did improve colonic transport times in constipated patients.[44–46]

There are many studies that have evaluated probiotic therapy as part of constipation management; however, overall, the results are varied. One systematic review evaluated 9 studies comparing nonpharmacologic means of therapy, such as fiber, probiotics, behavioral therapy, and some forms of alternative medicine. This study found that there was no evidence for any effect of probiotics when compared with placebo; however, a limitation is that the probiotic regimens compared across the different studies were not the same.[47] In a systematic review of RCTs by Chmielewska and Szajewska,[48] they evaluated 5 RCTs and found potential benefit but with not enough data to be considered more than investigational. In the review, it was noted that in the adult studies, treatment with *Bifidobacterium*, *E coli* Nissle 1917, and *Lactobacillus casei* did have favorable improvements in stool consistency and frequency. In pediatric cases, only *Lactobacillus casei rhamnosus* Lcr35 was found to have a beneficial improvement.[48] In a double-blinded study by Guerra and colleagues,[49] pediatric patients in Brazil with functional constipation were randomized to receive either yogurt supplemented with *Bifidobacterium longum* or only yogurt for 5 weeks. In this study, they noted improvement in defecation frequency and abdominal pain in both groups, but the probiotic group had additional improvement. Coccorullo and colleagues[45] completed a double-blinded randomized study on infants with constipation. They used *Lactobacillus reuteri* and found no effect on stool consistency or episodes of inconsolable crying but did note improvement in bowel frequency.

In summation, there is a variety of studies evaluating multiple different strains and dosing regimens of probiotics to be used in the functional constipation pediatric population. The NASGPHAN's clinical practice guideline review concluded that the current body of evidence does not support the use of probiotics in the treatment of childhood constipation. This conclusion is most likely due to the lack of consistent positive data and no standard regimens of probiotics that have been studied, which makes reviews challenging.

## IRRITABLE BOWEL DISEASE

Functional gastrointestinal disorders, including irritable bowel Syndrome (IBS), are quite common and comprise a significant population of patients managed by pediatric gastroenterologists. Irritable bowel syndrome is present in 10% to 20% of adolescents and affects females more often than males.[50] It is unfortunately commonly associated with poor quality of life and can be costly both in health care burden as well as in decreased function; one study found that IBS was second only to cold symptoms for work absenteeism.[51] Based on Rome III criteria, IBS is defined as abdominal pain with 2 or more of the following symptoms: improvement of the pain with defecation, onset of pain associated with change in frequency of stooling, or onset of pain associated with a change in stool appearance/texture. To meet diagnostic criteria for IBS, patients' symptoms should be present at least weekly for 2 months, without any clinical evidence for other organic causes.[14] There are 4 subtypes of IBS, based primarily on the type of stool change, including diarrhea predominant (IBS-D), constipation predominant (IBD-C), mixed phenotype (IBS-M), or unsubtyped IBS (inconsistent stool pattern that does not meet the criteria for IBS-D/C/M).[52] The pathophysiology of IBS is not fully understood; there is some suggestion that motility disruptions and visceral hypersensitivity are primary factors. There is also recent thought that diet, postinfectious changes, and alterations in the gastrointestinal microbiome may play a role.[14]

In regard to the microbiome contribution, there is some thought that the motility changes in IBS may result in changes to the bacterial flora via stasis and bacterial overgrowth; the changes in the underlying flora may contribute to increased gas via fermentation of nutritional byproducts.[53] Pimentel and colleagues[54] completed a double-blinded RCT in patients with IBS (who met Rome I criteria). In the study, patients with IBS were given rifaximin (an antibiotic commonly used to treat small intestinal bacterial overgrowth) at 400 mg 3 times a day for a 10-day course or placebo. The treated cohort of patients had greater improvement in their IBS symptoms (36%) compared with the placebo group (21%). In addition to evaluating antimicrobial therapy, there have been data to evaluate the use of probiotics to modify IBS symptoms. There is variation as to the results of how efficacious probiotic therapy is for IBS across different studies. Two studies by Kim and colleagues[55,56] evaluated VSL#3 on IBS symptoms in adult patients; both found some improvement in symptoms, specifically bloating and reduced flatulence. A separate study by Drigidi and colleagues[57] found that VSL-3 was effective as a therapy for adults with IBS. Lactobacillus GG has also been evaluated, with mixed results. A study by Bausserman and Michail[58] evaluated this probiotic in pediatric patients and found improvement in the reported abdominal distention (otherwise no change in symptoms). However, a study by O'Sullivan and O'Morain[59] demonstrated no effect in Lactobacillus GG therapy for adult patients with IBS. Other strains of Lactobacillus have also been evaluated. Lactobacillus plantarum 299v (LP299v) has been studied by multiple research groups as well. Niedzielin and colleagues[60] completed an open trial in adults with IBS using LP299v as a therapy; they found that for their patients it was an effective intervention. However, Sen and colleagues[61] completed a double-blinded controlled study with LP299v also in adult patients with IBS and found no effect.

The NASPGHAN's Nutrition Report Committee completed a review in 2006 and made the assessment that efficacy in ameliorating IBS symptoms with probiotics is possible. Overall, there does seem to be an ever-increasing amount of data that supports the use, more so than data that do not; however, as with other pathologies, it is challenging to make stronger recommendations given the differences in probiotic strain, dose, and duration of therapy as well as differences in study design.[40] Reviews are challenging give the lack of consistent positive data, as well as having no definitive standard probiotic regimens that have been studied. It is clear in this category of patients that, although probiotics may have a role in IBS therapy, there should be further evaluation as to which strains and dosing regimens are most appropriate as well as if they should be used for all of the IBS subsets or possibly only certain groups.

## DIARRHEAL ILLNESS

Diarrhea is an encompassing term that describes a condition associated with the passage of frequent, loose stools. The World Health Organization defines diarrhea as more than 3 loose or watery stools per day; however, the clinical presentation may be quite varied depending on the underlying cause of symptoms. There are many causes of diarrhea, including autoimmune (celiac disease, inflammatory bowel disease, autoimmune enteropathy), genetic (congenital secretory diarrheas), malabsorption (cystic fibrosis, pancreatic insufficiencies), and antibiotic-associated diarrhea (AAD). Infectious diarrhea is the most common subtype of the disease. Globally, diarrhea is a large problem with nearly 1.7 billion cases of childhood diarrhea per year and is the second leading cause of death in children younger than 5 years.[62] In the United States, acute viral infectious gastroenteritis accounts for more than 1.5 million outpatient visits and 200,000 hospitalizations per year.[63] The role of probiotics in the management of diarrheal illnesses varies depending on the underlying cause of symptoms. There are several proposed mechanisms as to how probiotics alter a course of diarrhea, and they vary depending on the underlying source of symptoms (antibiotic associated, viral, or bacterial). Potential suggested mechanisms of effect include activation of the immune system[64] and priming the intestines by competing for local binding sites.[65,66] There is also some thought that probiotics inhibit the ability of organisms to adhere to epithelial cells by increasing intestinal mucins.[67]

There are some data to suggest improvement in the duration of infectious diarrhea with the use of probiotics. A Cochrane review was completed in 2010; this review of 63 studies, 56 of which were in children or infants, found that probiotics reduced the risk of diarrhea lasting greater than 4 days by 59% and decreased the duration of diarrhea by 25 hours. The two most commonly studied probiotics were *Lactobacillus* GG and *Saccharomyces boulardii*.[68] In a meta-analysis by Van Niel and colleagues,[69] it was noted that several strains of lactobacilli reduced the duration of diarrhea by 0.7 days and improved the frequency of diarrhea on day 2 of symptoms by 1.6 stools per day. In this review, it was noted that a minimum of 10 billion colony-forming units were required in the first 48 hours to reduce the duration of diarrhea by more than a half day. The probiotic that has showed a benefit most consistently across studies is *Lactobacillus* GG.[70] However, although probiotics have shown improvement in mild to moderate diarrhea, they have not proven to be helpful in severe cases of diarrhea.[71–73] There have also been studies evaluating the utility of probiotics in preventing diarrhea. A randomized controlled study by Hatakka and colleagues[74] evaluated healthy children in Finland and the effects of consumption of milk with and without *Lactobacillus* GG. They found that the children who consumed *Lactobacillus* GG milk had a 16% reduction in absences due to gastrointestinal and respiratory illnesses. Weizman and colleagues[75] also completed a study to evaluate the effect of probiotics on diarrhea. Their study was a double-blinded, controlled, randomized study completed in Israel and included healthy infants in 14 day care centers. The infants were randomized to receive formula with *Bifidobacterium lactis* (BB-12), *Lactobacillus reuteri*, or no probiotics. The control group had more and longer episodes of diarrhea than either probiotic group; the *L reuteri* group, compared with BB-12 or controls, had a significant decrease of number of days with fever, clinic visits, childcare absences, and antibiotic prescriptions. Based on the available data, the NASPGHAN clinical practice guidelines for probiotic use in mild to moderate acute diarrhea are that efficacy is clearly shown, mostly with lactobacilli, in shortening diarrheal course and that there is a modest effect at preventing diarrhea.[40]

Diarrhea is known to be a potential side effect of antibiotics. Johnston and colleagues[76] completed a Cochrane review in 2011 evaluating the efficacy of probiotics for the prevention of AAD. They compared 16 RCTs and found that despite the variation in the probiotic strains used across studies, there was a protective effect of probiotics in preventing AAD. The review also investigated the effect of probiotic dose on symptom improvement and found that the effects were credible at doses greater than 5 billon colony-forming units per day. In the high-dose group, the number needed to treat to prevent one case of ADD was 7. The overall conclusion of the study was that high-dose therapy with *Lactobacillus rhamnosus* and *Saccharomyces boulardii* may be safe and effective in preventing AAD in healthy children. Another meta-analysis evaluating *Saccharomyces boulardii* use in adults and children found a similar number needed to treat; they cited that for every 10 patients treated with probiotics, one would avoid developing AAD.[77] In a systemic review by Hempel and colleagues,[78] 82 RCTs were compared; most of these studies used *Lactobacillus* therapy. They concluded that the pooled data suggested a reduction in AAD; however, there was a significant amount of heterogeneity regarding probiotic strain, dose, and course throughout the different trials. Although the preliminary suggestion is one of benefits, further study to elucidate the most effective probiotic regimen should be undertaken. There have been 2 other meta-analyses that also support this finding, with an approximate reduction of AAD by 60% with the use of *Saccharomyces boulardii* (in adults) and *Lactobacillus* GG (in children).[79,80] However, there are also data that do not suggest a true benefit. One study administered a combination of *Lactobacillus acidophilus* and *Lactobacillus bulgaricus*, which was not effective in preventing AAD in children who were taking amoxicillin.[81,82] In an adult study by the Mayo Clinic, *Lactobacillus* GG was equivalent to placebo for preventing diarrhea in hospitalized adults on antibiotics. These findings may be due to differences in probiotic strains selected for therapy as well as antibiotic administered. Overall, the NASPGHAN's clinical practice guidelines for AAD are that efficacy is clearly shown, but not all probiotics are effective; most of the data support the use of *Lactobacillus* GG and *Saccharomyces boulardii*.[40]

Although there are many bacteria that result in diarrhea, the authors focus on probiotic use in *Clostridium difficile* infection here, as this is a common complication of antibiotic use and hospitalization that has been evaluated specifically in the literature. As fecal transplant has been shown effective for recurrent *Clostridium difficile* infections,[83] using probiotics to alter the gastrointestinal microbiome is a similar proposition. In another systematic review by Johnston and colleagues,[84] 20 RCTs of adults and children with *Clostridium difficile*–associated diarrhea (CDAD) were evaluated.

The conclusion was that probiotics reduced the incidence of CDAD by 66%, without an increase in clinically relevant adverse effects. A Cochrane review in 2013 compared 23 RCTs evaluating the efficacy and safety of probiotic therapy in the prevention of CDAD. They suggested that probiotics reduce the risk of CDAD by 64% and reduce the risk of adverse events by 20% as compared with placebo. The conclusion was that for patients who are not immunocompromised or severely debilitated, the use of a short course of probiotics has moderate evidence to suggest this is both a safe and effective therapy for the prevention of CDAD.[85] A study by McFarland and colleagues[86] compared *Saccharomyces boulardii* plus standard antimicrobial therapy to placebo in adults with recurrent *Clostridium difficile* infection; they found that the probiotic group had a recurrence rate of 34.6%, as compared with the placebo group with a recurrence rate of 64.7%. Surawicz and colleagues[87] also studied *Saccharomyces boulardii*, used in conjunction with oral vancomycin in patients with recurrent *Clostridium difficile*; they also found a reduction of recurrence of 16.7% compared with 50.0% in the placebo group. A pediatric trial evaluating *Lactobacillus* GG suggested a benefit in preventing recurrent *Clostridium difficile* infections as well.[88] The NASPGHAN's clinical practice guidelines for probiotic use in *Clostridium difficile* infections note that efficacy is clearly shown but primarily in severe recurrent disease using *Saccharomyces boulardii* and *Lactobacillus* GG.[40]

## AUTISM

Autism is a neurodevelopmental disorder and is categorized as one of the pervasive developmental disorders of childhood. The *Diagnostic and Statistical Manual of Mental Disorders* has diagnostic criteria for autism as follows: patients with persistent deficits in social interactions as well as restricted and repetitive behaviors and interests. This definition describes autism spectrum disorder (ASD), which encompasses multiple phenotypes, including Asperger syndrome and pervasive developmental delay not otherwise specified, in addition to classic autism.[89] Gastrointestinal complaints are quite common in patients with ASD and are present approximately 3 to 4 times as often as in healthy patients.[90] The incidence of autism has increased steadily over the past 2 decades. There is some evidence to suggest this is in part due to changes in the criteria required for diagnosis as well as improvement in recognition of the disease. The prevalence for ASD is approximately 20.6 per 1000 children, with a male/female ratio of 4:1.[91] Despite the increasing amounts of pediatric patients affected by the disorder, there is still debate as to the underlying cause of symptoms. There are several factors that have been found to contribute to this complex and wide-ranging disease process. Genetic contributions from multiple loci, including chromosomes 16p11.2, 15q24, 11p12-p13, and many others, in addition to other gene variations like translocations, duplications, and microdeletions are thought to correlate with the development of autism. An inheritance pattern of 60% for monozygotic twins, but no concordance in dizygotic twins, speaks to the fact that, although genetics clearly plays a role in the cause, there are other environmental factors involved as well.[91] At present, the goal of treatment is to improve patients' ability to function. Early intervention for patients with initiation of supportive therapies has been shown to be more effective; there are some data to suggest that early management may reduce behavioral problems later on in life.[92–95] The primary focus in treatment is behavioral and educational interventions, which may be augmented with medications. After diagnosis, patients are often cared for by a variety of providers, including a developmental pediatrician, a psychologist, possibly a geneticist, speech and occupational therapists, and a psychiatrist; therapeutic plans are tailored to meet a patient's individual needs. In addition to mainstream standard of care, there is a relatively high use of complementary and alternative medicine (CAM) for these patients. In one study by Perrin and colleagues,[96] 28% of families with patients with ASD reported using CAM therapies; the highest rates of CAM use are in patients with severe disease and those with gastrointestinal symptoms or seizures. One such intervention is probiotic therapy. At this time, their proposed efficacy is based on the thought that alterations in the gastrointestinal microbiome and the enteric nervous system (ENS) may contribute and affect individuals with ASD.

The ENS is an essential component of the gastrointestinal tract and serves as a conduit between the gastrointestinal system and the central nervous system (CNS). The ENS begins to develop as early at 12 weeks into gestation and is derived from neural crest cells that migrate from the sacral and vagal segments of the fetal CNS.[14] Once developed, the ENS controls gastrointestinal motility and secretion and comprises one of the 3 divisions of the autonomic nervous system.[90] It is composed of 2 subtypes: myenteric (Auerbach) plexus and submucosal (Meissner) plexus. Together these systems allow the ENS to control gastrointestinal motility and secretion via a complex network of chemosensitive and mechanosensitive neurons.[14] The human ENS contains more than 100 million neurons; although it works closely with the CNS to modulate gastrointestinal function, it is capable of functioning without input from the CNS. It is the most complex component of the peripheral nervous system, and essentially all classes of neurotransmitter activity that are found in the CNS can be found in the ENS.[90] Although the CNS was once thought to be captain of the ship as a directive force for controlling neurologic activity, it has come to be realized that the ENS-CNS interplay is much more of an interactive interplay. Interestingly, 90% of vagal nerve fibers are afferent, which indicates that the brain may be receiving a significant amount of information from the ENS.[97] There is some suggestion that this continuous feedback of the bowel may also contribute to brain functions, such as mood and memory. There are data from animal models that the gastrointestinal microbiome provides signaling via the vagus nerve, with resultant CNS signaling that induces an anxiogenic or anxiolytic effect depending on the stimulus.[97] In humans, there has also been a relationship between vagal stimulation and mood. A study by Rush and colleagues[98] found that vagal nerve stimulation had an antidepressant effect in adults with treatment-resistant depression. Vagal nerve stimulation has also proven efficacious for the treatment of treatment-resistant forms of epilepsy, and this modality has been used in both adults and children.[99]

The microbiome is thought to play a role in the gut-nervous system behavior dynamic. There are many proposed mechanisms in which this may occur, including direct activation of the vagus nerve via the ENS in response to the local microbiome, metabolites produced locally by the gut flora that cross into systemic circulation and possibly through the blood-brain barrier, and interaction between microbial activation of cytokines with a systemic effect.[100,101] The leaky-gut hypothesis is one of these proposals, which suggests that gut permeability and abnormal translocation of microbial products and toxins result in the development of ASD. In line with this, several animal models do show alterations in behavior patterns with changes in host microbiome. One study by Sudo and colleagues[102] demonstrated that germ-free mice have an elevated response to stress that occurs because of force immobilization; this was thought to be due to higher levels of corticosterone in mice without microbiota. They also found that this behavioral pattern could be partially reversed with recolonization with *Bifidobacterium infantis*. In another study by Savignac and colleagues,[103] they noted that *Bifidobacteria* ingestion by mice was associated with improved learning abilities and improved cognition in an anxious mouse population.

There have been differences noted in the microbiome of autistic patients as compared with controls. A study by Kang and colleagues[104] compared the gastrointestinal microbiome of 20 autistic children with 20 controls; they found lower abundance of *Prevotella*, *Coprococcus*, and *Veillonellaceae* species, which are fermenting bacteria. They also noted that in general the children with ASD had a lower bacterial diversity as compared with controls. Hsiao and colleagues[105] also demonstrated alterations in the microbiome in mice with autismlike features. They treated these mice with *Bacteroides fragilis*, which corrected the gut permeability and improved the defects in the stereotypic, anxietylike, and sensorimotor behaviors. A study by Yano and colleagues[106] demonstrated the relationship between the gastrointestinal microbiome and serotonin regulation. They noted that indigenous spore-forming bacteria from mouse and human microbiota promoted serotonin synthesis in the colonic enterochromaffin cells. They also found that elevating luminal concentrations of certain microbial metabolites increased colonic and blood serotonin levels in mice. Interestingly, elevated levels of serotonin have been found in one-third of patients with ASD and has been correlated with gastrointestinal symptoms, such as abdominal pain and constipation.[107,108] As the gastrointestinal tract is the main site of serotonin production, the elevation in serotonin found in patients with ASD suggests that the gastrointestinal system plays a role in ASD pathogenesis as well. A study by Veenstra-VanderWeele and colleagues[109] discussed the correlation between an abnormality in a serotonin transporter gene (SLC6A4), which results in elevated serum serotonin levels, and an association with ASD. The study evaluated mice with transporter mutations and found that they did indeed have hyperserotonemia; they also noted that these mice displayed alterations in social function, communication, and repetitive behaviors.[110] These findings provide further evidence of the relationship between gut microbiome and subsequent biochemical changes within the body that correlate to changes in the neuropsychiatric state and behavior.

With the documented differences in the microbiome of patients with ASD, there has also been investigation as to whether probiotics could provide a therapeutic opportunity for this population. A study by Buffington and colleagues[111] studied the effects of a high-fat diet and probiotic therapy on mice pups. In the study, pregnant mice were given a high-fat diet that resulted in changes in the hypothalamus neurotransmission, with subsequent abnormal behavior in the mice pups comparable with autism-type behaviors. They found that administering *Lactobacillus reuteri* reversed the aberrant antisocial behaviors. A human study, completed by Pärtty and colleagues,[112] evaluated probiotic use in humans. In the study, 75 infants were given either placebo or *Lactobacillus rhamnosus* GG for the first 6 months of life; the group evaluated microbiota findings and psycho-behavioral diagnoses at 2 and 13 years of age. They found no major changes in the microbiota; however, at 13 years of age, 17% of children in the placebo group had attention-deficit disorder or Asperger syndrome, as opposed to none who received the probiotic.[112] Another study in Slovakian children, completed by Tomova and colleagues,[113] focused on evaluation of the role of the intestinal microbiome in autism. They found a decreased *Bacteroides/Firmicutes* ratio and an increased amount of *Desulfovibrio* species in the autistic population. A strong association between the amount of *Desulfovibrio* species present and the severity of autism reported was identified. During the study the children were given "Children Dophilus," which contains 3 strains of *Lactobacillus* (60%), 2 strains of *Bifidumbacteria* (25%), and one strain of *Streptococcus* (15%), given orally 3 times a day for 4 months. After the probiotic course, they noted improvement in the dysbiosis with increase in the *Bacteroidetes/Firmicutes* ratio to the level found in healthy children. *Desulfovibrio*, which they noted as a suspected etiopathogenetic agent of autism, decreased significantly after therapy as well. There is also conjecture that as many of the gastrointestinal symptoms experienced by children with ASD mirror those of patients with irritable bowel syndrome; as IBS also has alterations in the microbiome, and probiotics have been shown to be efficacious in IBS, then perhaps probiotics may be of use in ASD as well, given the similarities. Clearly, ASD is a multifactorial disease process; increasing amounts of data indicate that the gastrointestinal tract and its microbiome likely play a role in the disease process. There is potential for probiotics to play a role in therapy, but further investigation including patient trials should be pursued to illuminate this area further.

## SUMMARY

As evidenced earlier, there is a large volume of data available that alludes to the importance of the microbiome and its effects on systemic health and disease. In that vein, there has been an ever-growing interest in probiotics as a means to alter the disease course. This interest has been facilitated in part by marketing by the probiotic industry, with claims that probiotic therapy is an effect means of both prevention and treatment of disease. However, the efficacy of probiotic therapy varies widely depending on the strain used and the underlying disease process. Although probiotics have been found to be quite effective for some disease processes, they are not useful in others. It is also important to note that, although uncommon, there have been reports of patient harm due to probiotic use; as with other interventions, the use of probiotics may not be wholly benign depending on the patient population. One of the largest challenges to making generalized recommendations is the variation of colony-forming units and strains within different brands of probiotics. Overall, this is an area that does show great promise for certain conditions. Probiotic therapy should continue to be further investigated, with specific focus on the most useful strains and dosing for effect. As probiotics are used more and more for disease-altering purposes, it may also be time to classify them as medications or drugs to subjugate them to more stringent regulatory oversight.

## REFERENCES

1. Hill C, Guarner F, Reid G, et al. Expert consensus document. The International Scientific Association for Probiotics and Prebiotics consensus statement on the scope and appropriate use of the term probiotic. Nat Rev Gastroenterol Hepatol 2014;11:500–14.
2. Reid G. Probiotics: definition, scope and mechanisms of action. Best Pract Res Clin Gastroenterol 2016;30:17–25.
3. Neu J, Walker WA. Necrotizing enterocolitis. N Engl J Med 2011;364:255–64.
4. Mshvildadze M, Neu J, Schuster J, et al. Intestinal microbial ecology in premature infants assessed with non-culture-based techniques. J Pediatr 2010;156: 20–5.
5. Ardissone AN, de la Cruz DM, Davis-Richardson AG, et al. Meconium microbiome analysis identifies bacteria correlated with premature birth. PLoS One 2014;9:e90784.
6. Jimenez E, Marin ML, Martin R, et al. Is meconium from healthy newborns actually sterile? Res Microbiol 2008;159:187–93.
7. Collado MC, Cernada M, Neu J, et al. Factors influencing gastrointestinal tract and microbiota immune interaction in preterm infants. Pediatr Res 2015;77: 726–31.

8. Reuman PD, Duckworth DH, Smith KL, et al. Lack of effect of Lactobacillus on gastrointestinal bacterial colonization in premature infants. Pediatr Infect Dis 1986;5:663–8.

9. Deshpande G, Rao S, Patole S, et al. Updated meta-analysis of probiotics for preventing necrotizing enterocolitis in preterm neonates. Pediatrics 2010; 125(5):921–30.

10. Tarnow-Mordi WO, Wilkinson D, Trivedi A, et al. Probiotics reduce all-cause mortality in necrotizing enterocolitis: it is time to change practice. Pediatrics 2010; 125(5):1068–70.

11. AlFaleh K, Anabrees J. Probiotics for prevention of necrotizing enterocolitis in preterm infants. Cochrane Database Syst Rev 2014;(4):CD005496.

12. Costeloe K, Hardy P, Juszczak E, et al. Bifidobacterium breve BBG-001 in very preterm infants: a randomised controlled phase 3 trial. Lancet 2016;387(10019): 649–60.

13. Centers for Disease Control and Prevention. Fungal disease, Centers for Disease Control and Prevention 2015. Available at: http://www.cdc.gov/fungal/outbreaks/rhizopus-investigation.html. Accessed September 9, 2017.

14. Wyllie R, Hyams J. Pediatric gastrointestinal and liver disease. 5th edition. Philadelphia: Elsevier; 2016.

15. Hold GL. Western lifestyle: a "master" manipulator of the intestinal microbiota? Gut 2014;63(1):5–6.

16. Russell RK, Satsangi J. IBD: a family affair. Best Pract Res Clin Gastroenterol 2004;18(3):525–39.

17. Kronman MP, Zaoutis TE, Haynes K, et al. Antibiotic exposure and IBD development among children: a population-based cohort study. Pediatrics 2012;130(4): e794–803.

18. Shaw SY, Blanchard JF, Bernstein CN. Association between the use of antibiotics in the first year of life and pediatric inflammatory bowel disease. Am J Gastroenterol 2010;105(12):2687–892.

19. Virta L, Auvinen A, Helenius H, et al. Association of repeated exposure to antibiotics with the development of pediatric Crohn's disease–a nationwide, register-based Finnish case-control study. Am J Epidemiol 2012;175(8):775–84.

20. Mouli VP, Ananthakrishnan AN. Review article: vitamin D and inflammatory bowel diseases. Aliment Pharmacol Ther 2014;39(2):125–36.

21. Kaser A, Zeissig S, Blumberg RS. Inflammatory bowel disease. Annu Rev Immunol 2010;28:573–621.

22. Jostins L, Ripke S, Weersma RK, et al. Host-microbe interactions have shaped the genetic architecture of inflammatory bowel disease. Nature 2012;491(7422): 119–24.

23. Morgan XC, Tickle TL, Sokol H, et al. Dysfunction of the intestinal microbiome in inflammatory bowel disease and treatment. Genome Biol 2012;13:R79.

24. Michail S, Durbin M, Turner D, et al. Alterations in the gut microbiome of children with severe ulcerative colitis. Inflamm Bowel Dis 2012;18:1799–808.

25. Swidsinski A, Weber J, Loening-Baucke V, et al. Spatial organization and composition of the mucosal flora in patients with inflammatory bowel disease. J Clin Microbiol 2005;43(7):3380–9.

26. Hansen R, Russell RK, Reiff C, et al. Microbiota of de-novo pediatric IBD: increased Faecalibacterium prausnitzii and reduced bacterial diversity in Crohn's but not in ulcerative colitis. Am J Gastroenterol 2012;107(12):1913–22.

27. Gevers D, Kugathasan S, Denson LA, et al. The treatment-naive microbiome in new-onset Crohn's disease. Cell Host Microbe 2014;15(3):382–92.

28. Hold GL, Smith M, Grange C, et al. Role of the gut microbiota in inflammatory bowel disease pathogenesis: what have we learnt in the past 10 years? World J Gastroenterol 2014;20(5):1192–210.

29. Darfeuille-Michaud A, Boudeau J, Bulois P, et al. High prevalence of adherent-invasive Escherichia coli associated with ileal mucosa in Crohn's disease. Gastroenterology 2004;127(2):412–21.

30. Rolhion N, Darfeuille-Michaud A. Adherent-invasive Escherichia coli in inflammatory bowel disease. Inflamm Bowel Dis 2007;13(10):1277–83.

31. Rolfe VE, Fortun PJ, Hawkey CJ, et al. Probiotics for maintenance of remission in Crohn's disease. Cochrane Database Syst Rev 2006;(4):CD004826.

32. Zocco MA, Zileri Dal Verme L, Armuzzi A, et al. Comparison of Lactobacillus GG and mesalamine in maintaining remission of ulcerative colitis and Crohn's disease. Gastroenterology 2003;124(4 Suppl 1):A201.

33. Bousvaros A, Guandalini S, Baldassano RN, et al. A randomized, double-blind trial of Lactobacillus GG versus placebo in addition to standard maintenance therapy for children with Crohn's disease. Inflamm Bowel Dis 2005;11(9):833–9.

34. Butterworth AD, Thomas AG, Akobeng AK. Probiotics for induction of remission in Crohn's disease. Cochrane Database Syst Rev 2008;(3):CD006634.

35. Doherty GA, Bennett GC, Cheifetz AS, et al. Meta-analysis: targeting the intestinal microbiota in prophylaxis for post-operative Crohn's disease. Aliment Pharmacol Ther 2010;31:802.

36. Guslandi M, Giollo P, Testoni PA. A pilot trial of Saccharomyces boulardii in ulcerative colitis. Eur J Gastroenterol Hepatol 2003;15:607–98.

37. Huynh HQ, deBruyn J, Guan L, et al. Probiotic preparation VSL#3 induces remission in children with mild to moderate acute ulcerative colitis: a pilot study. Inflamm Bowel Dis 2009;15:760–8.

38. Miele E, Pascarella F, Giannetti E, et al. Effect of a probiotic preparation (VSL#3) on induction and maintenance of remission in children with ulcerative colitis. Am J Gastroenterol 2009;104:437–43.

39. Vahabnezhad E, Mochon AB, Wozniak LJ, et al. Lactobacillus bacteremia associated with probiotic use in a pediatric patient with ulcerative colitis. J Clin Gastroenterol 2013;47:437–9.

40. Michail S, Sylvester F, Fuchs G, et al. Clinical efficacy of probiotics: review of the evidence with focus on children. NASPGHAN clinical practice guidelines. J Pediatr Gastroenterol Nutr 2006;43:550–7.

41. Van den Berg MM, Benninga MA, Di Lorenzo C. Epidemiology of childhood constipation: a systematic review. Am J Gastroenterol 2006;101(10):2401.

42. Loening-Baucke V. Prevalence, symptoms and outcome of constipation in infants and toddlers. J Pediatr 2005;146:359.

43. Zoppi G, Cinquetti M, Luciano A, et al. The intestinal ecosystem in chronic functional constipation. Acta Paediatr 1998;87:836.

44. Agrawal A, Houghton LA, Morris J, et al. Clinical trial: the effects of a fermented milk product containing Bifidobacterium lactis DN-173 010 on abdominal distension and gastrointestinal transit in irritable bowel syndrome with constipation. Aliment Pharmacol Ther 2009;29:104.

45. Coccorullo P, Strisciuglio C, Martinelli M, et al. Lactobacillus reuteri (DSM 17938) in infants with functional chronic constipation: a double-blind, randomized, placebo-controlled study. J Pediatr 2010;157:598–602.

46. Tabbers MM, DiLorenzo C, Berger MY, et al. Evaluation and treatment of functional constipation in infants and children: evidence based recommendations

from ESPGHAN and NASPGHAN. J Pediatr Gastroenterol Nutr 2014;58(2): 258–74.

47. Tabbers MM, Boluyt N, Berger MY, et al. Nonpharmacologic treatments for childhood constipation: systematic review. Pediatrics 2011;128:753–61.

48. Chmielewska A, Szajewska H. Systematic review of randomized controlled trials: probiotics for functional constipation. World J Gastroenterol 2010;16:69–75.

49. Guerra PV, Lima LN, Souza TC, et al. Pediatric functional constipation treatment with Bifidobacterium-containing yogurt: a crossover, double-blind, controlled trial. World J Gastroenterol 2011;17:3916–21.

50. Saito YA, Schoenfeld P, Locke GR 3rd. The epidemiology of irritable bowel syndrome in North America: a systematic review. Am J Gastroenterol 2002;97: 1910–5.

51. Maxion-Bergemann S, Thielecke F, Abel F, et al. Costs of irritable bowel syndrome in the UK and US. Pharmacoeconomics 2006;24:21–37.

52. Shih DQ, Kwan LY. All roads lead to Rome: update on Rome III criteria and new treatment options. Gastroenterol Rep 2007;1(2):56–65.

53. Lin HC. Small intestinal bacterial overgrowth: a framework for understanding irritable bowel syndrome. JAMA 2004;292:852–8.

54. Pimentel M, Park S, Mirocha J, et al. The effect of a nonabsorbed oral antibiotic (rifaximin) on the symptoms of the irritable bowel syndrome: a randomized trial. Ann Intern Med 2006;145:557–63.

55. Kim HJ, Vazquez Roque MI, Camilleri M, et al. A randomized controlled trial of a probiotic combination VSL# 3 and placebo in irritable bowel syndrome with bloating. Neurogastroenterol Motil 2005;17:687–96.

56. Kim HJ, Camilleri M, McKinzie S, et al. A randomized controlled trial of a probiotic, VSL#3, on gut transit and symptoms in diarrhoea-predominant irritable bowel syndrome. Aliment Pharmacol Ther 2003;17:895–904.

57. Brigidi P, Vitali B, Swennen E, et al. Effects of probiotic administration upon the composition and enzymatic activity of human fecal microbiota in patients with irritable bowel syndrome or functional diarrhea. Res Microbiol 2001;152:735–41.

58. Bausserman M, Michail S. The use of Lactobacillus GG in irritable bowel syndrome in children: a double-blind randomized control trial. J Pediatr 2005; 147:197–201.

59. O'Sullivan MA, O'Morain CA. Bacterial supplementation in the irritable bowel syndrome. A randomised double-blind placebo controlled crossover study. Dig Liver Dis 2000;32:294–301.

60. Niedzielin K, Kordecki H, Birkenfeld B. A controlled, double blind, randomized study on the efficacy of Lactobacillus plantarum 299V in patients with irritable bowel syndrome. Eur J Gastroenterol Hepatol 2001;13:1143–7.

61. Sen S, Mullan MM, Parker TJ, et al. Effect of Lactobacillus plantarum 299v on colonic fermentation and symptoms of irritable bowel syndrome. Dig Dis Sci 2002;47:2615–20.

62. World Health Organization. Diarrhoeal disease. World Health Organization; 2017.

63. King CK, Glass R, Bresee JS, et al. Managing acute gastroenteritis among children: oral rehydration, maintenance, and nutritional therapy. MMWR Recomm Rep 2003;52:1.

64. Perdigon G, Alvarez S, Rachid M, et al. Immune system stimulation by probiotics. J Dairy Sci 1995;78:1597–606.

65. Duffy LC, Zielezny M, Riepenhoff-Talty M, et al. Reduction of virus shedding by B. bifidum in experimentally induced MRV infection. Dig Dis Sci 1994;39: 2334–40.

66. Duffy LC, Zielezny M, Riepenhoff-Talty M, et al. Effectiveness of Bifidobacterium bifidum in mediating the clinical course of murine rotavirus diarrhea. Pediatr Res 1994;35:690–5.

67. Mack DR, Michail S, Wei S, et al. Probiotics inhibit enteropathogenic E. coli adherence in vitro by inducing intestinal mucin gene expression. Am J Physiol 1999;276:G941–50.

68. Allen SJ, Martinez EG, Gregorio GV, et al. Probiotics for treating acute infectious diarrhoea. Cochrane Database Syst Rev 2010;(11):CD003048.

69. Van Niel CW, Feudtner C, Garrison MM, et al. Lactobacillus therapy for acute infectious diarrhea in children: a meta-analysis. Pediatrics 2002;109:678.

70. Szajewska H, Mrukowicz JZ. Probiotics in the treatment and prevention of acute infectious diarrhea in infants and children: a systematic review of published randomized, double-blind, placebo controlled trials. J Pediatr Gastroenterol Nutr 2001;33(Suppl 2):S17–25.

71. Costa-Ribeiro H, Ribeiro TC, Mattos AP, et al. Limitations of probiotic therapy in acute, severe dehydrating diarrhea. J Pediatr Gastroenterol Nutr 2003;36: 112–5. J Pediatr Gastroenterol Nutr 2006;43(4).

72. Salazar-Lindo E, Miranda-Langschwager P, Campos-Sanchez M, et al. Lactobacillus casei strain GG in the treatment of infants with acute watery diarrhea: a randomized, double-blind, placebo controlled clinical trial [ISRCTN67363048]. BMC Pediatr 2004;4:18.

73. Sarker SA, Sultana S, Fuchs GJ, et al. Lactobacillus paracasei strain ST11 has no effect on rotavirus but ameliorates the outcome of nonrotavirus diarrhea in children from Bangladesh. Pediatrics 2005;116:e221–8.

74. Hatakka K, Savilahti E, Pönkä A, et al. Effect of long term consumption of probiotic milk on infections in children attending day care centres: double blind, randomised trial. BMJ 2001;322:1327.

75. Weizman Z, Asli G, Alsheikh A. Effect of a probiotic infant formula on infections in child care centers: comparison of two probiotic agents. Pediatrics 2005;115: 5–9.

76. Johnston BC, Goldenberg JZ, Vandvik PO, et al. Probiotics for the prevention of pediatric antibiotic-associated diarrhea. Cochrane Database Syst Rev 2011;(11):CD004827.

77. Szajewska H, Mrukowicz J. Meta-analysis: non-pathogenic yeast Saccharomyces boulardii in the prevention of antibiotic-associated diarrhoea. Aliment Pharmacol Ther 2005;22:365–72.

78. Hempel S, Newberry SJ, Maher AR. Probiotics for the prevention and treatment of antibiotic-associated diarrhea: a systematic review and meta-analysis. JAMA 2012;307:1959–69.

79. Cremonini F, Di Caro S, Nista EC, et al. Meta-analysis: the effect of probiotic administration on antibiotic-associated diarrhoea. Aliment Pharmacol Ther 2002;16:1461–7.

80. D'Souza AL, Rajkumar C, Cooke J, et al. Probiotics in prevention of antibiotic associated diarrhoea: meta-analysis. BMJ 2002;324:1361.

81. Tankanow RM, Ross MB, Ertel IJ, et al. A double-blind, placebo-controlled study of the efficacy of Lactinex in the prophylaxis of amoxicillin induced diarrhea. DICP 1990;24:382–4.

82. Thomas MR, Litin SC, Osmon DR, et al. Lack of effect of Lactobacillus GG on antibiotic-associated diarrhea: a randomized, placebo-controlled trial. Mayo Clin Proc 2001;76:883–9.

83. Kassam Z, Lee CH, Yuan Y, et al. Fecal microbiota transplantation for Clostridium difficile infection: systematic review and meta-analysis. Am J Gastroenterol 2013;108:500–8.

84. Johnston BC, Ma SS, Goldenberg JZ, et al. Probiotics for the prevention of Clostridium difficile-associated diarrhea: a systematic review and meta-analysis. Ann Intern Med 2012;157:878–88.

85. Goldenberg JZ, Ma SS, Saxton JD, et al. Probiotics for the prevention of Clostridium difficile-associated diarrhea in adults and children. Cochrane Database Syst Rev 2013;(5):CD006095.

86. McFarland LV, Surawicz CM, Greenberg RN, et al. A randomized placebo-controlled trial of Saccharomyces boulardii in combination with standard antibiotics for Clostridium difficile disease. JAMA 1994;271:1913–8.

87. Surawicz CM, McFarland LV, Greenberg RN, et al. The search for a better treatment of recurrent Clostridium difficile disease: use of high-dose vancomycin combined with Saccharomyces boulardii. Clin Infect Dis 2000;31:1012–7.

88. Biller JA, Katz AJ, Flores AF, et al. Treatment of recurrent Clostridium difficile colitis with Lactobacillus GG. J Pediatr Gastroenterol Nutr 1995;21:224–6.

89. American Psychiatric Association. Autism spectrum disorder. In: Diagnostic and statistical manual of mental disorders. 5th edition. Arlington (VA): American Psychiatric Association; 2013. p. 50.

90. Rao M, Gershon M. The bowel and beyond: the enteric nervous system in neurological disorders. Nat Rev Gastroenterol Hepatol 2016;13(9):517–28.

91. Kliegman R, Stanton B, St Geme JW, et al. Nelson textbook of pediatrics. 19th edition. Philadelphia: Elsevier; 2016. Print.

92. Dawson G, Osterling J. Early intervention in autism: effectiveness and common elements of current approaches. In: Guralnick MJ, editor. Effectiveness of early intervention: second generation research. Baltimore (MD): Paul Brookes; 1997. p. 307.

93. Volkmar F, Siegel M, Woodbury-Smith M, et al. Practice parameter for the assessment and treatment of children and adolescents with autism spectrum disorder. J Am Acad Child Adolesc Psychiatry 2014;53:237.

94. Howlin P. Practitioner review: psychological and educational treatments for autism. J Child Psychol Psychiatry 1998;39:307.

95. Durand VM, Carr EG. Functional communication training to reduce challenging behavior: maintenance and application in new settings. J Appl Behav Anal 1991;24:251.

96. Perrin JM, Coury DL, Hyman SL, et al. Complementary and alternative medicine use in a large pediatric autism sample. Pediatrics 2012;130(Suppl 2):S77.

97. Forsythe P, Bienenstock J, Kunze WA. Vagal pathways for microbiome–brain–gut axis communication. Adv Exp Med Biol 2014;817:115–33.

98. Rush AJ, George MS, Sackeim HA, et al. Vagus nerve stimulation (VNS) for treatment-resistant depressions: a multicenter study. Biol Psychiatry 2000;47:276–86.

99. George MS, Sackeim HA, Rush AJ, et al. Vagus nerve stimulation: a new tool for brain research and therapy. Biol Psychiatry 2000;47:287–95.

100. Sampson TR, Mazmanian SK. Control of brain development, function, and behavior by the microbiome. Cell Host Microbe 2015;17:565–76.

101. Mayer EA, Knight R, Mazmanian SK, et al. Gut microbes and the brain: paradigm shift in neuroscience. J Neurosci 2014;34:15490–6.
102. Sudo N, Chida Y, Aiba Y, et al. Postnatal microbial colonization programs the hypothalamic-pituitary-adrenal system for stress response in mice. J Physiol 2004;558:263–75.
103. Savignac HM, Tramullas M, Kiely B, et al. Bifidobacteria modulate cognitive processes in an anxious mouse strain. Behav Brain Res 2015;287:59–72.
104. Kang DW, Park JG, Ilhan ZE, et al. Reduced incidence of Prevotella and other fermenters in intestinal microflora of autistic children. PLoS One 2013;8:e68322.
105. Hsiao EY, McBride SW, Hsien S, et al. Microbiota modulate behavioral and physiological abnormalities associated with neurodevelopmental disorders. Cell 2013;155:1451–63.
106. Yano JM, Yu K, Donaldson GP, et al. Indigenous bacteria from the gut microbiota regulate host serotonin biosynthesis. Cell 2015;161:264–76.
107. Marler S, Ferguson BJ, Lee EB, et al. Brief report: whole blood serotonin levels and gastrointestinal symptoms in autism spectrum disorder. J Autism Dev Disord 2016;46:1124–30.
108. Matondo RB, Punt C, Homberg J, et al. Deletion of the serotonin transporter in rats disturbs serotonin homeostasis without impairing liver regeneration. Am J Physiol Gastrointest Liver Physiol 2009;296:G963–8.
109. Veenstra-VanderWeele J, Muller CL, Iwamoto H, et al. Autism gene variant causes hyperserotonemia, serotonin receptor hypersensitivity, social impairment and repetitive behavior. Proc Natl Acad Sci USA 2012;109(14):5469–74.
110. Navarro F, Liu Y, Rhoads JM. Can probiotics benefit children with autism spectrum disorders? World J Gastroenterol 2016;22(46):10093–102.
111. Buffington SA, Di Prisco GV, Auchtung TA, et al. Microbial reconstitution reverses maternal diet-induced social and synaptic deficits in offspring. Cell 2016;165:1762–75.
112. Pärtty A, Kalliomäki M, Wacklin P, et al. A possible link between early probiotic intervention and the risk of neuropsychiatric disorders later in childhood: a randomized trial. Pediatr Res 2015;77:823–8.
113. Tomova A, Husarova V, Lakatosova S, et al. Gastrointestinal microbiota in children with autism in Slovakia. Physiol Behav 2015;138:179–87.

# Drug Treatment of Seizures and Epilepsy in Newborns and Children

Louis T. Dang, MD, PhD[a],*, Faye S. Silverstein, MD[b]

## KEYWORDS

- Anticonvulsant • Antiepileptic • Anti-seizure medication • Epilepsy • Pediatric

## KEY POINTS

- Many new antiepileptic drugs (AEDs) are available.
- Few AEDs are systematically evaluated in children and even fewer in neonates and infants.
- Off-label AEDs use is frequent in children.
- Minimal comparative efficacy data are available.
- Identification of specific genetic epilepsy mechanisms may enable future development of a precision medicine approach to guide drug treatment.

## INTRODUCTION

Epilepsy is a common and heterogeneous pediatric disorder characterized as a chronic predisposition to seizures. The estimated lifetime prevalence of epilepsy is approximately 1%, with onset mostly in early childhood and in the elderly.[1] Epilepsy has been traditionally diagnosed based on a history of 2 or more unprovoked seizures spaced greater than 24 hours apart. Recently, the definition has been expanded to include individuals who have had a single unprovoked seizure but who have a greater than 60% chance of additional seizures occurring over the next 10 years.[2] In clinical practice, risk prediction for additional seizures is most commonly based on identification of specific electroencephalography (EEG) patterns.

Disclosure: Both authors receive salary support from NIH (NIH HD028820, NIH HL094345). Neither has any conflict of interest with materials in this article.
[a] Division of Pediatric Neurology, Department of Pediatrics, University of Michigan, C.S. Mott Children's Hospital, Room 12-733, 1540 East Hospital Drive, Ann Arbor, MI 48109-4279, USA; [b] Division of Pediatric Neurology, Department of Pediatrics, University of Michigan, 8301 MSRB3, 1150 West Medical Center Drive, Ann Arbor, MI 48109-5646, USA
* Corresponding author.
E-mail address: louisdan@med.umich.edu

Epilepsies are classified by their associated seizure types (eg, focal vs generalized) and etiology.[3] At times, the constellation of seizure types, EEG findings, and age-dependent features (onset and remission) fit a recognized epilepsy syndrome. Readers are referred to standard texts and relevant review articles for detailed discussions of epilepsy classification, etiology, diagnostic evaluation, and prognosis.[4–7] Acute symptomatic seizures, febrile seizures, and status epilepticus may be associated with epilepsy but are distinct entities and treatment of these conditions is not covered in this article; they are covered in other reviews.[8]

The mainstay of medical treatment of epilepsy is prophylactic administration of medications, collectively described as antiepileptic drugs (AEDs), that can reduce the risk of seizure recurrence.[4,9–11] In 1993, there were approximately 7 AEDs that were commonly used to treat epilepsy; since then, many additional drugs have been developed and Food and Drug Administration (FDA) approved. These new-generation AEDs are broadly viewed as better than older AEDs with respect to having fewer adverse effects and drug interactions while retaining efficacy similar to older AEDs, such as carbamazepine and phenytoin. The goal of this article is to provide pediatricians with an overview of AEDs currently used to treat epilepsy in children, with a focus on guiding principles for drug therapy and recently introduced medications.

## OVERVIEW
### Starting Antiepileptic Drug Treatment

The history, neurologic examination, results of EEG and other neurodiagnostic tests, medical comorbidities, patient and family preference, and physician perspective all influence a decision to start AED treatment after a single unprovoked seizure, because estimates vary regarding the recurrence risk.[12] A recent Cochrane review concluded, "treatment of the first unprovoked seizure reduces the risk of a subsequent seizure but does not affect the proportion of patients in remission in the long-term," and there is no evidence of reduced mortality with AED treatment.[13] After a second unprovoked seizure, however, clinicians usually recommend starting an AED.[4,14,15]

Although more than 20 AEDs are currently FDA approved (**Tables 1** and **2**), in clinical practice, initial treatment options for infants and children include fewer agents (discussed later). Factors that influence drug selection include seizure and EEG classification (generalized vs focal vs specific epilepsy syndrome), drug formulation (liquid or chewable tablet vs capsule, convenience of dosing, **Table 3**), adverse-effect profile (**Table 4**), and clinician preferences.

Many of the older agents (see **Table 1**) are now prescribed less frequently in the United States, although they remain in wide use, particularly in low-resource settings. Perceived advantages of the newer drugs include greater convenience (no routine blood testing), broader spectrum (in particular for levetiracetam), fewer serious adverse effects, and fewer drug interactions.

As is the case for treatment of many of the pediatric disorders discussed in this issue, off-label treatment is common for children with epilepsy. Clinicians are generally comfortable extrapolating efficacy results from studies performed in adults to predict treatment responses in children; safety concerns and adverse effect profiles limit extrapolation to the youngest age groups.

Generic AED substitution has become a hot-button topic for clinicians and patients.[16] Although bioequivalence is difficult to document, recent studies and clinical experience suggest that generic substitution is feasible for many patients. Prescribers commonly recommend against switching among generic preparations, but this goal is sometimes challenging to attain in practice.

**Table 1**
**Antiepileptic drugs commonly used in children prior to 1993**

| Generic Name | Brand Names | Some Pros and Cons |
|---|---|---|
| Phenobarbital | Luminal | Pros: broad-spectrum efficacy, widely available, cheap, predictable pharmacokinetics<br>Cons: adverse behavioral effects, frequent drug interactions |
| Phenytoin | Dilantin | Pros: broad-spectrum efficacy, widely available<br>Cons: substantial risk of allergic reactions, variable absorption in infants, unpredictable pharmacokinetics, frequent drug interactions |
| Valproic Acid | Depakene, Depakote | Pros: broad-spectrum efficacy, widely available<br>Cons: broad range of severe and mild adverse systemic effects |
| Carbamazepine | Tegretol Tegretol XR | Pros: efficacy for focal seizures, widely available, cheap<br>Cons: need to introduce slowly, significant risk of severe allergic reaction/SJS, no intravenous formulation |
| Ethosuximide | Zarontin | Pros: efficacy for absence seizures, few adverse neurobehavioral effects<br>Cons: lack of efficacy for convulsive seizures |
| Clonazepam | Klonopin | Pros: broad-spectrum efficacy, widely available, no serious systemic adverse effects<br>Cons: sedation, increased oral secretions, tachyphylaxis |
| Primidone | Mysoline | Pros: metabolized to phenobarbital and has broad spectrum of efficacy (including for generalized tonic-clonic and focal seizures)<br>Cons: frequent and diverse adverse effects (similar to other barbiturates) |

### Adding or Switching to a Second Drug

Two factors commonly influence the decision to add a second AED or switch to an alternate agent: lack of efficacy and adverse effects. In some instances, lack of efficacy reflects nonadherence (ie, inconsistent administration of prescribed AED)[17] or inadequate dosing (and dose adjustment for most newer AEDs is based on clinical response rather than target drug levels). In some cases, selection of an inappropriate medication can result in more frequent seizures; one example of this phenomenon is when carbamazepine is prescribed for a child with generalized epilepsy.

Appropriately selected AEDs can also elicit a broad range of adverse reactions (see **Table 4**). Irritability and personality changes are common in children treated with levetiracetam. Severe allergic reactions, including Stevens-Johnson syndrome (SJS), have been reported with many AEDs, including phenytoin, lamotrigine, clobazam, carbamazepine, and oxcarbazepine. Changes in appetite (higher with valproate and lower with topiramate and zonisamide) are also common.

A general principle for AED prescribers is avoidance of polypharmacy, in view of risks of cumulative adverse reactions. Yet in a substantial minority of children with complex epilepsy, concurrent treatment with multiple AEDs improves seizure control.

### Duration of Treatment

When AED treatment is implemented, one of the first questions families ask is anticipated duration of therapy. Again, although many patient-specific factors influence this decision, a common answer is, "when seizure-free for 2 years." A recent Cochrane review[18] provided support for this approach and concluded, "there is evidence to support waiting for at least two seizure-free years before discontinuing AEDs in children,

**Table 2**
**Antiepileptic drugs Food and Drug Administration approved 1993–2016**

| Generic Name | Brand Names | Approval Date and Indications |
|---|---|---|
| Drugs approved from 1993 to 2005 | | |
| Gabapentin | Neurontin | 1993 adjunctive therapy for ages >12 y with focal epilepsy<br>2000 extended to ages 3–12 y |
| Felbamate | Felbatol | 1993 adjunctive or monotherapy for ages >14 y with focal epilepsy and as adjunctive therapy for ages 2–14 with LGS; withdrawn in 1994 and subsequently reintroduced with new risk labeling |
| Lamotrigine | Lamictal<br>Lamictal XR | 1994 adjunctive therapy for ages ≥16 y with epilepsy<br>1998 adjunctive therapy for ages ≥2 y with LGS<br>1998 conversion to monotherapy in ages ≥16 y receiving an enzyme-inducing AED<br>2010 extended-release tablets for adjunctive therapy for generalized epilepsy for ages ≥13 y |
| Topiramate | Topamax<br>Trokendi XR | 1996 adjunctive therapy for ages ≥16 with focal epilepsy<br>1999 adjunctive therapy for ages ≥2 with generalized or focal-onset epilepsy<br>2001 adjunctive therapy for ages ≥2 with LGS<br>2005 initial monotherapy for ages ≥10 y with focal or generalized-onset epilepsy<br>2011 monotherapy indication extended to ages 2–9 y<br>2013 extended release tablets as initial monotherapy for ages ≥10 y with focal or generalized epilepsy and as adjunctive therapy for ages ≥6 y with focal or generalized epilepsy or LGS. |
| Tiagabine | Gabatril | 1997 adjunctive therapy for ages >12 y with focal epilepsy |
| Levetiracetam | Keppra<br>Keppra XR | 1999 adjunctive therapy for adults with focal epilepsy<br>2005 expanded indication to include adjunctive therapy for ages ≥4 y with focal epilepsy<br>2006 adjunctive therapy for ages ≥12 y with juvenile myoclonic epilepsy and for adults with myoclonic seizures<br>2007 adjunctive therapy for ages ≥6 y with generalized epilepsy<br>2008 extended release tablets as adjunctive therapy for ages ≥16 y with focal epilepsy<br>2011 expanded indication to include adjunctive therapy for ages ≥1 mo with focal epilepsy |
| Oxcarbazepine | Trileptal<br>Oxtellar XR | 2000 adjunctive and monotherapy for adults with focal epilepsy and adjunctive therapy for children ages 4–16 y with focal epilepsy<br>2003 monotherapy for ages ≥4 y with focal epilepsy<br>2005 expanded indication to include adjunctive therapy for ages ≥2 y with focal epilepsy<br>2012 extended-release tablets for adjunctive treatment for ages ≥6 y with focal epilepsy |
| Zonisamide | Zonegran | 2000 adjunctive therapy for ages ≥16 y with focal epilepsy |
| Pregabalin | Lyrica | 2005 adjunctive therapy for adults with focal epilepsy |
| Drugs approved since 2005 | | |
| Lacosamide | Vimpat | 2008 adjunctive therapy for ages ≥17 y with focal epilepsy |

(continued on next page)

**Table 2**
**(continued)**

| Generic Name | Brand Names | Approval Date and Indications |
|---|---|---|
| Rufinamide | Banzel | 2008 adjunctive therapy for ages ≥4 y with LGS<br>2015 additional approval for ages 1–4 years old with LGS |
| Vigabatrin | Sabril | 2009 adjunctive therapy in ages ≥10 y with refractory focal seizures, and as monotherapy in ages 1–24 mo with epileptic spasms |
| Clobazam | Onfi | 2011 adjunctive therapy for ages ≥2 y with LGS |
| Perampanel | Fycompa | 2012 adjunctive therapy for ages ≥12 y with focal epilepsy<br>2015 adjunctive therapy for ages ≥12 y with generalized epilepsy |
| Eslicarbazepine | Aptiom | 2013 adjunctive and monotherapy for adults with focal epilepsy |
| Brivaracetam | Briviact | 2016 adjunctive therapy for ages ≥16 y with focal epilepsy |

particularly in individuals who have an abnormal EEG, partial seizures, or both." As a note of caution, however, the investigators also concluded, "there is insufficient evidence to establish when to withdraw AEDs in children with generalized seizures," and clinician practice varies for these patients. Treatment duration can also be guided by diagnosis of specific epilepsy syndromes (eg, life-long treatment of juvenile myoclonic epilepsy).

## ADVERSE EFFECTS OF ANTIEPILEPTIC DRUGS
### Central Nervous System–Related Adverse Effects

An important consideration when considering AED options is the potential for adverse effects. All AEDs can cause nonspecific symptoms, such as dizziness, behavioral/ mood changes, and somnolence; the frequency and severity of these symptoms vary substantially among agents and among patients. These symptoms may be mild, transient, and dose related but may also be unpredicted and severe. Susceptibility to adverse central nervous system (CNS) effects in individual patients is often difficult to anticipate (see **Table 4**).

In children, levetiracetam is commonly implicated as a cause of worsening mood and personality changes; supplementation with pyridoxine, anecdotally, may attenuate behavioral adverse effects. Clobazam can also cause agitation and irritability. On the other hand, lamotrigine and valproic acid may have positive psychotropic effects. Although sedation and somnolence can complicate treatment with any AED, these symptoms are infrequent with some drugs (eg, levetiracetam, lamotrigine, and lacosamide). AED-related cognitive impairment is a frequent concern and may be difficult to distinguish from declines in function as a result of sedation and personality changes and/or recurrent seizures; topiramate is more frequently implicated as contributing to neuropsychological impairment. A meta-analysis of placebo-controlled trials found an association between suicidal thoughts and attempts in patients treated with an AED (0.43%) compared with patients receiving placebo (0.24%), and the FDA issued a black box warning for a risk of suicidality associated with taking any AED.[19]

### Systemic Adverse Effects

Pediatricians are frequently asked to evaluate and manage systemic adverse effects of AEDs. All AEDs, in particular phenytoin and carbamazepine, can cause a rash

**Table 3**
**Pediatric dosing for selected antiepileptic drugs**

| Drug | Liquid Formulations (mg/mL) | Tablets or Capsules | Practical Guidelines for Starting and Maintenance Dose Ranges |
|------|------|------|------|
| Phenobarbital | 4 | 15, 30, 60, 100, 16.2, 32.4, 64.8, 97.2 | Initial: 15–20 mg/kg<br>Maintenance: 4–6 mg/kg/d (infant), 3–5 mg/kg/d (child)<br>Maximum: limited by sedation |
| Valproic acid | 50 | 125, 250, 500 | Initial: 10–15 mg/kg/d divided BID or TID<br>Increase by 5–10 mg/kg/d each week<br>Maintenance: 20–30 mg/kg/d divided BID or TID<br>Maximum: 60 mg/kg/d |
| Carbamazepine | 20 | 100, 200, 300, 400 | Initial: 5–15 mg/kg/d, divided BID or TID<br>Increase by 5 mg/kg/d every 3–7 d<br>Maintenance: 15–20 mg/kg/d<br>Maximum: 35 mg/kg/d |
| Ethosuximide | 50 | 250 | Initial: 250 mg/d<br>Increase 250 mg/d every week to 500–1500 mg/d divided BID<br>Maximum: 30–40 mg/kg/d |
| Levetiracetam | 100 | 250, 500, 750, 1000 | Initial: 10–20 mg/kg/d divided BID<br>Increase by 10 mg/kg/d every week<br>Maintenance: 20–60 mg/kg/d<br>Maximum: 60 mg/kg/d |
| Oxcarbazepine | 60 | 150, 300, 600 | Initial: 5 mg/kg/d<br>Increase by 5 mg/kg/d every 5 d<br>Maintenance: 15–30 mg/kg/d<br>Maximum: 60 mg/kg/d |
| Lamotrigine | — | 2, 5, 25, 50, 100, 150, 200, 250, 300 | Initial: 0.3 mg/kg/d × 2 wk<br>0.6 mg/kg/d × 2 wk<br>1 mg/kg/d × 1 wk<br>1.5 mg/kg/d × 1 wk<br>2 mg/kg/d × 1 wk, then increase by 1 mg/kg/d every week<br>Doses usually divided BID<br>Maintenance: 5–10 mg/kg/d divided BID<br>Maximum: 15–20 mg/kg/d<br>If co-administered with valproic acid, lamotrigine dosages are halved and maximum dose is 5 mg/kg/d |

*(continued on next page)*

**Table 3**
**(*continued*)**

| Drug | Liquid Formulations (mg/mL) | Tablets or Capsules | Practical Guidelines for Starting and Maintenance Dose Ranges |
|---|---|---|---|
| Topiramate | variable | 15, 25, 50, 100, 150, 200 | Initial: 1 mg/kg/d divided BID/TID<br>Increase by 0.5–1 mg/kg/d every week<br>Maintenance: 5–9 mg/kg/d<br>Maximum: 15 mg/kg/d |
| Clobazam | 2.5 | 5, 10, 20 | Initial: 0.25 mg/kg/d divided BID<br>Increase by 0.25 mg/kg/d every week<br>Maintenance: 0.5–1 mg/kg/d<br>Maximum: 1–2 mg/kg/d |
| Lacosamide | 10 | 50, 100, 150, 200 | Not FDA approved in children<br>Initial: 1 mg/kg/d<br>Increase by 1 mg/kg/d every week<br>Maintenance: 2–10 mg/kg/d<br>Maximum: 10 mg/kg/d |
| Zonisamide | Variable | 25, 50, 100 | Not FDA approved in children<br>Initial: 2 mg/kg/d divided daily or BID<br>Increase 1 mg/kg/d every week<br>Maintenance: 8–10 mg/kg/d<br>Maximum: 12 mg/kg/d |

soon after initiation of treatment. Several medications, most frequently lamotrigine, phenytoin, and carbamazepine but also oxcarbazepine, clobazam, and zonisamide, can cause SJS, which can be fatal if the offending agent is not stopped quickly. Timely evaluation of rashes in children who recently began treatment with a new AED is important; mucous membrane lesions should raise concern for SJS, and if there is suspicion for a drug-reaction, the AED should be stopped immediately. The need for urgent alternative AED therapy depends on the epilepsy history.

Pediatricians should be aware of potential effects of AED on appetite and nutrition. Valproic acid, gabapentin, and vigabatrin can stimulate appetite and lead to weight gain, whereas topiramate and zonisamde can suppress appetite and result in weight loss. AEDs can lower vitamin D levels by inducing its cytochrome P450 (CYP450)-mediated metabolism as well as other ill-defined mechanisms.[20] Even the newer AEDs that do not induce CYP450 pathways are associated with low vitamin D levols.

Another important health concern in girls of childbearing age is the potential teratogenicity of AEDs.[21] Of the older AEDs, risks of congenital malformation are highest with gestational exposure to valproate; intermediate with exposure to phenytoin, phenobarbital (PB), and topiramate; and lower in individuals treated with carbamazepine and lamotrigine. Other AEDs have not been studied well enough to stratify their risk. Supplemental folate (0.4–4 mg/day), which reduces teratogenic potential of valproate, should be recommended to girls of childbearing age with epilepsy.

**Table 4**
**Practical tidbits about commonly used antiepileptic drugs**

| More Common Adverse Effects | | | | |
|---|---|---|---|---|
| On Mood or Behavior | Allergic Reaction/ Stevens-Johnson Syndrome | Appetite Modulation | Drug Interactions | Intravenous Formulation |
| Phenobarbital | Phenytoin | Valproic acid (increase) | Contraceptives | Phenobarbital |
| Levetiracetam | Carbamazepine | Topiramate (decrease) | Tacrolimus and cyclosporin A | Fosphenytoin |
| Topiramate | Oxcarbazepine | | | Levetiracetam |
| Clobazam | Lamotrigine | | | Lacosamide |
| Perampanel | Zonisamide (*sulfonamide cross-reaction) | | | Valproic acid |
| | Clobazam | | | |

## Drug Interactions

Many AEDs (most potently, phenytoin, PB, carbamazepine, and primidone) induce enzymes involved in CYP450-based metabolism, whereas others (eg, valproate) inhibit CYP450 enzymes.[22] Because CYP450 enzymes metabolize many AEDs, drug interactions are common. For example, in a patient receiving valproic acid, upward-dose titration of lamotrigine must be slowed and target dose reduced to minimize adverse effects. Primary physicians should be aware that multiple AEDs might attenuate oral contraceptive efficacy, typically by CYP450 induction (eg, carbamazepine, clobazam, eslicarbazepine, oxcarbazepine, PB, phenytoin, topiramate, perampanel, primidone, felbamate, and lamotrigine). The interaction can be bidirectional, and estrogen-containing contraception can decrease lamotrigine and valproic acid levels, causing large fluctuations in drug levels with cyclical oral contraceptive administration.

Many other medications, including antineoplastic, antimicrobial, cardiovascular, and immunosuppressant agents, can interact with AEDs. For example, the enzyme-inducing AEDs can decrease drug levels of cyclosporin A, sirolimus, and tacrolimus as well as many antineoplastic agents, such as cyclophosphamide, etoposide, ifosfamide, and methotrexate. Furthermore, many AED levels can be altered by coadministration with other medications or by systemic illness. For example, nasogastric feeds drastically decrease oral phenytoin absorption, and erythromycin can lead to carbamazepine toxicity through inhibition of CYP450-3A4 metabolism. Finding appropriate AEDs in patients with hepatic or renal failure can be difficult because of the altered metabolism of AEDs, and toxicities of AEDs (eg, valproate and hepatotoxicity). In critically ill patients, levetiracetam has become a popular choice because of the rarity of severe systemic adverse effects, lack of drug interactions, and intravenous formulation.

## Improving Antiepileptic Drug Tolerability

Several strategies can improve AED tolerability. If a second AED is prescribed, the cause of prior drug failures should be considered. For example, in a patient with a history of a phenytoin-related allergic reaction, drugs with a high risk for cross-reactions, such as carbamazepine, should be avoided. If CNS adverse effects were encountered with prior AED treatment, slowed introduction of a new agent (eg, half the typical starting dose) and slowed upward-dose titration may improve tolerability of the new medication.

Families may request AED discontinuation at the first sign of an adverse effect. Providing anticipatory guidance that some adverse behavioral effects resolve, either spontaneously or with a slowed-dose titration schedule, may encourage medication adherence around the time of AED initiation.

### Intractability

Approximately 10% to 20% of children with epilepsy have pharmacoresistance, usually defined as the failure to control seizures by 2 well-tolerated and appropriately chosen and dosed AEDs.[23] Although accurate prediction of pharmacoresistance is challenging, abnormal neuroimaging portends a higher risk for poor prognosis. A majority of children who develop pharmacoresistance do so in the first 3 years after onset of their epilepsy. Because additional AEDs in intractable epilepsy have only a small chance of significant benefit, other therapies, such as the ketogenic diet, epilepsy surgery, and vagal nerve stimulation, should be considered.

## THE NEWER ANTIEPILEPTIC DRUGS

Readers are referred to standard textbooks for more detailed information about the older AEDs, listed in **Table 1**.[24] These medications are still widely used, particularly in low-resource settings, because they are cheap and often effective, although the risks of side effects and drug interactions are generally higher compared with newer drugs.

It is important to emphasize that there is limited postmarketing data regarding AED efficacy, adverse reactions, optimal combination strategies, and comparative drug efficacy for treatment of pediatric epilepsy. Similarly, there are few systematic data to guide AED selection related to important neurologic (cognitive and neuromotor), psychiatric (mood, attention, and impulsivity), and systemic comorbidities, and choices are often determined by individual clinician experiences and preferences.

This section highlights important characteristics of the newer AEDs (FDA approved after 1992) with which primary care physicians may be less familiar; they are listed here in alphabetical order and in **Table 2** in the order they were FDA-approved.

### Brivaracetam

Brivaracetam has a similar molecular structure to levetiracetam and was developed to more potently bind synaptic vesicle glycoprotein 2A (SV2A), the proposed distinctive mechanism underlying the antiepileptic efficacy of both drugs. Brivaracetam is currently only FDA approved in patients ages 16 and older for adjunctive therapy for focal epilepsy. Initial experience suggests that brivaracetam can be effective in patients who have failed levetiracetam treatment.

### Clobazam

Clobazam is a long-acting benzodiazepine, with a broad spectrum of efficacy. Although it has been available as an anxiolytic and antiepileptic medication since the 1970s, it was only approved by the FDA in the United States for adjunctive treatment of Lennox-Gastaut syndrome (LGS), a difficult to treat pediatric epilepsy syndrome characterized by tonic, atonic, and absence seizures, in 2011. It is now widely used, particularly in young children with refractory epilepsy. Clobazam is usually well tolerated, with the most common side effects drowsiness and irritability; rarely, it can elicit SJS.

### Eslicarbazepine

Eslicarbazepine is related to oxcarbazepine, a commonly used drug for focal epilepsy that is similar to carbamazepine. Although oxcarbazepine is converted to the active (S) and the inactive enantiomers of licarbazepine in a 4:1 ratio, eslicarbazepine is exclusively converted to the active metabolite, S-licarbazepine. Therefore, the mechanism of action and spectrum of efficacy are the same as carbamazepine and oxcarbazepine, but adverse effects are less frequent. In view of the substantially higher cost of this agent and the paucity of pediatric data, however, oxcarbazepine is currently preferable to eslicarbazepine as initial therapy in focal epilepsy.

### Felbamate

Felbamate has multiple mechanisms of action, including excitatory (N-methyl-D-aspartate [NMDA]-glutamate) receptor antagonism, positive modulation of inhibitory (γ-aminobutyric acid [GABA] type A) receptors, and sodium channel blockade. It is typically prescribed only for children with intractable, severe epilepsies because in a small proportion of cases it can elicit potentially lethal adverse effects, such as aplastic anemia and hepatic failure.[25] It can be effective, however, in focal and generalized epilepsies, including LGS. Common side effects include decreased appetite with nausea and insomnia.

### Gabapentin

Gabapentin binds to a subunit of the voltage-gated calcium channel, decreasing calcium influx. The main advantages of gabapentin are its benign safety profile and lack of drug interactions. The main disadvantage is its modest efficacy, particularly when used as monotherapy in children. It can be used as adjunctive therapy for focal seizures and may attenuate chronic unexplained irritability in children with severe neurologic impairment. Its chief adverse effect is somnolence.

### Lacosamide

Lacosamide is a sodium channel blocker, similar in its mechanism of action to phenytoin. Initial experience indicates that it has a more benign side-effect profile (particularly with regard to systemic adverse effects) than phenytoin. Lacosamide can cause cardiac arrhythmias, such as heart block, bradycardia, and a prolonged PR interval; both baseline EKG and follow-up EKGs at higher doses are often recommended. It is available as tablets, oral suspension, and intravenous formulations. Lacosamide is effective for treatment of focal seizures[26] but does not exacerbate generalized seizures, as does carbamazepine.

### Lamotrigine

Lamotrigine is also a sodium channel blocker and likely also has other mechanisms of action. It is a commonly used AED because of its tolerability, wide spectrum of efficacy, generally benign side-effect profile, and potential for mood stabilization. Although lamotrigine can cause potentially fatal SJS, titrating the dose upward very slowly (typically over 10–12 weeks) and providing anticipatory guidance for families and patients can mitigate this risk. In view of the need for a slow upward-dose titration, it is not optimal for patients who need rapid-onset treatment. Although lamotrigine is used to treat both focal and generalized epilepsies, it can increase myoclonic seizures in some patients.

### Levetiracetam

The mechanism of action for levetiracetam is putatively through its binding of the presynaptic vesicle glycoprotein SV2A. It is a frequently used medication for initial monotherapy in all age groups because of its wide spectrum of efficacy against focal and generalized seizures, benign side-effect profile, lack of drug interactions, and ease of administration as intravenous, liquid, or tablet formulations. Treatment can also be started and the dose titrated upward more quickly than for many other AEDs. The most common side effect is irritability, and, anecdotally, vitamin $B_6$

(pyridoxine) can counteract the irritability. Brivaracetam, a chemical analogue of leve-tiracetam, has recently become available on the market.

### Oxcarbazepine

Oxcarbazepine is a sodium channel blocker, similar to carbamazepine. It is the only well-established medication for initial monotherapy in children with focal-onset epi-lepsy for which randomized controlled trials demonstrated efficacy (although levetira-cetam was not compared in those trials). Oxcarbazepine is usually well tolerated but can cause SJS, drowsiness, fatigue, headaches, and hyponatremia.

### Perampanel

Perampanel, an AMPA glutamate receptor antagonist, has broad-spectrum efficacy and is approved by the FDA for adjunctive treatment of focal seizures and generalized tonic-clonic seizures in patients ages 12 years and older. It is typically well tolerated but can cause aggression and irritability, particularly at higher doses, in addition to typical AED side effects of dizziness, somnolence, and headache.[27]

### Pregabalin

Pregabalin is similar in structure, mechanism, and efficacy to gabapentin but is only FDA-approved in adults.

### Rufinamide

Rufinamide is a sodium channel blocker, likely with additional mechanisms of action. It has a broad spectrum of efficacy but is FDA approved only for adjunctive treatment of LGS. It is available as a tablet and liquid but has no intravenous formulation. Rufina-mide can shorten the QT interval and is, therefore, contraindicated in patients with fa-milial short QT syndrome. Prescribers should use lower doses of rufinamide dose in patients who are also on valproic acid because valproic acid impedes clearance of rufinamide.

### Tiagabine

Tiagabine inhibits reuptake of synaptic GABA. It is seldom used, because of its narrow spectrum of efficacy against focal seizures and its potential to exacerbate generalized seizures. It may cause nonconvulsive status epilepticus.

### Topiramate

Topiramate also has several mechanisms of action, including glutamate (AMPA/kai-nate subtype) receptor antagonism, enhanced GABA activity, and sodium channel blockade. It has a wide spectrum of anticonvulsant efficacy and may also be of benefit for migraine prophylaxis and tic suppression. Although it has many potential systemic side effects, including acute glaucoma and kidney stones, few are life threatening. The most common side effects include cognitive slowing, decreased appetite, and paraes-thesias. Oligohydrosis (impaired sweating) can also occur, and therefore it is important for families to be especially vigilant of hyperthermia when treated children have febrile illnesses or are active during hot weather. This medication is available in tablets and sprinkle capsules and may be compounded at specialized pharmacies into a liquid.

### Vigabatrin

Vigabatrin selectively and irreversibly inhibits GABA transaminase, the enzyme that degrades the inhibitory neurotransmitter, GABA; the resultant increase in brain GABA is hypothesized to underlie anticonvulsant efficacy. It was approved in the

United States in 2009 as adjunctive therapy for refractory focal epilepsy in older children and as monotherapy for infantile spasms (discussed later). Vigabatrin has a distinctive adverse effect profile, including an ill-defined risk of irreversible retinal injury, and transient, asymptomatic (but pronounced) subcortical MRI abnormalities of uncertain significance.

### Zonisamide

Zonisamide is a sodium and calcium channel blocker and inhibits carbonic anhydrase. It has a wide spectrum of efficacy and has a similar side-effect profile to topiramate (sedation, cognitive slowing, anorexia, kidney stones, and oligohydrosis) and risk of SJS, but cognitive impairment risk is less pronounced than with topiramate. It is structurally related to sulfonamides and is contraindicated for children with sulfonamide allergy. Although it is currently available as a liquid from compounding pharmacies, insurance coverage for liquid preparations can be limited. It is not currently FDA approved in children but is widely used off-label.

### Non–Food and Drug Administration–Approved Agents

Particularly in cases where available AEDs are ineffective, families seek alternative treatments. Substantial enthusiasm has been generated about anticonvulsant properties of both plant-based and synthetic formulations of cannabidiol, a compound found in marijuana.[28] Cannabidiol formulations are under study for epileptic spasms, LGS, Dravet syndrome, and other treatment-resistant pediatric epilepsies (NCT02318602, NCT02324673, NCT02318537, NCT02318563, and NCT02551731).

The final section of this article highlights 3 important pediatric topics: treatment of seizures in neonates, treatment of epileptic spasms, and emerging evidence for precision medicine-based AED selection.

## ANTICONVULSANT THERAPY IN NEONATES

In the pediatric age group, seizure incidence peaks in the neonatal period. Most seizures in neonates are symptomatic, that is, a result of acute brain injury or metabolic derangement rather than a manifestation of epilepsy. Gestational age adds complexity in terms of understanding mechanisms, etiologies, and possibly responsiveness to therapy for neonatal seizures. In neonates, seizures are often difficult to clinically diagnose at the bedside, and EEG monitoring represents the most reliable method both for diagnosis and assessment of treatment efficacy. Neurodiagnostic tests (in particular brain imaging) reveal the seizure etiology more commonly than in older children and the underlying cause of neonatal seizures is a major determinant of neurodevelopmental outcome. Hypoxic-ischemic encephalopathy remains the most common cause of neonatal seizures; other common etiologies include ischemic stroke, intracerebral hemorrhage, infection, and metabolic abnormalities.[29,30] In neonates, single, isolated seizures are unusual; neonatal seizures are often recurrent and may be refractory to conventional anticonvulsant drug therapy.

Scientific explanations for this developmental susceptibility to seizures have emerged and include properties and expression patterns of excitatory (glutamate) and inhibitory (GABA) receptors; moreover, GABA receptor activation may be paradoxically excitatory in the immature brain.[29] Factors that influence treatment efficacy include seizure etiology, maturational determinants of pharmacokinetic and pharmacodynamic properties of anticonvulsant drugs, and concurrent treatments (medications and interventions, such as therapeutic hypothermia). Although it remains challenging to document that effective seizure treatment improves neurodevelopmental outcomes, there is substantial impetus to identify drugs that safely and rapidly suppress neonatal seizures.[31]

In the neonatal intensive care unit, an intravenous loading dose of PB (20–30 mg/kg) represents the most common initial treatment of seizures. A classic study, performed more than 20 years ago, showed that PB (40 mg/kg) stopped seizures in less than 50% of treated neonates, as did an equivalent dose of phenytoin.[32] Modest efficacy, coupled with concerns about potential deleterious effects of PB in the developing brain, has resulted in increasing utilization of levetiracetam in this age group (despite limited evidence of its safety and efficacy in neonates). Since publication of a study of levetiracetam pharmacokinetics in term neonates showed that more frequent dosing was needed to maintain serum concentrations in the range seen in children and adults,[33] higher doses (loading doses of 40–60 mg/kg vs initial utilization of 20 mg/kg) have been more commonly used to treat neonates. Whether levetiracetam should be used as a first-line agent in neonates is currently uncertain; an ongoing clinical trial (NCT01720667) is comparing the efficacy of intravenous levetiracetam and PB as first-line therapy for neonatal seizures.

There is no consensus regarding optimal treatment of neonatal seizures that are refractory to PB, fosphenytoin (a prodrug of phenytoin that has much lower risk of tissue damage with extravasation), and levetiracetam. Options include midazolam infusion, topiramate (enteral administration), and lidocaine (contraindicated with preceding phenytoin exposure).

In cases of refractory neonatal seizures without an apparent etiology, consideration of an underlying metabolic encephalopathy is warranted; these rare disorders, which may have specific treatments, are highlighted in a recent review.[34]

Yet, because most neonatal seizures do not reflect epilepsy but rather are provoked by acute brain injury or metabolic abnormality, a particularly important question for pediatricians is whether AEDs need to be continued after seizures stop. It is challenging to weigh the risks and benefits of continued drug treatment in infants for whom seizure recurrence is uncertain; clinical practice varies widely. A recent multicenter observational cohort study of more than 300 neonates, treated at 7 US centers, found that a majority who had symptomatic neonatal seizures were discharged home on AED therapy; yet, after adjustment for potential confounding factors, only study site and seizure etiology were significant determinants of continued treatment.[35] Their findings highlight the need for future studies that clarify the optimal duration of AED treatment in this unique population.

## TREATMENT OF EPILEPTIC SPASMS

Epileptic spasms are a unique seizure type, characterized as flexor, extensor, or mixed flexor-extensor spasms, and typically manifesting as brief, symmetric contractions of the muscles of the neck, trunk, or extremities, lasting only a few seconds each but often occurring in clusters around transitions between sleep and wakefulness. Although spasms typically manifest at approximately 3 months to 7 months of age, onset in older children has been reported, and this prompted the recent shift from the previous terminology of infantile spasms to epileptic spasms. Structural brain abnormalities, such as cerebral malformations and perinatal brain injury, are the most common etiologies. Genetic and metabolic etiologies also are identified in a significant portion of infants, but approximately a quarter of infants with spasms have an unknown cause.

West syndrome is a triad of epileptic spasms, a chaotic, high-amplitude EEG background termed hypsarrhythmia, and developmental delay/arrest. Epileptic spasms represent the prototypic epileptic encephalopathy, where the seizures and epileptiform activity likely contribute to or exacerbate underlying brain dysfunction. Although it is often difficult to discern whether preexisting neurologic abnormalities or the spasms themselves underlie long-term neurodevelopmental deficits in affected children, there is some evidence that rapid diagnosis and treatment of spasms may result in better long-term outcomes.

A US consortium established a multicenter, prospective database to examine the natural history and responses to treatment in infants with newly diagnosed infantile spasms.[36] Children were considered responders if there was clinical remission and resolution of hypsarrhythmia that was sustained at 3 months after first treatment initiation. Standard treatments evaluated included corticotropin, oral corticosteroids, and vigabatrin. Of 230 infants enrolled, 46% receiving standard therapy responded to initial treatment (55% receiving corticotropin as initial treatment, 39% for oral corticosteroids, and 36% for vigabatrin). Neither etiology nor development significantly modified the response pattern by treatment group. Corticotropin seemed more effective than other standard therapies.

A recent international study concluded, however, that combination treatment incorporating corticotropin with vigabatrin was more effective than hormonal therapy alone.[37] An intriguing clinical observation that remains unexplained is that in cases of spasms in association with tuberous sclerosis, vigabatrin is often remarkably and rapidly effective and represents first-line treatment.

## PRECISION MEDICINE STRATEGIES FOR EPILEPSY TREATMENT

Precision medicine involves using knowledge of a patient's specific genotype to tailor therapies and may include targeting the specific pathogenic molecular pathway. Successful application of this strategy for treatment of epilepsy has emerged from expanding genomic research in epilepsy, multicenter efforts to study genotype-phenotype correlations and improving affordability and availability of genetic diagnosis.[38] Identification of several specific genetic abnormalities in patients with epilepsy can influence therapeutic decisions (**Table 5**), and this number is rapidly growing.

Several of these diseases (eg, pyridoxine-dependent epilepsy) had defined treatments even before the specific genetic mutations were identified. Some genetic abnormalities suggest modification of therapies, such as general avoidance of sodium channel blockers in SCN1A-related Dravet syndrome. Conversely, in other sodium channelopathies, such as SCN2A-related and SCN8A-related epileptic encephalopathies, patients often respond well to high-dose phenytoin (a sodium channel blocker). Other diseases, such as mechanistic target of rapamycin (mTOR) pathway abnormalities in tuberous sclerosis[39] and gain-of-function or loss-of function mutations in potassium channels,[40,41] can implicate treatments that target the biology of the genetic dysfunction.

Pharmacogenetics also have increasing applicability in therapeutic choices. For example, testing should be considered to identify the HLA-B1502 allele in individuals of Asian descent prior to starting carbamazepine or oxcarbazepine, because this allele results in a high risk for SJS with exposure to these drugs. In another example, patients with a mutation in the mitochondrial DNA polymerase gamma have a significantly increased risk of hepatic failure if exposed to valproic acid.

## FUTURE DIRECTIONS

The plethora of new AEDs, highlighted in this article, illustrates the remarkable advances attained in the treatment of pediatric epilepsy. Yet many important questions

**Table 5**
**Precision medicine and pediatric epilepsy: targeted treatments**

| Disease | Genetic Abnormality | Epilepsy Syndromes | Treatment Implications |
|---------|---------------------|--------------------|------------------------|
| Tuberous sclerosis | mTOR pathway gene mutations | Epileptic spasms | Vigabatrin = first-line treatment |
| | | Refractory epilepsy | Consider everolimus |
| Dravet syndrome | SCN1A | Mixed | Usually avoid sodium channel blockers (lamotrigine and phenytoin) |
| SCN2A-related epileptic encephalopathy | SCN2A | West syndrome, LGS, Ohtahara syndrome | High-dose phenytoin |
| SCN8A-related epileptic encephalopathy | SCN8A | Epileptic encephalopathy | High-dose phenytoin |
| Familial epilepsy syndromes with potassium channel mutations | KCNQ2 | Benign familial neonatal convulsions Neonatal epileptic encephalopathy | Carbamazepine, oxcarbazepine may help with de novo heterozygous missense variants |
| Migrating partial seizures of infancy | KCNT1 | Epilepsy of infancy with migrating focal seizures | Quinidine may be effective for gain-of-function variants |
| GLUT1 deficiency syndrome | SLC2A1 | GLUT1-related epilepsy | Ketogenic diet |
| Benign familial infantile seizures | PRRT2 | Benign familial infantile seizures | Carbamazepine |
| Pyridoxine-dependent epilepsy | ALDH7A1 | Neonatal seizures | Pyridoxine |
| Pyridoxal 5'-phosphate-dependent epilepsy | PNPO | Neonatal seizures | Pyridoxal-5-phosphate |

about optimal drug therapy for seizures and epilepsy across the pediatric age range remain unanswered.

There are major gaps in knowledge about developmental stage–specific efficacy and toxicity of AEDs, particularly for neonates and young infants. Few systematic studies directly compare the efficacy and tolerability of the newer AEDs, and information that can help clinicians individualize drug therapy is greatly needed. Data are lacking to support strategies for optimizing combination drug therapy—with respect to gaining insights about positive and negative interactions between AEDs and also between AEDs and other drugs commonly used in pediatric practice (including those discussed in other articles in this issue). Although it is attractive to speculate that personalized genetic data will provide clinicians with mechanistic insights to guide drug selection, particularly for children with complex epilepsy syndromes, this goal has yet to be attained beyond the rare cases described previously in the precision medicine section.

It is also important to emphasize the critical distinction between drug therapy to prevent seizure recurrence in individuals with established epilepsy and drug treatment to prevent the development or progression of epilepsy (epileptogenesis). The AEDs discussed in this article can be of substantial benefit to limit risks of seizure recurrence, but none has been shown to prevent the development of epilepsy. An essential prerequisite to achieve this goal is delineation of the cellular and molecular mechanisms that underlie epileptogenesis, a priority for many investigators in this field. The next era of pediatric AED therapy will hopefully incorporate agents to target these pivotal mechanisms and thereby prevent or attenuate risk for epilepsy, particularly after early-life brain injury.

**REFERENCES**

1. Bell GS, Neligan A, Sander JW. An unknown quantity - the worldwide prevalence of epilepsy. Epilepsia 2014;55(7):958–62.
2. Fisher RS, Acevedo C, Arzimanoglou A, et al. A practical clinical definition of epilepsy. Epilepsia 2014;55(4):475–82.
3. Fisher RS, Cross JH, French JA, et al. Operational classification of seizure types by the international league against epilepsy. Epilepsia 2017;58(4):522–30.
4. Glauser TA, Loddenkemper T. Management of childhood epilepsy. Continuum 2013;19(3 Epilepsy):656–81.
5. St Louis EK, Cascino GD. Diagnosis of epilepsy and related episodic disorders. Continuum 2016;22(1 Epilepsy):15–37.
6. Wirrell E. Infantile, childhood, and adolescent epilepsies. Continuum 2016;22(1 Epilepsy):60–93.
7. Camfield P, Camfield C. Childhood epilepsy: what is the evidence for what we think and what we do? J Child Neurol 2003;18(4):272–87.
8. Glauser T, Shinnar S, Gloss D, et al. Evidence-based guideline: treatment of convulsive status epilepticus in children and adults: report of the guideline committee of the American Epilepsy Society. Epilepsy Curr 2016;16(1):48–61.
9. Abou-Khalil BW. Antiepileptic drugs. Continuum 2016;22(1 Epilepsy):132–56.
10. Rosati A, De Masi S, Guerrini R. Antiepileptic drug treatment in children with epilepsy. CNS Drugs 2015;29(10):847–63.
11. French JA, Gazzola DM. Antiepileptic drug treatment: new drugs and new strategies. Continuum 2013;19(3 Epilepsy):643–55.
12. Sander JW. The use of antiepileptic drugs—principles and practice. Epilepsia 2004;45:28–34.
13. Leone MA, Giussani G, Nolan SJ, et al. Immediate antiepileptic drug treatment, versus placebo, deferred, or no treatment for first unprovoked seizure. Cochrane Database Syst Rev 2016;(5):CD007144.
14. Arya R, Glauser TA. Pharmacotherapy of focal epilepsy in children: a systematic review of approved agents. CNS Drugs 2013;27(4):273–86.
15. Glauser T, Ben-Menachem E, Bourgeois B, et al. Updated ILAE evidence review of antiepileptic drug efficacy and effectiveness as initial monotherapy for epileptic seizures and syndromes. Epilepsia 2013;54(3):551–63.
16. Yamada M, Welty TE. Generic substitution of antiepileptic drugs: a systematic review of prospective and retrospective studies. Ann Pharmacother 2011;45(11):1406–15.
17. Modi AC, Wu YP, Rausch JR, et al. Antiepileptic drug nonadherence predicts pediatric epilepsy seizure outcomes. Neurology 2014;83(22):2085–90.
18. Strozzi I, Nolan SJ, Sperling MR, et al. Early versus late antiepileptic drug withdrawal for people with epilepsy in remission. Cochrane Database Syst Rev 2015;(2):CD001902.

19. US Food and Drug Administration. Information for healthcare professionals: suicidal behavior and ideation and antiepileptic drugs. 2008. Available at: https://www.fda.gov/Drugs/DrugSafety/PostmarketDrugSafetyInformationforPatientsandProviders/ucm100192.htm. Accessed April 30, 2017.

20. Shellhaas RA, Joshi SM. Vitamin D and bone health among children with epilepsy. Pediatr Neurol 2010;42(6):385–93.

21. Pennell PB. Pregnancy, epilepsy, and women's issues. Continuum 2013;19(3 Epilepsy):697–714.

22. Zaccara G, Perucca E. Interactions between antiepileptic drugs, and between antiepileptic drugs and other drugs. Epileptic Disord 2014;16(4):409–31.

23. Wirrell EC. Predicting pharmacoresistance in pediatric epilepsy. Epilepsia 2013; 54(Suppl. S2):19–22.

24. Wyllie E, Cascino GD, Gidal BE, et al. Wyllie's treatment of epilepsy: principles and practice. Philadelphia: Lippincott Williams & Wilkins; 2012.

25. Shah YD, Singh K, Friedman D, et al. Evaluating the safety and efficacy of felbamate in the context of a black box warning: a single center experience. Epilepsy Behav 2016;56:50–3.

26. Toupin J-F, Lortie A, Major P, et al. Efficacy and safety of lacosamide as an adjunctive therapy for refractory focal epilepsy in paediatric patients: a retrospective single-centre study. Epileptic Disord 2015;17(4):436–43.

27. Singh K, Shah YD, Luciano D, et al. Safety and efficacy of perampanel in children and adults with various epilepsy syndromes: a single-center postmarketing study. Epilepsy Behav 2016;61:41–5.

28. O'Connell BK, Gloss D, Devinsky O. Cannabinoids in treatment-resistant epilepsy: a review. Epilepsy Behav 2017;70(Pt B):341–8.

29. Silverstein FS, Jensen FE. Neonatal seizures. Ann Neurol 2007;62(2):112–20.

30. Glass HC, Shellhaas RA, Wusthoff CJ, et al. Contemporary profile of seizures in neonates: a Prospective Cohort Study. J Pediatr 2016;174:98–103.e1.

31. Donovan MD, Griffin BT, Kharoshankaya L, et al. Pharmacotherapy for neonatal seizures: current knowledge and future perspectives. Drugs 2016;76(6):647–61.

32. Painter MJ, Scher MS, Stein AD, et al. Phenobarbital compared with phenytoin for the treatment of neonatal seizures. N Engl J Med 1999;341(7):485–9.

33. Sharpe CM, Capparelli EV, Mower A, et al. A seven-day study of the pharmacokinetics of intravenous levetiracetam in neonates: marked changes in pharmacokinetics occur during the first week of life. Pediatr Res 2012;72(1):43–9.

34. Pearl PL. Amenable treatable severe pediatric epilepsies. Semin Pediatr Neurol 2016;23(2):158–66.

35. Shellhaas RA, Chang T, Wusthoff CJ, et al. Treatment duration after acute symptomatic seizures in neonates: a multicenter cohort Study. J Pediatr 2017;181: 298–301.e1.

36. Knupp KG, Coryell J, Nickels KC, et al. Response to treatment in a prospective national infantile spasms cohort. Ann Neurol 2016;79(3):475–84.

37. O'Callaghan FJK, Edwards SW, Alber FD, et al. Safety and effectiveness of hormonal treatment versus hormonal treatment with vigabatrin for infantile spasms (ICISS): a randomised, multicentre, open-label trial. Lancet Neurol 2017;16(1): 33–42.

38. Berkovic SF, Scheffer IE, Petrou S, et al. A roadmap for precision medicine in the epilepsies. Lancet Neurol 2015;14(12):1219–28.

39. French JA, Lawson JA, Yapici Z, et al. Adjunctive everolimus therapy for treatment-resistant focal-onset seizures associated with tuberous sclerosis

(EXIST-3): a phase 3, randomised, double-blind, placebo-controlled study. Lancet 2016;388(10056):2153–63.

40. Sands TT, Balestri M, Bellini G, et al. Rapid and safe response to low-dose carbamazepine in neonatal epilepsy. Epilepsia 2016;57(12):2019–30.

41. Bearden D, Strong A, Ehnot J, et al. Targeted treatment of migrating partial seizures of infancy with quinidine. Ann Neurol 2014;76(3):457–61.

# Therapeutic Drug Monitoring in Inflammatory Bowel Disease
## History and Future Directions

Elizabeth A. Spencer, MD, Marla C. Dubinsky, MD*

## KEYWORDS

- Inflammatory bowel disease • Therapeutic drug monitoring
- Thiopurine metabolite monitoring • Biologics

## KEY POINTS

- The roots of therapeutic drug monitoring (TDM) in IBD lie in thiopurines and the tenet of titrating metabolite levels to achieve 6-TGN>235 and 6-MMP<5700.
- TDM for biologic drugs involves measuring drug concentrations and anti-drug antibodies with a subsequent change in therapy to achieve desired levels and prevent antibody formation.
- Proactive TDM with biologics is gaining popularity given its ability to reduce drug costs and improve patient outcomes, but this still requires further validation.
- There is still debate over ideal trough concentrations for each biologic given that patient-specific factors can influence the concentration required for desired end-points, like mucosal or fistula healing.
- Drug concentrations and anti-drug antibody levels should be carefully interpreted given the variability between types of assays.

*Variability is the law of life, and as no two faces are the same, so no two bodies are alike, and no two individuals react alike and behave alike under the abnormal conditions which we know as disease.*

—Sir William Osler in 1903

Disclosures: M.C. Dubinsky consults for AbbVie, Boehringer Ingelheim, Celgene, Genentech, Janssen, Pfizer, Prometheus, Salix, Shire, Takeda, and UCB.
Pediatric Gastroenterology and Hepatology, Department of Pediatrics, Susan and Leonard Feinstein IBD Clinical Center, Icahn School of Medicine, Mount Sinai, Mt. Sinai Hospital, 1 Gustave L Levy Place, Box 1656, New York, NY 10029, USA
* Corresponding author.
*E-mail address:* marla.dubinsky@mssm.edu

pediatric.theclinics.com

# INTRODUCTION

Inflammatory bowel disease (IBD), comprising mainly the 2 entities Crohn disease (CD) and ulcerative colitis (UC), is a chronic inflammatory disease of the digestive tract. Pharmacotherapy for IBD has focused on dampening this inflammation with agents to both induce remission and then provide durable maintenance, all while avoiding the use of steroids. However, the steroid-sparing regimens are still limited in number and do not lead to adequate disease control in all patients. Clinical trials in IBD have, in general, shown only a 50% to 60% response, and this decreases to 30% in the maintenance phase as patients start to lose response.[1–4] These trials are limited by the use of label dosing, which is either fixed or based on simple weight cutoffs. Label dosing does not take into account individual variability in metabolism and clearance and can be suboptimal, leading to lack of clinical response and development of antidrug antibodies (ADAs). Current clinical practice is designed to optimize response to available medications via tailored dosing regimens, which can be achieved through therapeutic drug monitoring (TDM).

TDM is based on the assumption that the response of a drug is tied to a clinical laboratory measure, such as the unbound concentration of drug in plasma at the end of a dosing interval. This measurement ideally reflects the influence of patient-specific factors such as demographics, disease activity, and drug interactions. The goal of TDM is to then optimize this measure within a target range for each unique individual to maximize benefit while avoiding toxicity. It can also be used to monitor compliance and elucidate the root cause of treatment failures.[5,6]

TDM started its evolution in the IBD space with thiopurines, 6-mercaptopurine (6-MP) and azathioprine (AZA), which were the cornerstone of steroid-sparing maintenance regimens until the advent of monoclonal antibodies (mAbs).[7–9] Despite their prominence in the 1990s and 2000s, there were several concerns over thiopurines' safety profile, leading to the first application of TDM in IBD to achieve a better balance between reaping thiopurines' therapeutic effects without the concomitant adverse effects of severe leukopenia and hepatotoxicity.

IBD specialists were then able to turn their knowledge of TDM to biologics as they increased in prominence with the introduction of infliximab (IFX). TDM is now commonplace in clinical practice, and there has been a compendium of research showing that careful monitoring to achieve sufficient mAb concentrations and to avoid ADA leads to better outcomes.

Although TDM is widely recognized as beneficial to maximize response to, and minimize cost from, mAbs, it is debated whether it should be practiced in a reactive way when a patient is symptomatic and a loss of response is suspected or if it should be practiced in a proactive way to stay abreast of this loss of response. This debate is driving ongoing research in the utility of proactive monitoring with more and more sophisticated systems of dose adjustment under development, such as dashboard-driven dosing systems. This article reviews TDM in IBD from its inception with thiopurines to its active evolution with biologics.

# THIOPURINES
## *Thiopurine Metabolism and Thiopurine Methyltransferase*

The origin of TDM with thiopurines is rooted in their unique metabolism. After absorption, AZA is converted quickly and nonenzymatically to 6-MP and S-methyl-4-nitro-5-thioimidazole. 6-MP is then further processed via competing catabolic and anabolic pathways with extensive first-pass metabolism via xanthine oxidase, which is found in the intestine as well as the liver. It subsequently undergoes further catabolism by thiopurine methyltransferase (TPMT) before eventually being anabolized to the active metabolites, 6-

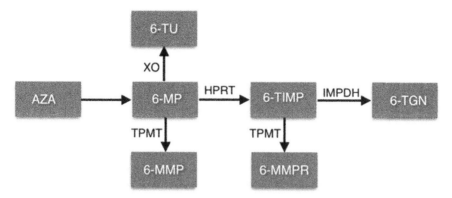

**Fig. 1.** Thiopurine metabolism. HPRT, hypoxanthine phosphoribosyltransferase; IMPDH, inosine monophosphate dehydrogenase; 6-MMP, 6-methylmercaptopurine; 6-TIMP, 6-thioinosine monophosphate; 6-TU, 6-thiouric acid; XO, xanthine oxidase. (*Adapted from* Singh N, Dubinsky MC. Therapeutic drug monitoring in children and young adults with inflammatory bowel disease: a practical approach. Gastroenterol Hepatol (N Y) 2015;11(1):48–55.)

thioguanine nucleotides (6-TGNs) and 6-methyl-mercaptopurine ribonucleotides (6-MMPRs). A simplified schema of thiopurines' metabolism is shown in **Fig. 1**.[10,11]

It was established that the TPMT enzyme has a genetically determined activity level with variable myelosuppression.[10] Those homozygous for TPMT[L] have very low to absent activity, although this variant is found in only 0.3% of the population; however, at standard doses, people with this variant can have life-threatening myelosuppression. The same severe myelosuppression can occur in those who are heterozygous, TPMT[L]/TPMT[H], because they have intermediate activity, and this genotype is more common, found in 11% of the population.[12,13] In several large series, there was good concordance of ~95% between genotyping and phenotyping with a TPMT enzyme activity level.[14] However, Colombel and colleagues,[15] who reported on this association between TPMT and myelosuppression, also noted that most cases of myelosuppression were not caused by low TPMT activity, making it clear that just TPMT alone is not sufficient to tailor therapy to prevent leukopenia; more recently, genotyping of the most common TPMT variants was shown to explain only 16% of cases of leukopenia.[16] At any rate, these data led to the common practice of checking TPMT before the initiation of therapy, and, since that time, it has been shown to be a useful test. In a large Dutch study, TPMT variant carriers with an a priori dose reduction had a 10-fold reduction in leukopenic events (relative risk, 0.11; 95% confidence interval [CI], 0.01–0.85).[16]

Based on this pharmacogenomic knowledge, the current recommendation is to initiate therapy with AZA 2 to 3 mg/kg/d or 6-MP 1 to 1.5 mg/kg/d in normal metabolizers. A patient heterozygous for TPMT[L]/TPMT[H] or with intermediate activity should be given half the standard dose, and thiopurines are contraindicated in the rare patients who are homozygous for TPMT[l] or with a low activity level[3] (**Box 1**).

### Thiopurine Metabolite Monitoring

A clue to the utility of metabolite measurements could be found in TPMT methylation itself because it competes with the activation pathway of thiopurines, leading to patients with low or intermediate activity having higher levels of 6-TGN. In the same articles examining the TPMT activity, there was a noted linear association between 6-TGN and bone marrow suppression. These same findings were seen in the childhood acute lymphoblastic leukemia literature, which reported an association between

---

**Box 1**
**Screening with thiopurine initiation**

Measure TPMT before starting therapy:
- Low or absent activity: contraindicated
- Intermediate activity: initiation with 50% of usual dose
- Normal activity: 6-MP 1 to 1.5 mg/kg/d or AZA 2 to 3 mg/kg/d

Frequent complete blood count monitoring in first 12 weeks then every 3 months (every 2 weeks ×2, every 4 weeks ×2, every 8 weeks ×2, then every 3 months)

Thiopurine level monitoring at 6 to 8 weeks and as needed thereafter to achieve 6-TGN level greater than 235 pmol/8 × $10^8$ red blood cells (RBCs) and 6-methylmercaptopurine level less than 5700 pmol/8 × $10^8$ RBCs

Recommend use of sunscreen and hats; annual skin checks

Annual pap smears

Check Epstein-Barr virus status

Vaccinate with live vaccines 4 weeks before starting immunomodulator

---

higher 6-TGN level and chemotherapy response, and it is this literature that led to its exploration within IBD.[17,18]

### Interpretation of Levels

The ideal level of 6-TGN was defined to be greater than 235 pmol/8 × $10^8$ red blood cells (RBCs) after a series of studies.[19–21] In pediatrics, Cuffari and colleagues[22] reported higher rates of clinical remission in patients with higher 6-TGN levels in CD. This finding was further supported by a pediatric study (N = 92) in 2000 that suggested that the odds of a therapeutic response were 5 times higher in patients with 6-TGN levels greater than 235 pmol/8 × $10^8$ RBCs (95% CI, 2.6–9.7; P<.001).[10] Osterman and colleagues'[23] 2006 meta-analysis of 12 studies, which included these 2 studies, crystallized this tenet, showing that patients with 6-TGN levels greater than 230 to 260 pmol/8 × $10^8$ RBCs were more likely to be in clinical remission (odds ratio [OR], 3.27 [1.7–6.3]; P<.001).

In contrast, the metabolite 6-methylmercaptopurine (6-MMP) has been linked to hepatotoxicity in a dose-dependent fashion, usually observed with levels greater than 5700 pmol/8 × $10^8$ RBCs.[24] Thiopurine metabolism in up to 20% of patients has been shown to be skewed toward excessive production of 6-MMP,[25] and a high 6-MMP/6-TGN ratio can be used to determine a patient's risk profile. One study described a markedly increased hepatotoxicity risk with a 6-MMP/6-TGN ratio greater than 24 (OR, 5.35; 95% CI, 3.43–8.43; P = .001), and their reported ideal ratio for response was between 4 and 24.[26] Another study reported that only 67% of patients with mild ultramethylation (ratios of 20–50) were forced to discontinue treatment, and that a ratio greater than 50 was the cut point that led to more frequent discontinuation of thiopurines (P<.03).[27]

Thus, this balance between 6-TGN and 6-MMP can be used to tease out drug inefficiency and intolerance. The metabolites reach steady state about 4 to 8 weeks after the initiation of therapy, and they can be drawn at that point.[28] If the patient has 6-TGN and 6-MMP levels that are both low, it is justified to consider patient compliance, and, if good compliance is verified, then dose escalation is warranted. If a patient has a therapeutic 6-TGN level, a 6-MMP level greater than 5700 pmol/8 × $10^8$ RBCs, and normal liver enzymes, then the liver enzymes should simply be monitored more frequently. If the 6-MMP level is greater than 5700 pmol/8 $\times$ $10^8$ RBCs and the 6-TGN is greater than 400 pmol/8 $\times$ $10^8$ RBCs, then dose deescalation should be undertaken. The eventual possible, or thiopurine-resistant, group has 6-MMP level greater than 5700 pmol/8 $\times$ $10^8$ RBCs with 6-TGN level less than 235 pmol/8 $\times$ $10^8$ RBCs[24]; some clinicians use allopurinol to preferentially shunt the metabolism toward 6-TGN in this group, but this carries a significant risk of toxicity, namely leukopenia[25] (**Table 1**).

## MONOCLONAL ANTIBODIES TARGETING TUMOR NECROSIS FACTOR ALPHA
### Infliximab

Infliximab (IFX) (Remicade, Janssen Biotech) is a chimeric mouse-human immuno-globulin G1 mAb to tumor necrosis factor alpha (TNF$\alpha$) that was first US Food and Drug Administration (FDA) approved for adult IBD in 1998 with subsequent approval in pediatrics in 2006.[29,30] The standard, FDA-approved dose is 5 mg/kg at 0, 2, and 6 weeks followed by a maintenance regimen of 5 mg/kg every 8 weeks. IFX revolution-ized IBD therapy, improving quality of life as well as short-term and long-term out-comes.[31,32] However, it still remains an imperfect medication with between 10% and 40% of patients never responding (primary nonresponders)[33,34] and with an addi-tional 12% per patient-year having a secondary loss of response (SLR).[35]

SLR is thought to be caused by humoral immune sensitization, although it is unclear whether this is from the production of antiinfliximab antibodies (ATIs) leading to faster drug clearance or lower drug concentration for patient-specific reasons (high inflam-matory burden and/or individual differences in clearance) producing the necessary environment for ATI formation. However, avoidance of this immune sensitization, namely through obtaining appropriate trough concentrations and avoiding ATI forma-tion, is the cornerstone of TDM in mAbs.[36]

There are several known covariates (**Table 2**) that can be in flux in ill patients and that affect IFX pharmacokinetics. It is unclear whether these need to be included in a larger overarching TDM algorithm. Fasanmade and colleagues[37] revealed an asso-ciation between low serum albumin level and faster clearance of IFX. In addition, increased systemic inflammation (high baseline C-reactive protein [CRP] or TNF$\alpha$ level) can lead to increased clearance through the reticuloendothelial system as well as a proposed target-mediated drug deposition AKA antigen sink.[38] Brandse and col-leagues[39] also showed that IFX can be lost in stool; endoscopic nonresponders at week 8 had higher fecal IFX concentrations compared with endoscopic responders (median [interquartile range (IQR)], 4.66 µg/mL [1.49–16.29 µg/mL] vs 1.16 µg/mL [0.0–4.82 µg/mL]; $P = .0588$). These factors, low albumin level, antigen sink, and stool

| Table 1 Interpretation of thiopurine metabolite levels | |
|---|---|
| **6-TGN and 6-MMP Scenario (pmol/8 $\times$ $10^8$ RBCs)** | **Action** |
| 6-TGN <235, 6-MMP <5700 | Check for compliance; if compliant, dose escalate |
| 6-TGN >235, 6-MMP >5700, normal LFTs | Maintain dose and monitor LFTs |
| 6-TGN >400, 6-MMP >5700 | Dose deescalate |
| 6-TGN <235, 6-MMP >5700 | Consider switching therapy |

*Abbreviation:* LFTs, liver function tests.

**Table 2**
**Covariates that affect monoclonal antibody clearance**

| | Impact on Pharmacokinetics |
|---|---|
| Presence of ADAs | • Decreases serum mAb levels<br>• Three-fold-increased clearance<br>• Worse clinical outcomes |
| Concomitant use of IMM | • Reduces formation<br>• Increases serum mAb levels<br>• Decreases mAb clearance<br>• Better clinical outcomes |
| High baseline TNF-$\alpha$ | • May decrease mAb levels by increasing clearance |
| Low albumin level | • Increases clearance<br>• Worse clinical outcomes |
| High baseline CRP level | • Increases clearance |
| Body size | • High BMI may increase clearance |
| Gender | • Men have higher clearance |

*Abbreviations:* BMI, body mass index; CRP, C-reactive protein; IMM, immunomodulator.

*Adapted from* Ordas I, Mould DR, Feagan BG, et al. Anti-TNF monoclonal antibodies in inflammatory bowel disease: pharmacokinetics-based dosing paradigms. Clin Pharmacol Ther 2012;91(4):635–46.

loss, have led to the common clinical practice of initiating induction on hospitalized patients with UC with a dose of 10 mg/kg, and it follows that they are given consideration in an IFX dosing algorithm. Other covariates shown to affect IFX pharmacokinetics are high body mass index and male sex.[38]

### Exposure Response: Establishment of Trough Concentrations

Maser and colleagues[40] in 2006 reported that, in CD, detectable trough concentrations, with or without ATI, correlated with higher rates of clinical remission (82% vs 6%; $P<.001$), lower CRP levels (2.0 vs 11.8 μg/L; $P<.001$), and higher rates of endoscopic improvement (88% vs 33%; $P<.001$). Similarly, Seow and colleagues[41] showed improved rates of clinical remission and endoscopic improvement in UC and, furthermore, showed that undetectable IFX concentrations were associated with a higher rate of colectomy (55% vs 7%; OR, 9.3; 95% CI, 2.9–29.9; $P<.001$). Maintenance infliximab for luminal Crohn's disease (ACCENT 1), a clinical trial evaluating IFX induction in active CD, showed that patients who failed to respond to IFX had lower serum IFX concentrations than those who had a sustained response (1.9 vs 4.0 μg/mL; $P = .03$).[42]

Efforts were then directed to determining the exact trough concentrations required to best achieve clinical and endoscopic response (**Table 3**). A post-hoc analysis of ACT-1 and ACT-2 (Active Ulcerative Colitis Trials 1 and 2) defined trough concentrations of 3.7 μg/mL, 5.1 μg/mL, and 41 μg/mL at weeks 30, 14, and 8, respectively, as predictors of optimal outcomes.[43] This finding was similarly shown in the ACCENT I post-hoc analysis with trough concentrations greater than or equal to 3.5 μg/mL at week 14 in the 5-mg/kg dose group (OR, 3.5; CI, 1.1–11.4) and a greater than or equal to 60% decrease in CRP level (OR, 7.3; CI, 1.4–36.7), both significantly associated with durable sustained response.[44]

However, clinical and endoscopic responses are likely not the ideal targets of therapy; mucosal healing (MH) is the newly proposed treat-to-target goal.[52–54] Ungar and colleagues'[45] retrospective study of 78 patients on IFX suggest that trough concentrations of IFX greater than 5 μg/mL (area under the curve (AUC), 0.75; $P<.0001$) identified

**Table 3**
**Proposed trough concentrations during maintenance**

| Drug | Proposed Trough[a] Concentrations During Maintenance |
|---|---|
| Infliximab | >5[45] µg/mL to achieve mucosal healing[b] |
| Adalimumab | >12[45] µg/mL to achieve mucosal healing |
| Golimumab | >1.5[46] µg/mL to achieve clinical remission and response; paucity of data for mucosal healing |
| Certolizumab pegol | >10–15[47] µg/mL at week 8[a] for endoscopic remission; however, general paucity of data |
| Vedolizumab | >10[48]–15[49] µg/mL for clinical remission; >40 µg/mL vedolizumab concentration at week 6 during induction has also been a proposed target concentration[50] |
| Ustekinumab | >5[51] µg/mL to achieve endoscopic response |

[a] With the exception of certolizumab pegol.
[b] Higher does may be required for those with perianal disease.

patients with MH with 85% specificity. Increasing trough concentrations to greater than 8 µg/mL only minimally increases rates of MH.[45] Papamichael and colleagues[55] used multiple logistic regression analysis and identified greater than or equal to 15 µg/mL IFX concentration at week 6 (OR, 4.6; 95% CI, 1.2–17.1; $P$ = .025) and greater than or equal to 2.1 µg/mL at week 14 (OR, 5.6; 95% CI, 1.7–18; $P$ = .004) to be associated with short-term MH, which was defined as a Mayo endoscopic sub-score less than or equal to 1 during weeks 10 to 14.[55] The requirement of higher IFX concentrations for MH is likely tied to the need to overcome the phenomenon found by Yarur and colleagues[56] that tissue with severe inflammation has a lower concentration of anti-TNFα (mean normalized anti-TNFα in tissue: uninflamed, 0.93 µg/mL ; mild inflammation, 2.17 µg/mL; moderate inflammation, 13.71 µg/mL ; severe inflammation, 2.2 µg/mL ; $P$ = .0042 µg/mL).

Perianal disease might also require a higher target trough concentration. A recent study showed higher median IFX concentrations (15.8 µg/mL [IQR, 9.9–27] vs 4.4 µg/mL [IQR, 0–9.8]; $P$<.0001) in patients with fistula healing.[57] Likewise, Davidov and colleagues[58] showed that higher IFX concentrations during induction and at weeks 2, 6, and 14, were associated with improvement in, or total resolution of, fistula drainage.

### Antiinfliximab Antibodies

Surveillance and prevention of ATI formation are closely connected with trough concentration monitoring. Many clinicians initially questioned whether or not the simple presence of ATI at any trough concentration without an infusion reaction warranted the cessation of IFX therapy, especially given the limited treatment regimens for IBD. It has since been noted that ATI can be transient, and, currently, it is being proposed that, if ATI occurs in the first 6 months of therapy or if the ATI titer is greater than 9 µg/mL, then sustained ATI are more likely.[59]

Overcoming levels of ATI less than 9 can be accomplished by the addition of an immunomodulator (IMM), either methotrexate (MTX) or thiopurines, dose escalation and tighter monitoring of IFX serum concentrations, or both. A small case series from Ben-Horin and colleagues[60] suggested that using IMM with maintenance IFX increased IFX concentrations, decreased ATI titers, and improved patient outcomes. Alternatively, it may be possible to eschew concomitant IMMs and still avoid ATI by using close monitoring of serum concentrations with dose and/or frequency adjustments to sustain therapeutic concentrations with proactive TDM.[3]

### Combination Therapy (Monoclonal Antibodies Plus Immunomodulators)

Colombel and colleagues[61] and Feagan and colleagues[62] both established in adult IBD that combination therapy with IFX and an IMM led to higher IFX serum concentrations and lower rates of ATI. Within the Pediatric Inflammatory Bowel Disease Collaborative Research Group Registry, Grossi and colleagues[63] showed a greater likelihood of remaining on IFX for 5 years when concomitant IMMs were used for greater than 6 months compared with monotherapy with IFX or IMM for less than 6 months. They also directly compared the effect of thiopurines versus MTX on IFX durability in men receiving IMM for greater than 6 months, and they showed that durability of IFX was significantly greater with MTX than with thiopurines ($P<.01$).[63] Within pediatrics, the recently published DEVELOP registry findings could direct the choice between thiopurines and MTX because of the reported increased risk of malignancy with thiopurines. With 5766 participants and 24,543 patient-years of follow-up, Hyams and colleagues[64] reported that pediatric patients with IBD exposed to thiopurines either alone or in combination with biologics have a significantly increased risk of malignancy compared with a reference population (2.88-fold and 3.06-fold respectively). There were no increased rates of malignancy in those exposed to either biologics alone or with MTX (1.11-fold to 1.49-fold).

### Reactive or Proactive Therapeutic Drug Monitoring

Along with the debate about the proper therapeutic range of trough concentrations, there is a concurrent query regarding timing, especially with respect to the prevention of silent ATI formation that leads to an SLR. Should TDM be a reactive or proactive strategy, and, if proactive, when is the ideal time to obtain serum concentrations?

Afif and colleagues[65] performed a retrospective study of 155 patients receiving IFX and reported clinical response in 86% of patients who had dose escalations of IFX compared with 33% response in those who were switched to another anti-TNFα. Ben-Horin and Chowers[66] performed a review of PubMed literature to show that 50% to 70% of patients with an SLR were able to recapture response after dose intensification, but the follow-up time in the reviewed 11 studies was limited. Kopylov and colleagues[67] showed in 76 patients with CD that only 36% had a sustained clinical response at 12 months after a single IFX dose intensification; this percentage increased to 50% after a second dose intensification. In a multicenter retrospective study of 168 patients with CD, Katz and colleagues[68] found that dose intensification of IFX led to sustained, regained response in 47% of patients.

In a 2014 pediatric prospective observational study, Singh and colleagues[69] showed week 14 IFX concentrations of greater than 3, greater than 4, and greater than 7 µg/mL to have respective positive predictive values of 64%, 76%, and 100% for persistent remission at week 54. However, in another pediatric study (N = 50) of a dashboard-guided dosing system, 44% of patients had a week 14 IFX concentration less than 3 µg/mL.[70] Week 10 concentrations were then examined in a prospective cohort study of 77 children with CD. They showed higher week 10 IFX concentrations to be associated with ongoing IFX therapy at 12 months (median [IQR] concentrations in patients on therapy at 12 months: 20.40 [11.20–35.00] µg/mL vs 8.70 [0.90–16.90] µg/mL in those off therapy; $P = .01$), but they also showed that 4% of the patients had already formed ATI by week 10, raising the question of whether IFX concentration and ATI monitoring should begin even earlier than week 10 for a proactive TDM strategy.[71]

Proactive TDM for mAbs started to receive more attention following the Trough Level Adapted Infliximab Treatment (TAXIT) trial, and, despite clinical remission at

1 year being similar between the proactive maintenance TDM group and the group with dosing changes based on clinical symptoms (69% vs 72%; $P$ = .7), there were many secondary outcomes that were superior in the proactive group. These outcomes included less rescue therapy (7% vs 17%; $P$ = .004) and fewer patients with undetectable trough concentrations (OR, 3.7; $P$<.001).[72] In an observational study of 126 patients with IBD of whom 48 had proactive TDM, Vaughn and colleagues[73] showed an association between proactive dose adjustments to keep trough concentrations between 5 and 10 μg/mL and sustained remission compared with concentrations less than 5 μg/mL (hazard ratio [HR], 0.03; 95% CI, 0.01–0.1; $P$<.0001) or no TDM (HR, 0.3; 95% CI, 0.1–0.6; $P$ = .0006). In a recently published multicenter, retrospective study of 264 patients with IBD, Papamichael and colleagues[74] showed that proactive monitoring reduced the risk of treatment failure (HR, 0.16; 95% CI, 0.09–0.27; $P$<.001), IBD-related surgery and hospitalization (HR, 0.30; 95% CI, 0.11–0.80; $P$ = .017; and HR, 0.16; 95% CI, 0.07–0.33; $P$<.001, respectively), and ATI (HR, 0.25; 95% CI, 0.07–0.84; $P$ = .025).[74] However, a prospective study of 20 patients with IBD in deep remission who were dose deescalated to achieve IFX trough concentrations between 3 and 7 had 2 patients relapse at 8 months with trough concentrations of 5.5 and 4.9 μg/mL respectively, and, although a small study, this 10% relapse rate is not negligible.[75]

### Adalimumab

Adalimumab (Humira, AbbVie) is an anti-TNFα biologic delivered by subcutaneous injection with maintenance dosing of 20 to 40 mg every other week to weekly, giving fewer ways to adjust dosing compared with IFX. However, the general principles found to be true in IFX are, for the most part, echoed in adalimumab. Roblin and colleagues[76] found a trough concentration less than 4.9 μg/mL to be correlated with absence of MH in 40 patients with IBD (likelihood ratio, 4.3; sensitivity, 66%; specificity, 85%; positive predictive value, 88%; negative predictive value, 51%). Ungar and colleagues'[45] retrospective study of 67 patients on adalimumab showed that trough concentrations greater than 7.1 μg/mL (AUC, 0.7; $P$<.004) identified patients with MH with 85% specificity, with gains in MH plateauing at 12 μg/mL. Yarur and colleagues[77] found random, nontrough concentrations in patients with MH of 13 to 14 μg/mL.

Like IFX, adalimumab is immunogenic; in a retrospective study of 30 patients with CD, West and colleagues[78] showed that rates of clinical remission were improved in the absence of ADA (77% vs 20%), and the presence of ADA was correlated with lack of response ($P$ = .006). Dose escalation from biweekly to weekly can recapture those with SLR.[79]

### Other Anti–tumor Necrosis Factor Alpha Monoclonal Antibodies

The TDM data in anti-TNFα therapies other than IFX and adalimumab are limited but seem to follow the same tenets. Golimumab (GLM) (Symponi, Janssen Biotech) is a subcutaneous injectable for UC typically dosed at 100 mg every 4 weeks. The Efficacy and Safety of Golimumab in Moderately to Severely Active Ulcerative Colitis (PURSUIT) trial found higher serum concentrations to be associated with increasing rates of clinical response, clinical remission, and MH at weeks 6 and 54.[80,81] A small study (N = 21) stratified patients into responders and nonresponders and compared their 2-week (responder, 10.0 [7.8–10.5] μg/mL vs nonresponder, 7.4 [4.8–8.3] μg/mL; $P$ = .035) and 6-week (responder, 5.1 [4.0–7.9] μg/mL vs nonresponder, 2.1 [1.8–4.2] μg/mL; $P$ = .037) serum concentrations. They performed a receiver operating characteristic (ROC) analysis that suggested an association between a GLM concentration of 2.6 μg/mL at week 6 (90% specificity, 56% sensitivity; $P$ = .034) and clinical improvement at week 14.[82] Adedokun and colleagues[46] performed an ROC analysis on PURSUIT data to identify optimal serum GLM concentrations associated with clinical response at week 6 and clinical remission at weeks 30 and 54, and they identified concentrations of 2.5 μg/mL at week 6 and 1.4 μg/mL during maintenance. However, higher concentrations during induction may be needed to achieve mucosal healing because patients with MH had median concentrations of 3.14 μg/mL compared with 1.70 μg/mL in those without MH ($P<.001$). In contrast, the cutoff of 1.4 μg/mL during maintenance aligns with the median concentration of 1.22 μg/mL in patients with MH compared with 0.83 μg/mL in those without MH ($P = .005$) at weeks 30 and 54.

Certolizumab pegol (CZP) (Cimzia, UCB) is an injectable pegylated anti-TNFα mAb approved for CD. A post-hoc analysis of the MUSIC trial (89 patients with CD with active, severe endoscopic disease) showed higher plasma CZP concentration quartiles to be associated with endoscopic remission at both week 10 ($P = .0302$) and week 54 ($P<.0206$). Specifically, at week 10, the endoscopic remission and response rates were 20% and 30%, respectively, in the group with the lowest quartile of week 8 CZP concentrations. Patients in the top 3 quartiles had much better rates of endoscopic response and endoscopic remission with respective endoscopic response and remission of 60% and 50% of the second quartile (8.98 to <16.12), 56% and 56% of the third quartile (16.12 to <23.30), and 88% and 75% of the fourth quartile (>23.30).[47]

## BEYOND ANTI–TUMOR NECROSIS FACTOR ALPHA
### Vedolizumab

Vedolizumab (VDZ) (Entyvio, Takeda) is an anti-$\alpha^4\beta^7$ integrin that modulates lymphocyte trafficking to the intestine. Most of the TDM data for VDZ come from the GEMINI I (Vedolizumab in Moderate to Severe Ulcerative Colitis)[48] and GEMINI 2 (Vedolizumab in Moderate to Severe Crohn's Disease)[49] clinical trials. Post-hoc analysis of the GEMINI I data showed that higher concentrations of VDZ at week 6 were associated with MH (63% if >35.7 μg/mL vs 20% if <17.1 μg/mL).[83] This finding is similarly seen in their evaluation of clinical remission during induction because 37% of patients in the fourth quartile (VDZ 33.3–65.6 μg/mL) at week 6 were in remission compared with 5.6%, 11.3%, and 16.4% in the first 3 quartiles (which ranged from 0 to <33.3 μg/mL), respectively.[48] At week 52, clinical remission in the every-8-week dosing group was found in 42.1% of the first quartile (0 to <6.0 μg/mL), 78.9% of the second quartile (6.0 to <9.8 μg/mL), 63.2% of the third quartile (9.8 to <14.2 μg/mL), and 80% of the fourth quartile (14.2–42.8 μg/mL). GEMINI 2 showed similar percentages of clinical remission at both week 6 and week 52 in the second, third, and fourth quartiles (second to fourth quartile ranges: week 6, 15.2–142 μg/mL; week 52, 7.5–54.5 μg/mL with every-8-week dosing; and 20.8–70.8 μg/mL with every-4-week dosing).[49]

In a recent prospective study of 29 patients with IBD, those in clinical remission at week 28 were noted to have higher week 6 VDZ serum concentrations (41.7 vs 21.0 μg/mL; $P<.05$). An ROC analysis performed with this study suggested a target concentration of 40.1 μg/mL of VDZ at week 6 for sustained clinical remission (100% sensitivity, 70% specificity).[50] VDZ is minimally immunogenic with ADA found in at least 1 sample in 3.7% and 4.1% patients and greater than or equal to 2 consecutive samples in 1% and 0.4% patients in GEMINI I and II respectively.[48,49]

### Ustekinumab

Ustekinumab (UST) (Stelara, Janssen Biotech) is an anti-P40 mAb, blocking a subunit of interleukin (IL)-12 and IL-23. It was approved by the FDA for treatment of CD in September 2016.[84] TDM in UST is still in its infancy, but the UNITI studies, which included 1369 patients with moderate to severe CD, showed a higher likelihood of Crohn's Disease Activity Index consistent with clinical remission with higher concentrations (40% with >6.7 µg/mL vs 29% with <1.6 µg/mL; $P = .06$).[85] The greatest increase in clinical remission was seen when serum concentrations were more than 3.6 µg/mL, and only 2.3% of patients developed antibodies to UST at 1 year.[86] Battat and colleagues[51] recently published a prospective study of 62 patients with CD that suggested that UST greater than 4.5 µg/mL at week 26 was the optimal concentration for endoscopic response (AUC, 0.67; sensitivity, 67%; specificity, 70%) with 76% of patients with greater than 4.5 µg/mL with endoscopic response versus 41% with less than 4.5 µg/mL ($P = .008$). Battat and colleagues[51] had similar findings to UNITI regarding immunogenicity because zero patients were noted to have ADA by week 26.[51]

### Cost Saving and Therapeutic Drug Monitoring

Aside from patient outcomes, another driving force behind TDM is reduction in cost, which can be burdensome with mAbs. TAXIT found a 28% reduction in cost over their 1-year study period with proactive dose adjustments.[72,87] Three studies in CD that used modeling to perform dose adjustments by serum concentration showed savings from $5396 per patient over a 1-year period to €13,130 per patient over 5 years.[88–90]

It should also be noted that IFX allows for 2 types of adjustments: dose and frequency. Katz and colleagues[68] found that both forms of escalation (10 mg/kg every 8 weeks vs 5 mg/kg every 4 weeks) were equally effective, and the cost and inconvenience of having more frequent visits should be weighed.

### Assay Variability

Another complexity is the corrections that need to be made when comparing the results of various commercially available IFX concentration and ATI assays. Enzyme-linked immunosorbent assays (ELISAs) have less clinical utility in TDM, given that the detection of drug in the serum can compete with ATI, leading to inconclusive results; in conjunction with patient convenience, this was the origin of obtaining concentrations at trough in order to minimize confounding of drug with ATI. Homogeneous mobility shift assays (HMSAs) separate and quantify the drug and ATI concentrations independently using high-pressure liquid chromatography in combination with size-exclusion chromatography. Although there is a very good correlation between HMSA and ELISA or electrochemiluminescent immunosorbent assay for drug concentrations, the same is not seen for ATI.[3] Note that variability in assays could alter the desired target range for clinical outcomes.[91,92]

With the advent of biosimilars, the assays need to be further validated to prove their usefulness in assessing each new biosimilar.[93] Gils and colleagues[94] showed that the IFX ELISA quantifies ATI for two IFX biosimilars equally well as IFX.

### The Future of Therapeutic Drug Monitoring

Decision support tools, such as dashboards, are at the cutting edge of TDM's evolution. With the aid of computer modeling, they can predict ideal personalized dosing based on drug concentrations in conjunction with patient covariates and allow real-time adjustments.[95] A retrospective study from 2017 compared dose adjustments based on standard of care with an IFX dashboard's bayesian-forecasted recommendations.

Using week 14 clinical data only, the dashboard recommended dose or interval changes in 44% of the 50 patients. When week 14 IFX concentration and ATI status were used in conjunction with clinical data, the dashboard recommended that 96%

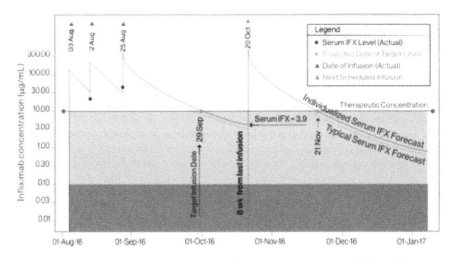

**Fig. 2.** Example of pharmacokinetics dashboard for IFX dosing for an individual with moderately to severely active IBD. The dashboard accounts for dose, IFX serum concentration, and laboratory values, and, in this case, is predicting rapid drug clearance. The ideal trough concentration can be set on a patient-by-patient basis, and the goal for this patient was set at 10 μg/mL. To achieve this trough, the patient would need to receive the fourth infusion 4 weeks earlier than the standard 8-week dosing. The model predicts that, if the patient waits the standard 8 weeks for the next infusion, the drug trough concentration would be 3.9 μg/mL.

of patients have a dose or interval adjustment. The blinded clinical decisions made based on standard of care aligned with the dashboard recommendations in only 22% of the patients.[70] This finding reflects the complexity of the pharmacokinetics of mAbs and shows that current standard-of-care dose adjustments are likely not sufficient to maximize the potential of biologics. Research is ongoing with this Precision IFX dashboard, shown in **Fig. 2**, and it is currently being prospectively used to guide dose adjustments in the hope of addressing whether sophisticated, computer-modeled, proactive adjustments lead to better clinical outcomes and improved therapy durability.

## SUMMARY

From its origin with thiopurines, TDM has been used in IBD to maximize patient outcomes and minimize adverse events. Special attention should be given to appropriately choosing dosing and target serum concentrations based on patient-specific factors to optimize each individual patient's care. TDM in IBD gives providers the opportunity to maximize response to available medications and advance the goals management to such lofty goals as mucosal and fistula healing.

## REFERENCES

1. Allez M, Karmiris K, Louis E, et al. Report of the ECCO pathogenesis workshop on anti-TNF therapy failures in inflammatory bowel diseases: definitions, frequency and pharmacological aspects. J Crohns Colitis 2010;4(4):355–66.
2. D'Haens GR, Panaccione R, Higgins PD, et al. The London Position Statement of the World Congress of Gastroenterology on biological therapy for IBD with the European Crohn's and Colitis Organization: when to start, when to stop, which

drug to choose, and how to predict response? Am J Gastroenterol 2011;106(2): 199–212 [quiz: 213].

3. Singh N, Dubinsky MC. Therapeutic drug monitoring in children and young adults with inflammatory bowel disease: a practical approach. Gastroenterol Hepatol 2015;11(1):48–55.

4. Van Assche G, Vermeire S, Rutgeerts P. Infliximab therapy for patients with inflammatory bowel disease: 10 years on. Eur J Pharmacol 2009;623(Suppl 1): S17–25.

5. Lesko LJ, Schmidt S. Individualization of drug therapy: history, present state, and opportunities for the future. Clin Pharmacol Ther 2012;92(4):458–66.

6. Kang JS, Lee MH. Overview of therapeutic drug monitoring. Korean J Intern Med 2009;24(1):1–10.

7. Present DH, Meltzer SJ, Krumholz MP, et al. 6-Mercaptopurine in the management of inflammatory bowel disease: short- and long-term toxicity. Ann Intern Med 1989;111(8):641–9.

8. Markowitz J, Grancher K, Kohn N, et al. A multicenter trial of 6-mercaptopurine and prednisone in children with newly diagnosed Crohn's disease. Gastroenterology 2000;119(4):895–902.

9. Candy S, Wright J, Gerber M, et al. A controlled double blind study of azathioprine in the management of Crohn's disease. Gut 1995;37(5):674–8.

10. Dubinsky MC, Lamothe S, Yang HY, et al. Pharmacogenomics and metabolite measurement for 6-mercaptopurine therapy in inflammatory bowel disease. Gastroenterology 2000;118(4):705–13.

11. Dubinsky MC. Azathioprine, 6-mercaptopurine in inflammatory bowel disease: pharmacology, efficacy, and safety. Clin Gastroenterol Hepatol 2004;2(9):731–43.

12. Weinshilboum RM, Sladek SL. Mercaptopurine pharmacogenetics: monogenic inheritance of erythrocyte thiopurine methyltransferase activity. Am J Hum Genet 1980;32(5):651–62.

13. Tai HL, Krynetski EY, Yates CR, et al. Thiopurine S-methyltransferase deficiency: two nucleotide transitions define the most prevalent mutant allele associated with loss of catalytic activity in Caucasians. Am J Hum Genet 1996;58(4):694–702.

14. Hindorf U, Appell ML. Genotyping should be considered the primary choice for pre-treatment evaluation of thiopurine methyltransferase function. J Crohns Colitis 2012;6(6):655–9.

15. Colombel JF, Ferrari N, Debuysere H, et al. Genotypic analysis of thiopurine S-methyltransferase in patients with Crohn's disease and severe myelosuppression during azathioprine therapy. Gastroenterology 2000;118(6):1025–30.

16. Coenen MJ, de Jong DJ, van Marrewijk CJ, et al. Identification of patients with variants in TPMT and dose reduction reduces hematologic events during thiopurine treatment of inflammatory bowel disease. Gastroenterology 2015;149(4): 907–17.e7.

17. Lennard L, Van Loon JA, Weinshilboum RM. Pharmacogenetics of acute azathioprine toxicity: relationship to thiopurine methyltransferase genetic polymorphism. Clin Pharmacol Ther 1989;46(2):149–54.

18. Lennard L, Lilleyman JS, Van Loon J, et al. Genetic variation in response to 6-mercaptopurine for childhood acute lymphoblastic leukaemia. Lancet 1990; 336(8709):225–9.

19. Ooi CY, Bohane TD, Lee D, et al. Thiopurine metabolite monitoring in paediatric inflammatory bowel disease. Aliment Pharmacol Ther 2007;25(8):941–7.

20. Pozler O, Chladek J, Maly J, et al. Steady-state of azathioprine during initiation treatment of pediatric inflammatory bowel disease. J Crohns Colitis 2010;4(6): 623–8.

21. Grossman AB, Noble AJ, Mamula P, et al. Increased dosing requirements for 6-mercaptopurine and azathioprine in inflammatory bowel disease patients six years and younger. Inflamm Bowel Dis 2008;14(6):750–5.

22. Cuffari C, Theoret Y, Latour S, et al. 6-Mercaptopurine metabolism in Crohn's disease: correlation with efficacy and toxicity. Gut 1996;39(3):401–6.

23. Osterman MT, Kundu R, Lichtenstein GR, et al. Association of 6-thioguanine nucleotide levels and inflammatory bowel disease activity: a meta-analysis. Gastroenterology 2006;130(4):1047–53.

24. Dubinsky MC, Yang H, Hassard PV, et al. 6-MP metabolite profiles provide a biochemical explanation for 6-MP resistance in patients with inflammatory bowel disease. Gastroenterology 2002;122(4):904–15.

25. Gearry RB, Day AS, Barclay ML, et al. Azathioprine and allopurinol: a two-edged interaction. J Gastroenterol Hepatol 2010;25(4):653–5.

26. Kopylov U, Amre D, Theoret Y, et al. Thiopurine metabolite ratios for monitoring therapy in pediatric Crohn disease. J Pediatr Gastroenterol Nutr 2014;59(4): 511–5.

27. Kreijne JE, Seinen ML, Wilhelm AJ, et al. Routinely established skewed thiopurine metabolism leads to a strikingly high rate of early therapeutic failure in patients with inflammatory bowel disease. Ther Drug Monit 2015;37(6):797–804.

28. Derijks LJ, Gilissen LP, Engels LG, et al. Pharmacokinetics of 6-mercaptopurine in patients with inflammatory bowel disease: implications for therapy. Ther Drug Monit 2004;26(3):311–8.

29. Hyams J, Crandall W, Kugathasan S, et al. Induction and maintenance infliximab therapy for the treatment of moderate-to-severe Crohn's disease in children. Gastroenterology 2007;132(3):863–73 [quiz: 1165–6].

30. Hyams J, Damaraju L, Blank M, et al. Induction and maintenance therapy with infliximab for children with moderate to severe ulcerative colitis. Clin Gastroenterol Hepatol 2012;10(4):391–9.e1.

31. Sherman M, Tsynman DN, Kim A, et al. Sustained improvement in health-related quality of life measures in patients with inflammatory bowel disease receiving prolonged anti-tumor necrosis factor therapy. J Dig Dis 2014;15(4):174–9.

32. Casellas F, Rodrigo L, Nino P, et al. Sustained improvement of health-related quality of life in Crohn's disease patients treated with infliximab and azathioprine for 4 years. Inflamm Bowel Dis 2007;13(11):1395–400.

33. Papamichael K, Gils A, Rutgeerts P, et al. Role for therapeutic drug monitoring during induction therapy with TNF antagonists in IBD: evolution in the definition and management of primary nonresponse. Inflamm Bowel Dis 2015;21(1): 182–97.

34. Pouillon L, Bossuyt P, Peyrin-Biroulet L. Considerations, challenges and future of anti-TNF therapy in treating inflammatory bowel disease. Expert Opin Biol Ther 2016;16(10):1277–90.

35. Chaparro M, Panes J, Garcia V, et al. Long-term durability of infliximab treatment in Crohn's disease and efficacy of dose "escalation" in patients losing response. J Clin Gastroenterol 2011;45(2):113–8.

36. Papamichael K, Cheifetz AS. Therapeutic drug monitoring in IBD: the new standard-of-care for anti-TNF therapy. Am J Gastroenterol 2017;112(5):673–6.

37. Fasanmade AA, Adedokun OJ, Olson A, et al. Serum albumin concentration: a predictive factor of infliximab pharmacokinetics and clinical response in patients with ulcerative colitis. Int J Clin Pharmacol Ther 2010;48(5):297–308.

38. Ordas I, Mould DR, Feagan BG, et al. Anti-TNF monoclonal antibodies in inflammatory bowel disease: pharmacokinetics-based dosing paradigms. Clin Pharmacol Ther 2012;91(4):635–46.

39. Brandse JF, van den Brink GR, Wildenberg ME, et al. Loss of infliximab into feces is associated with lack of response to therapy in patients with severe ulcerative colitis. Gastroenterology 2015;149(2):350–5.e2.

40. Maser EA, Villela R, Silverberg MS, et al. Association of trough serum infliximab to clinical outcome after scheduled maintenance treatment for Crohn's disease. Clin Gastroenterol Hepatol 2006;4(10):1248–54.

41. Seow CH, Newman A, Irwin SP, et al. Trough serum infliximab: a predictive factor of clinical outcome for infliximab treatment in acute ulcerative colitis. Gut 2010; 59(1):49–54.

42. Hanauer SB, Feagan BG, Lichtenstein GR, et al. Maintenance infliximab for Crohn's disease: the ACCENT I randomised trial. Lancet 2002;359(9317):1541–9.

43. Reinisch W, Sandborn WJ, Rutgeerts P, et al. Long-term infliximab maintenance therapy for ulcerative colitis: the ACT-1 and -2 extension studies. Inflamm Bowel Dis 2012;18(2):201–11.

44. Cornillie F, Hanauer SB, Diamond RH, et al. Postinduction serum infliximab trough level and decrease of C-reactive protein level are associated with durable sustained response to infliximab: a retrospective analysis of the ACCENT I trial. Gut 2014;63(11):1721–7.

45. Ungar B, Levy I, Yavne Y, et al. Optimizing anti-TNF-alpha therapy: serum levels of infliximab and adalimumab are associated with mucosal healing in patients with inflammatory bowel diseases. Clin Gastroenterol Hepatol 2016;14(4): 550–7.e2.

46. Adedokun OJ, Xu Z, Marano CW, et al. Pharmacokinetics and exposure-response relationship of golimumab in patients with moderately-to-severely active ulcerative colitis: results from phase 2/3 PURSUIT induction and maintenance studies. J Crohns Colitis 2017;11(1):35–46.

47. Colombel JF, Sandborn WJ, Allez M, et al. Association between plasma concentrations of certolizumab pegol and endoscopic outcomes of patients with Crohn's disease. Clin Gastroenterol Hepatol 2014;12(3):423–31.e1.

48. Feagan BG, Rutgeerts P, Sands BE, et al. Vodolizumab ao induction and maintenance therapy for ulcerative colitis. N Engl J Med 2013;369(8):699–710.

49. Sandborn WJ, Feagan BG, Rutgeerts P, et al. Vedolizumab as induction and maintenance therapy for Crohn's disease. N Engl J Med 2013;369(8):711–21.

50. Paul S, Williet N, Claudez P, et al. Sa1939 serum vedolizumab assay at week 6 predicts sustained clinical remission and lack of recourse to optimisation in IBD. Gastroenterology 2017;150(4):S410.

51. Battat R, Kopylov U, Bessissow T, et al. Association between ustekinumab trough concentrations and clinical, biomarker, and endoscopic outcomes in patients with Crohn's disease. Clin Gastroenterol Hepatol 2017;15(9):1427–34.e2.

52. D'Haens G, Sandborn WJ, Feagan BG, et al. A review of activity indices and efficacy end points for clinical trials of medical therapy in adults with ulcerative colitis. Gastroenterology 2007;132(2):763–86.

53. Peyrin-Biroulet L, Sandborn W, Sands BE, et al. Selecting Therapeutic Targets in Inflammatory Bowel Disease (STRIDE): determining therapeutic goals for treat-to-target. Am J Gastroenterol 2015;110(9):1324–38.

54. Colombel JF, Rutgeerts P, Reinisch W, et al. Early mucosal healing with infliximab is associated with improved long-term clinical outcomes in ulcerative colitis. Gastroenterology 2011;141(4):1194–201.

55. Papamichael K, Van Stappen T, Vande Casteele N, et al. Infliximab concentration thresholds during induction therapy are associated with short-term mucosal healing in patients with ulcerative colitis. Clin Gastroenterol Hepatol 2016;14(4): 543–9.

56. Yarur AJ, Jain A, Sussman DA, et al. The association of tissue anti-TNF drug levels with serological and endoscopic disease activity in inflammatory bowel disease: the ATLAS study. Gut 2016;65(2):249–55.

57. Yarur AJ, Kanagala V, Stein DJ, et al. Higher infliximab trough levels are associated with perianal fistula healing in patients with Crohn's disease. Aliment Pharmacol Ther 2017;45(7):933–40.

58. Davidov Y, Ungar B, Bar-Yoseph H, et al. Association of induction infliximab levels with clinical response in perianal Crohn's disease. J Crohns Colitis 2016;11(5): 549–55.

59. Vande Casteele N, Gils A, Singh S, et al. Antibody response to infliximab and its impact on pharmacokinetics can be transient. Am J Gastroenterol 2013;108(6): 962–71.

60. Ben-Horin S, Waterman M, Kopylov U, et al. Addition of an immunomodulator to infliximab therapy eliminates antidrug antibodies in serum and restores clinical response of patients with inflammatory bowel disease. Clin Gastroenterol Hepatol 2013;11(4):444–7.

61. Colombel JF, Sandborn WJ, Reinisch W, et al. Infliximab, azathioprine, or combination therapy for Crohn's disease. N Engl J Med 2010;362(15):1383–95.

62. Feagan BG, McDonald JW, Panaccione R, et al. Methotrexate in combination with infliximab is no more effective than infliximab alone in patients with Crohn's disease. Gastroenterology 2014;146(3):681–8.e1.

63. Grossi V, Lerer T, Griffiths A, et al. Concomitant use of immunomodulators affects the durability of infliximab therapy in children with Crohn's disease. Clin Gastroenterol Hepatol 2015;13(10):1748–56.

64. Hyams JS, Dubinsky MC, Baldassano RN, et al. Infliximab not associated with increased risk of malignancy or hemophagocytic lymphohistiocytosis in pediatric patients with inflammatory bowel disease. Gastroenterology 2017;152(8): 1901–14.e3.

65. Afif W, Loftus EV Jr, Faubion WA, et al. Clinical utility of measuring infliximab and human anti-chimeric antibody concentrations in patients with inflammatory bowel disease. Am J Gastroenterol 2010;105(5):1133–9.

66. Ben-Horin S, Chowers Y. Review article: loss of response to anti-TNF treatments in Crohn's disease. Aliment Pharmacol Ther 2011;33(9):987–95.

67. Kopylov U, Mantzaris GJ, Katsanos KH, et al. The efficacy of shortening the dosing interval to once every six weeks in Crohn's patients losing response to maintenance dose of infliximab. Aliment Pharmacol Ther 2011;33(3):349–57.

68. Katz L, Gisbert JP, Manoogian B, et al. Doubling the infliximab dose versus halving the infusion intervals in Crohn's disease patients with loss of response. Inflamm Bowel Dis 2012;18(11):2026–33.

69. Singh N, Rosenthal CJ, Melmed GY, et al. Early infliximab trough levels are associated with persistent remission in pediatric patients with inflammatory bowel disease. Inflamm Bowel Dis 2014;20(10):1708–13.

70. Dubinsky MC, Phan BL, Singh N, et al. Pharmacokinetic dashboard-recommended dosing is different than standard of care dosing in infliximab-treated pediatric IBD patients. AAPS J 2017;19(1):215–22.
71. Stein R, Lee D, Leonard MB, et al. Serum infliximab, antidrug antibodies, and tumor necrosis factor predict sustained response in pediatric Crohn's disease. Inflamm Bowel Dis 2016;22(6):1370–7.
72. Vande Casteele N, Ferrante M, Van Assche G, et al. Trough concentrations of infliximab guide dosing for patients with inflammatory bowel disease. Gastroenterology 2015;148(7):1320–9.e3.
73. Vaughn BP, Martinez-Vazquez M, Patwardhan VR, et al. Proactive therapeutic concentration monitoring of infliximab may improve outcomes for patients with inflammatory bowel disease: results from a pilot observational study. Inflamm Bowel Dis 2014;20(11):1996–2003.
74. Papamichael K, Chachu KA, Vajravelu R, et al. Improved long-term outcomes of patients with inflammatory bowel disease receiving proactive compared with reactive monitoring of serum concentrations of infliximab. Clin Gastroenterol Hepatol 2017. In Press.
75. Paul S, Roblin X, Peyrin-Biroulet L. Letter: infliximab de-escalation based on trough levels in patients with inflammatory bowel disease. Aliment Pharmacol Ther 2015;42(7):939–40.
76. Roblin X, Rinaudo M, Del Tedesco E, et al. Development of an algorithm incorporating pharmacokinetics of adalimumab in inflammatory bowel diseases. Am J Gastroenterol 2014;109(8):1250–6.
77. Yarur AJ, Jain A, Hauenstein SI, et al. Higher adalimumab levels are associated with histologic and endoscopic remission in patients with Crohn's disease and ulcerative colitis. Inflamm Bowel Dis 2016;22(2):409–15.
78. West RL, Zelinkova Z, Wolbink GJ, et al. Immunogenicity negatively influences the outcome of adalimumab treatment in Crohn's disease. Aliment Pharmacol Ther 2008;28(9):1122–6.
79. Dubinsky MC, Rosh J, Faubion WA Jr, et al. Efficacy and safety of escalation of adalimumab therapy to weekly dosing in pediatric patients with Crohn's disease. Inflamm Bowel Dis 2016;22(4):886–93.
80. Sandborn WJ, Feagan BG, Marano C, et al. Subcutaneous golimumab induces clinical response and remission in patients with moderate-to-severe ulcerative colitis. Gastroenterology 2014;146(1):85–95 [quiz: e14–5]
81. Hibi T, Imai Y, Senoo A, et al. Efficacy and safety of golimumab 52-week maintenance therapy in Japanese patients with moderate to severely active ulcerative colitis: a phase 3, double-blind, randomized, placebo-controlled study-(PURSUIT-J study). J Gastroenterol 2017.
82. Detrez I, Dreesen E, Van Stappen T, et al. Variability in golimumab exposure: a 'real-life' observational study in active ulcerative colitis. J Crohns Colitis 2016;10(5):575–81.
83. Rosario M, French JL, Dirks NL, et al. Exposure-efficacy relationships for vedolizumab induction therapy in patients with ulcerative colitis or Crohn's disease. J Crohns Colitis 2017;11(8):921–9.
84. MacDonald JK, Nguyen TM, Khanna R, et al. Anti-IL-12/23p40 antibodies for induction of remission in Crohn's disease. Cochrane Database Syst Rev 2016;(11):CD007572.
85. Feagan BG, Sandborn WJ, Gasink C, et al. Ustekinumab as induction and maintenance therapy for Crohn's disease. N Engl J Med 2016;375(20):1946–60.

86. Adedokun OJ, Xu Z, Gasink C, et al. Sa1934 pharmacokinetics and exposure-response relationships of ustekinumab during IV induction and SC maintenance treatment of patients with Crohn's disease with ustekinumab: results from the UNITI-1, UNITI-2, and IM-UNITI studies. Gastroenterology 2016;150(4):S408.

87. Steenholdt C, Brynskov J, Thomsen OO, et al. Individualised therapy is more cost-effective than dose intensification in patients with Crohn's disease who lose response to anti-TNF treatment: a randomised, controlled trial. Gut 2014; 63(6):919–27.

88. Velayos FS, Kahn JG, Sandborn WJ, et al. A test-based strategy is more cost effective than empiric dose escalation for patients with Crohn's disease who lose responsiveness to infliximab. Clin Gastroenterol Hepatol 2013;11(6):654–66.

89. Roblin X, Attar A, Lamure M, et al. Cost savings of anti-TNF therapy using a test-based strategy versus an empirical dose escalation in Crohn's disease patients who lose response to infliximab. J Mark Access Health Policy 2015;3.

90. Martelli L, Olivera P, Roblin X, et al. Cost-effectiveness of drug monitoring of anti-TNF therapy in inflammatory bowel disease and rheumatoid arthritis: a systematic review. J Gastroenterol 2017;52(1):19–25.

91. Vande Casteele N, Gils A. Pharmacokinetics of anti-TNF monoclonal antibodies in inflammatory bowel disease: adding value to current practice. J Clin Pharmacol 2015;55(Suppl 3):S39–50.

92. Guiotto C, Daperno M, Frigerio F, et al. Clinical relevance and inter-test reliability of anti-infliximab antibodies and infliximab trough levels in patients with inflammatory bowel disease. Dig Liver Dis 2016;48(2):138–43.

93. Ben-Horin S, Yavzori M, Benhar I, et al. Cross-immunogenicity: antibodies to infliximab in remicade-treated patients with IBD similarly recognise the biosimilar Remsima. Gut 2016;65(7):1132–8.

94. Gils A, Van Stappen T, Dreesen E, et al. Harmonization of infliximab and anti-infliximab assays facilitates the comparison between originators and biosimilars in clinical samples. Inflamm Bowel Dis 2016;22(4):969–75.

95. Mould DR, Dubinsky MC. Dashboard systems: pharmacokinetic/pharmacodynamic mediated dose optimization for monoclonal antibodies. J Clin Pharmacol 2015;55(Suppl 3):S51–9.

# Non-steroidal Anti-inflammatory Drugs in Newborns and Infants

Jacob V. Aranda, MD, PhD, FRCPC[a],*, Fabrizio Salomone, PhD[b], Gloria B. Valencia, MD[a], Kay D. Beharry, BS[a]

## KEYWORDS

- NSAIDs • Ibuprofen • Indomethacin • Paracetamol • Acetaminophen • Ketorolac
- Cyclooxygenases • Newborns

## KEY POINTS

- Non-steroidal anti-inflammatory drugs (NSAIDs) (indomethacin, ibuprofen) and acetaminophen are used in neonates and infants for pain and fever control, for patent ductus arteriosus closure, for prevention of intraventricular hemorrhage, and potentially for retinopathy of prematurity.
- NSAIDs inhibit cyclooxygenases (COX-1, COX-2) and peroxidases, thus, blocking prostaglandin synthesis from arachidonic acid.
- Pharmacokinetic/pharmacodynamic profiles of indomethacin, ibuprofen, and acetaminophen allow effective and safe dosing guidelines.
- Various modifications around these guidelines continue, including the route of administration (oral, rectal, intravenous), duration of therapy, rate of dosing (bolus vs continuous), and the dose itself.
- Emerging evidence that NSAIDs also inhibit caspases and cell death presents a novel target for pharmacologic interventions in neonatal diseases.

## INTRODUCTION

Non-steroidal anti-inflammatory drugs (NSAIDs) are commonly used in newborns and children as antipyretic agents to control fever; as analgesic, anti-inflammatory, and vasoactive agents to manage pain and modulate inflammation; to close a symptomatic patent ductus arteriosus (PDA)[1]; and to prevent intraventricular hemorrhage

Disclosure Statement: Supported by grant number NIH/NICHD1U54HD071594-05. J.V. Aranda received donation of Investigational Drug (Neoprofen) from Recordati S p A for the conduct of the SPIPROP Trial (ClinTrials.Gov #NCT02344225).
a State University of New York Downstate Medical Center, 450 Clarkson Avenue, Box 49, Brooklyn, NY 11203, USA; b Neonatology and Pulmonary Rare Disease Unit, Corporate Pre-Clinical R and D, Chiesi Farmaceutici S.p.A, Largo Belloli 11/A, Parma IT-43122, Italy
* Corresponding author.
*E-mail address:* jacob.aranda@downstate.edu

Pediatr Clin N Am 64 (2017) 1327–1340
http://dx.doi.org/10.1016/j.pcl.2017.08.009
0031-3955/17/© 2017 Elsevier Inc. All rights reserved.

pediatric.theclinics.com

(IVH) and, potentially, retinopathy of prematurity (ROP). This review focuses on the mechanisms shared by the various NSAIDs and their clinical pharmacology profiles in newborns and young infants. Understanding the molecular and clinical pharmacology of these commonly used drugs may aid in their rational, safe, and effective uses as well as discovery of potential clinical applications besides antipyretics, analgesia, and ductal closure.

The NSAIDs are composed of several molecular entities with diverse chemical structures but with a shared and common mechanism of action directed to arachidonic acid (AA) metabolism and the biosynthesis of prostaglandins (PGs) (**Figs. 1** and **2**). These actions result in the blockade of PG biosynthesis resulting in the known effects of NSAIDs on inflammation, analgesia, antipyretics, vasodilatation, or vasoconstriction. These common and shared pharmacologic actions are also reflected on their observed and well-known adverse effects on gastrointestinal, hematologic, renal, and other organ systems. These pharmacodynamic (PD) and adverse effects have been extensively reviewed elsewhere[2] and are not repeated here.

Inflamed tissues substantially increase PG biosynthesis. $PGE_2$ and PG prostacyclin ($PGI_2$) are the major prostanoids that mediate inflammation[3] via activation of their respective receptors, EP2 and IP receptors. Both $PGE_2$ and $PGI_2$ also decrease the threshold of nociceptor stimulation producing peripheral sensitization as well as central sensitization and increased excitability of the spinal horn neurons leading to increased pain perception.[3] $PGE_2$ can cross the blood-brain barrier and acts on its receptors on thermosensitive neurons in the hypothalamus causing fever or elevation of body temperature with increased heat generation and decreased heat loss.[3] $PGE_2$ also promotes and helps maintain vascular dilatation of the PDA.[1,4] All of these processes are modulated or inhibited by NSAIDs via blocking of the biosynthesis of $PGE_2$ and other prostanoids (see **Figs. 1** and **2**).

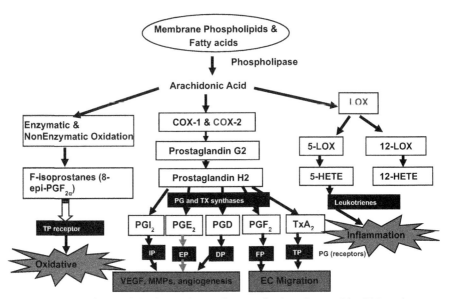

**Fig. 1.** AA metabolism and the biosynthesis of PGs and other eicosanoids. COX, cyclooxygenase; DP, Prostaglandin D Receptor; EC, endothelial cell; HETE, Hydroxyeicosatetraenoic acid; LOX, lipoxygenase; MMPs, matrix metalloproteinases; $TxA_2$, thromboxane $A_2$; VEGF, vascular endothelial growth factor.

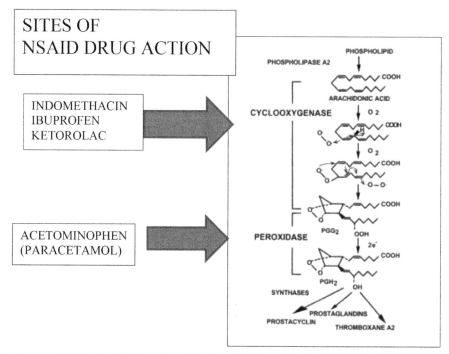

Fig. 2. Pharmacologic sites of NSAID action. (*Adapted from* Smith WL, DeWitt DL, Garavito RM. Cyclooxygenases: structural, cellular, and molecular biology. Annu Rev Biochem 2000;69:145–82.)

### *Arachidonic Acid Metabolites and Sites of Non-steroidal Anti-inflammatory Drug Action*

**Fig. 1** describes the biosynthesis of PGs and prostanoids from AA and the site of action of the NSAIDs (see **Fig. 2**). AA is a 20-carbon polyunsaturated fatty acid abundant in cell membranes phospholipids that is the precursor of a large family of bioactive compounds known as eicosanoids, including prostaglandins, thromboxane, and leukotrienes. Generally, AA is maintained at very low levels in the cell via esterification with membrane phospholipids.[5] In response to a wide variety of stimuli (physical, chemical, inflammatory, mitogenic), phospholipase $A_2$ enzyme is activated and hydrolyzes the phospholipids of the cell membranes to release AA into the cytoplasm.[6] Once released, free AA has 3 potential fates: (a) reincorporation into phospholipid, (b) diffusion outside the cell, and (c) metabolism.[7] Free AA is then converted to $PGG_2$, which is then converted by a peroxidase (POX) reaction (see **Fig. 2**) to the unstable PG endoperoxide ($PGH_2$) by cytosolic PG G/H synthase, which has cyclooxygenase (COX) and hydroperoxidase activities.[6] $PGH_2$ serves as a substrate for several cell-specific isomerases and synthases to produce biologically active PGs, $PGI_2$ and thromboxane ($TxA_2$), also known as prostanoids.[5,8] AA is also acted on by lipoxygenases, which belong to a class of non-heme iron–containing enzymes to form hydroperoxide products, leukotrienes and lipoxins, which are highly involved in inflammation, cardiovascular disease, and gastrointestinal damage,[5] and epoxygenases to form epoxyeicosatrienoic acids (cytochrome P450 metabolites). A parallel family of free radical catalyzed isomers, the isoeicosanoids, are formed by nonenzymatic peroxidation of AA[9] and are biomarkers of oxidative stress. Collectively, these lipid mediators are called eicosanoids and depend on the availability of AA. Eicosanoids regulate a wide variety of physiologic, pathologic, and cellular processes, including cell proliferation and migration, apoptosis, and metabolism.[10] They regulate constriction of blood vessels, constriction of smooth muscle, aggregation of platelets, sensitization of neurons to pain, regulation of intracellular calcium, cell division, and many other molecular events that are critical to the maintenance of physiologic homeostasis.[11] In the retina, eicosanoids and epi-eicosanoids play key roles in blood vessel responses to injury.

### Cyclooxygenase, Prostanoids, and Inhibition by Non-steroidal Anti-inflammatory Drugs

COX exists in 2 isoforms (COX-1 and COX-2) that regulate the production of prostanoids. COX enzymes are highly conserved evolutionarily and are encoded by 2 different genes. *COX-1* is constitutively expressed at high levels in cells and tissues and is the major isoform expressed in healthy tissue. It generates prostanoids for many functions, including vasomotor tone and platelet aggregation. COX-1 is present at a basal level in certain tissues, but its expression is induced in response to inflammatory and mitogenic stimuli. *COX-2* is also constitutively expressed and plays specific functions in reproduction, renal physiology, bone resorption, and neurotransmission.[12–14] COX-3 is a recently identified acetaminophen-sensitive COX isoform, highly abundant in astrocytes, endothelial cells, and pericytes, though absent in neurons.[15] It is a splice variant of the COX-1 isoform. The action of COX produces 5 biologically active prostanoids that include $PGD_2$, $PGE_2$, $PGF_{2\alpha}$, $PGI_2$, and $TxA_2$. These products act as secondary messengers by interacting with G-protein–coupled receptors.[16] Prostanoids are potent vasoconstrictors ($TxA_2$, $PGF_{2\alpha}$) or vasodilators ($PGE_2$, $PGD_2$, $PGI_2$). $TxA_2$ stimulates platelet aggregation, whereas $PGI_2$, expressed in the vascular endothelium, inhibits platelet aggregation. Released prostanoids are immediately released outside of the cell. Because they are chemically or metabolically unstable, they act only locally, near their site of production.[17] $PGE_2$ is one of the most abundant PGs produced in the body and exhibits differential biological activities via its various receptor subtypes. $PGE_2$ is synthesized from $PGH_2$ by cytosolic PGE synthase (cPGES) or microsomal PGES (mPGES) isozymes.[18] cPGES is constitutively and abundantly expressed in the cytosol of various tissues and cells, and it requires glutathione (GSH) as a cofactor.[19] After $PGE_2$ is formed, it is actively transported through the membrane by the ATP-dependent multidrug-resistance protein-4 or diffuses across the plasma membrane to act at or nearby its site of secretion.[20] $PGE_2$ then acts locally through binding one or more of its 4 receptors (EP1, EP2, EP3, and EP4).[21] EP3 and EP4 receptors are the most widely distributed with their mRNAs being expressed in almost all tissues and have the highest affinity for binding $PGE_2$. In contrast, the distribution of EP1 mRNA is restricted to certain organs. EP2 is the least abundant of the EP receptors. Both EP1 and EP2 bind $PGE_2$ with lower affinity.[22] COX-2 prefers mPGES and mPGES-derived $PGE_2$, in cooperation with vascular endothelial growth factor (VEGF), seems to play a critical role in angiogenesis and tissue remodeling,[17] thus, demonstrating a link between COX-2 and VEGF to promote angiogenesis. $PGE_2$ signaling to EP1 and EP3 receptors mediates vasoconstriction, whereas $PGE_2$ signaling to EP2 and EP4 receptors mediates vasodilation. Multiple isoforms of the EP3 receptor are generated through alternative mRNA splicing. *$PGI_2$* is one of the most important prostanoids that regulates cardiovascular homeostasis. Vascular cells, including endothelial cells, vascular smooth muscle cells (VSMCs), and endothelial progenitor cells, are the major source of $PGI_2$.[23] $PGI_2$ is generated by the action of COX, preferentially COX-2, and PGI synthase (PGIS), a member of the cytochrome P450 superfamily that specifically converts PGH2 to $PGI_2$.[17] $PGI_2$ exerts its effects locally via the IP receptor, is not stored, and is rapidly converted by nonenzymatic processes to an inactive hydrolysis product, 6-keto-PGF1$\alpha$.[24] $PGI_2$ is a potent vasodilator and an inhibitor of platelet aggregation, leukocyte adhesion, and VSMC proliferation.[25] $PGF_{2\alpha}$ is synthesized from PGH2 via PGF synthase (PGFS), and it acts via the FP receptor (FPA and FPB) to elevate the intracellular free calcium concentration to mediate vasoconstriction. $TxA_2$, an unstable AA metabolite with a half-life (t½) of about 30 seconds, is synthesized from $PGH_2$ via TXS and is nonenzymatically degraded into biologically inactive $TXB_2$.[17] $TxA_2$ is predominantly derived from platelet COX-1 but can also be produced by other cell types, including by macrophage COX-2.[26] $TxA_2$ activity is principally mediated through the TP receptor of which there are 2 splice variants, TP$\alpha$ and TP$\beta$, in humans. $TxA_2$ signaling to the TP receptor mediates several physiologic and pathophysiologic responses, including platelet adhesion and aggregation, smooth muscle contraction and proliferation, and activation of endothelial inflammatory responses.[27] $PGD_2$ is a major eicosanoid; is synthesized in both the central nervous system and peripheral tissues by 2 $PGD_2$-synthesizing enzymes, hematopoietic and lipocalin, respectively; and signals to the FP receptor to mediate vasodilation.[28] Of all prostanoids, COX-1 couples preferentially, but not exclusively, with TXS, PGFS, and the cPGES isozymes,[29] whereas COX-2 prefers PGIS and mPGES isozymes, both of which are often coinduced along with COX-2 by cytokines and tumor promoters.[9] COX-2 is the dominant source of PGs that mediate pain and inflammation, whereas COX-1 is the dominant source of PGs that maintain normal functions.[29] $PGE_1$ maintains the patency of patent ductus, and its inhibition leads to ductal constriction and closure.[30] Recently, Smith and colleagues[31] have shown that NSAIDs, such as ibuprofen, naproxen, and ketorolac, inhibit catalytic activity of cysteine-aspartic proteases (caspases) at physiologic concentrations. During inflammation, these NSAIDs inhibit caspases leading to reduced cell death and decreased proinflammatory cytokines. This novel target of NSAIDs may also lead to further modulation of inflammatory responses.[31] Familiarity with these mechanisms underlying the effects of NSAIDs in newborns optimizes their effective use and allows prediction and avoidance of expected adverse effects of these drugs as well as discovering new indications. Commonly used NSAIDs, ibuprofen, indomethacin including acetaminophen, and ketorolac, are further discussed later. Although their use for some specific indications, such as PDA closure, is a matter of intense debate, knowledge and familiarity of their pharmacologic actions and profiles promote safe and effective pharmacotherapeutics in newborns and young infants.

### Ibuprofen

Ibuprofen is an aryl propionic acid derivative used in newborns and young infants for pain and fever management and for PDA closure. Ibuprofen and acetaminophen together are the most commonly used NSAIDs in newborns and young children given via intravenous, oral, or rectal routes. Ibuprofen is a racemate, having R and S chiral enantiomers with the pharmacologic activity attributed to the S enantiomer. Its use in newborns increased following a phase 1 study showing safety and efficacy for ductal closure in preterm neonates[32] given ibuprofen lysine. Subsequent randomized trials showed increased ductal closure in ibuprofen-treated infants compared with non-treated infants, which confirmed efficacy for PDA closure with reasonable safety.[4,33,34] Ibuprofen lysine was approved by the Food and Drug Administration (FDA) for PDA closure in 2006 and ibuprofen-tromethamine (THAM) was approved by the European Medication Agency in 2004. Systematic reviews[35] and a recent meta-analysis,[37] which reviewed 33 randomized and quasi randomized studies comparing intravenous ibuprofen with oral or intravenous indomethacin, oral ibuprofen, oral or intravenous paracetamol, have shown comparable efficacy on ductal closure. Compared with indomethacin, ibuprofen is associated with less renal adverse effects.[35,36]

Ibuprofen is highly protein bound (94%) in newborns.[37] Possible bilirubin displacement from the albumin binding site is a consideration in significant hyperbilirubinemia. Ibuprofen is mainly excreted in the urine after extensive metabolism in the liver to pharmacologically inactive oxidative metabolites, hydroxyl-ibuprofen and carboxy-ibuprofen, via cytochrome P450 isoenzymes CYP2C9 and CYP2C8[38] followed by acyl-glucuronidation. However, CYP2C8 and CYP2C9 are deficient in preterm newborns, decreasing drug metabolism. Polymorphisms of these CYPs have been identified in preterm newborns; however, they do not affect ductal closure response.[39]

Pharmacokinetic (PK) studies of intravenous ibuprofen showed a delayed elimination in preterm newborns whereby plasma t½ was 22 hours with slow plasma clearance.[37] Population PK studies on ibuprofen enantiomers show a substantially prolonged t½ for S ibuprofen (t½ = 34.3 hours) compared with R ibuprofen (t½ = 8.3 hours) and a slower clearance rate for S ibuprofen (3.5 mL/h/kg) versus R ibuprofen (25.5 mL/h/kg), which increased with postnatal age.[40] The effect of the enantiomers PK profile on ductal closure and adverse effects remains to be studied because the pharmacologic effects of ibuprofen are attributed to S ibuprofen. PK studies of orally administered ibuprofen showed excellent absorption with peak plasma concentrations at 8 hours, which remained at plateau for about 24 hours.[41] PK profiles and ibuprofen plasma concentrations in 72 preterm neonates following rectal administration was similar to those following the oral route.[42]

The usual loading dose of 10 mg/kg followed by 5 mg/kg/d for 2 days was based on the initial efficacy studies, dose finding, and PK studies.[32,37,43] However, there are many practice variations in dosing around these recommendations. Ibuprofen's use in pain and fever control in newborns and young infants remains to be studied. Ibuprofen's role in modulating inflammation due to infections or noninfectious causes remains to be studied.

### Acetaminophen (paracetamol)

Acetaminophen (N-acetyl-p-aminophenol, APAP, or paracetamol) is very commonly used worldwide in young infants as an analgesic and antipyretic drug and more recently for ductal closure. It is generally preferred as an analgesic because of its better tolerance notwithstanding its weaker analgesic activity compared with other NSAIDs. Its activity is similar to selective COX-2 inhibitors, such as poor antiplatelet activity ($TxA_2$) and good gastrointestinal tolerance.[44] The mechanism by which acetaminophen inhibits COX-1, COX-2, and COX-3 (splice variant of COX-1) has been debated[44–46]; but inhibition of the POX site downstream of the cyclooxygenases (see **Fig. 2**) is well accepted. POX inhibition results in phenoxy radical formation from a critical tyrosine residue that is essential for COX resynthesis and activity.[44–46] COX depends on POX activity. However, POX is independent from COX.[16]

Oral, rectal, and intravenous acetaminophen formulations are used for management of pain in newborns and young infants from a variety of painful procedures, such as heel stick, circumcision,[47] eye examinations, postoperative pain, and others.[48] Studies to establish evidence of efficacy in newborn pain have shown inconsistent results[49] partly because of the various types of pain sources and the differences in pain assessment tools. Despite the paucity of evidence, acetaminophen in newborns and young infants remains an important pharmacologic agent for pain management.

Following the observational report of successful PDA closure in 5 preterm neonates,[50] at least 14 nonrandomized and 2 randomized trials as reviewed by Terrin and colleagues[51] were reported and collectively demonstrated that the efficacy of acetaminophen was comparable with that reported for ibuprofen.[52] Like the other NSAIDs, the efficacy of APAP partly depends on gestational and postnatal age.[53] The 2 randomized trials of oral paracetamol versus oral ibuprofen included in the review[52,53] showed equivalent efficacy and reasonable safety and also a lower risk of hyperbilirubinemia with paracetamol.[52]

### Pharmacokinetics, drug disposition, and dosing

APAP is metabolized by the liver and, to a lesser extent, the kidney and intestine. Following a therapeutic dose in adults, APAP undergoes conjugation with glucuronide (APAP- glucuronide, 52%–57% of urinary metabolites) by glucuronyl transferase (UGT1A1, UGT1A6, UGT1A9, and UGT2B15) and sulfation (APAP sulfate, 30%–44%) by sulfotransferases.[54] The same biotransformation pathway occurs in newborns, but APAP sulfation is 5.5 times higher than glucuronide formation.[55] Glucuronide conjugation increases with postnatal age and is independent of multiple drug exposure.[55] This postnatal change is expected, as sulfation is very active in the fetal liver but glucuronidation is not. A minor fraction of APAP is oxidized to a highly reactive toxic metabolite N-acetyl-p-benzoquinone imine or NAPQI (5%–10%) via CYP2E1, which has low activity in the immediate postnatal period. Less than 5% of APAP is excreted unchanged. APAP and metabolites are excreted via renal and fecal routes. NAPQI is highly reactive and is primarily responsible for acetaminophen-induced hepatotoxicity. NAPQI is detoxified by binding to the sulfhydryl group of GSH to form APAP-GSH, which is ultimately excreted in the urine as cysteine and mercapturic acid conjugates. Despite increasing use of APAP in the preterm, very few toxicities have been reported, which may be attributed to low activity of the cytochromes P450 in the immediate postnatal thereby minimizing formation of the toxic metabolite NAPQI. However, there are toxicity reports of APAP in newborn and young infants; these were treated successfully with N-acetyl cysteine.[56,57]

The PK/PD profiles of APAP following a single dose or multiple doses have been described in preterm and term newborns.[58,59] The serum t½ was 4.6 hours in preterm infants and 2.9 hours in term infants, with slower drug clearance rates in preterm neonates. Population PK modeling in preterm and term newborns showed that body weight predicted the APAP PK profile.[60] From the published PK data, a suggested dose regimen of intravenous APAP in neonates and infants at gestational ages of 32 to 44 weeks is a loading dose of 20 mg/kg (or 2 mL/kg) followed by a maintenance dose of 10 mg/kg (or 1 mL/kg) every 6 hours.[61] This dose would achieve steady-state plasma concentrations associated with reasonable analgesia. In older infants, the suggested dose is 15 mg/kg (or 1.5 mL/kg) every 6 hours.[61] The interval between 2 maintenance doses should be increased up to 12 hours if the neonates' gestational age is between 28 and 31 weeks.[61] Rectally administered APAP has variable absorption, and the usual dose of 20 mg/kg rectally achieves low subtherapeutic plasma concentrations.[62–65]

### Indomethacin

Indomethacin is a methylated indole acetic acid derivative approved by the FDA for closure of PDA in preterm newborns in 1985. Currently, it is not usually used for fever or analgesia but mainly for PDA closure and prevention of IVH. Following initial observational studies of PDA closure in 6 neonates given indomethacin,[66] subsequent controlled trials showed higher PDA closure in treated neonates compared with placebo.[67,68] Indomethacin also decreased the risk of IVH compared with placebo-treated neonates.[68–70] Meta-analyses confirmed efficacy on ductal closure but with significant renal, gastrointestinal, hematologic, and other adverse effects.[2,71] Prophylactic indomethacin has short-term benefits for preterm infants, including a reduction in the incidence of symptomatic PDA, PDA surgical ligation, and severe IVH. However, there is no evidence of an effect on mortality or neurodevelopment.[68]

Indomethacin has been administered via intravenous, oral, or rectal routes. Oral indomethacin is poorly absorbed, with only 20% bioavailability.[72] It is highly protein bound (98%); but because of relatively small doses, the drug is unlikely to achieve plasma drug concentrations that may produce bilirubin displacement.[73] Indomethacin undergoes metabolism via O-demethylation followed by N-deacylation[74] producing desmethyl, desbenzoyl, and desmethyl-desbenzoyl metabolites and their respective conjugates along with acid labile p-chlorobenzoic acid.[75] At least 58% of newborn infants demethylate indomethacin; half of the unchanged and demethylated drug was found as conjugates in urine; 14% deacylated the drug. Indomethacin is slowly eliminated by newborn infants compared with adults.[76–79] The drug elimination t½ is about 20 hours,[79] ranging from 10 to 25 hours, which is 3 times longer than adults, with slow clearance rates that are about 7 times slower than adults. Drug elimination significantly depends on gestational age.

Usual dosing is an initial 0.2 mg/kg intravenously followed by 0.1 mg/kg/d intravenously for at least 2 days. However, there have been many variations around dosing regimens, including continuous versus bolus infusions, short (<3 days) or longer treatment (>4 days), and even higher doses[80] with increased ROP risk associated with increased dose.[81] Sufficient pharmacologic data allow dose manipulations targeted to a desired plasma drug concentration, which remains debatable.

### Ketorolac

*Ketorolac tromethamine* is a racemic mixture of (-)S- and (+)R-enantiomeric forms in equal portions with pharmacologic activity almost all attributed to S ketorolac. In newborns and young infants (<6 months of age), ketorolac is used mainly for analgesia following congenital heart surgery,[82,83] abdominal surgery, and other pain sources.[84] Ketorolac eye drops have been suggested to potentially prevent ROP.[85–87] Avila-Vazquez and colleagues[85] treated 59 neonates with ketorolac eye drops and had significantly fewer babies with ROP compared with a historical control. Although far from establishing efficacy for ROP prevention, 2 studies in preterm newborns showed that ocular ketorolac was not associated with any adverse effects.[85,80] More recently, Aranda and colleagues[87] have shown that ocular ketorolac exerts a synergistic pharmacologic effect with caffeine in preventing oxygen-induced retinopathy in the neonatal rat model exposed to intermittent hypoxia akin to a newborn baby with frequent oxygen desaturation or apnea.

The PK/PD profile of ketorolac in newborn and young infants in the first few postnatal days and weeks remains to be studied. Zuppa and colleagues[88] reported the population PK profile of ketorolac (0.5 mg/kg) in 3 neonates and 9 infants aged 0.4 to 32.0 weeks. The plasma clearance (2.6 mL/kg/min) in these infants was greater than older children and adults,[88] which has been described with other drugs. In children aged 4 to 8 years given 0.5 mg/kg of ketorolac intravenously, the plasma t½ was 6.1 hours with a mean plasma clearance of 0.70 mL/kg/min.[89]

Ketorolac ocular PK in newborn infants has not yet been studied. However, the ocular PK/PD in neonatal rats showed that ocular ketorolac eye drops were rapidly transferred (within 1 hour) into the systemic circulation and other ocular tissues, including the lens and the choroid and posterior segment of the eyes (Aranda and colleagues unpublished data, 2015), and inhibited $PGE_1$ plasma levels. Ketorolac is highly protein bound (99%) and, therefore, should be carefully used when hyperbilirubinemia is present. In adults, ketorolac has excellent bioavailability (100%), undergoes hepatic metabolism via hydroxylation and conjugation, and is excreted mainly in urine (92%) as drug metabolites (40%) and unchanged parent drug (60%).[90,91]

The PK profile of the R(+) and S(−) racemates differs; because the pharmacologic effect is exclusively due to the S enantiomer, the PK differences would impact on the drug action. Hayball and colleagues[92] administered a bolus intramuscular injection of 30 mg/kg of ketorolac racemate to 4 young, healthy volunteers and showed a twice greater volume of distribution at steady state of S(−) ketorolac compared with R(+) ketorolac and the shorter t½ of S(−) compared with R(+) ketorolac (2.3 ±0.2 hours and 3.6 ±0.7 hours, $P = .03$). These data indicate that the distribution of ketorolac is enantioselective in men as well as in pregnant and postpartum women.[93] Like ibuprofen, there is no inversion of R(+) form to S(−) form in adult humans and is unlikely to occur in the newborn. Kauffman and colleagues[94] showed that the plasma clearance of racemic ketorolac in 50 children aged 3 to 18 years was 2 times faster than adults. Plasma t½ was 4 hours and clearance was 1.1 mL/min/kg. The plasma clearance of the S(−) enantiomer was 4 times that of the R(+) enantiomer. Terminal t½ of S(−) ketorolac was 40% that of the R(+) enantiomer, and the apparent volume of distribution of the S(−) enantiomer was greater than that of the R(+) form. Recovery of S(−) ketorolac glucuronide was 2.3 times greater than R(+) enantiomer.[94] PK behavior of these enantiomers in the newborn needs to be defined.

Ketorolac is yet a poorly studied drug in newborns and young infants. The role of this drug in pain management and in prevention of ROP deserves to be explored more intensely to establish the rational and appropriate dose guidelines based on PK/PD and other requisite studies. Discovery of a safe and effective dose and appropriate formulation will allow for required clinical trials to establish efficacy and safety.

## SUMMARY AND FUTURE DIRECTIONS

NSAIDs and acetaminophen are commonly used in infants and newborns for pain and fever control, for pharmacologic closure of the PDA, and prevention of IVH. They are also being evaluated for potential use in the prevention of ROP. NSAIDs and acetaminophen inhibit COX-1, COX-2, and POX, thus, blocking and decreasing PG synthesis from AA. PGs are part of the eicosanoids, which regulate a wide variety of physiologic, pathologic, and cellular processes, including cell proliferation and migration, apoptosis, and metabolism. They regulate constriction of blood vessels, constriction of smooth muscle, aggregation of platelets, sensitization of neurons to pain, regulation of intracellular calcium, cell division, and many other molecular events that are critical to the maintenance of physiologic homeostasis. In the retina, eicosanoids and epi-eicosanoids play key roles in blood vessel responses to injury. Emerging evidence that NSAIDs also inhibit caspases and cell death presents a novel target for pharmacologic interventions in neonatal diseases. Although their use for specific indications (eg, PDA) remains a matter of intense and heated debate, familiarity of the clinical pharmacology profiles of indomethacin, ibuprofen, acetaminophen, and ketorolac allow relatively effective and safe dosing guidelines. However, various modifications around these guidelines continue, including route of administration, duration of therapy, rate of dosing (bolus vs continuous), and the dose itself. Studies on the efficacy and safety of ocular NSAID (ketorolac) for prevention of retinopathy of prematurity are ongoing. The opioid-sparing effects of NSAIDs need to be studied further to minimize neonatal exposure to opiates while providing pain control. Pharmacologic synergisms with other drugs like caffeine should be studied further. Increasing knowledge of how these molecular entities work may foster and promote targeted development and rational, safe, effective, and intelligent uses of these drugs to prevent or minimize neonatal morbidities and improve long-term outcomes.

## REFERENCES

1. Liebowitz M, Clyman RI. Prophylactic indomethacin compared with delayed conservative management of the patent ductus arteriosus in extremely preterm infants: effects on neonatal outcomes. J Pediatr 2017;187:119–26.e1.
2. Johnston PG, Gillam-Krakauer M, Fuller MP, et al. Evidence-based use of indomethacin and ibuprofen in the neonatal intensive care unit. Clin Perinatol 2012; 39:111–36.
3. Grosser T, Smyth E, Fitzgerald GA. Anti-inflammatory, antipyretic and analgesic agents: pharmacotherapy of gout. Chapter 34. In: Brunton L, Chabner B, Knollman B, editors. Goodman and Gilman- The pharmacologic basis of therapeutics. 12th edition. McGraw Hill Professionals; 2011.
4. Aranda JV, Clyman R, Cox B, et al. A randomized, double-blind, placebo-controlled trial on intravenous ibuprofen L-lysine for the early closure of nonsymptomatic patent ductus arteriosus within 72 hours of birth in extremely low-birth-weight infants. Am J Perinatol 2009;26:235–45.
5. Rao PNP, Knaus EE. Evolution of nonsteroidal anti-inflammatory drugs (NSAIDs): cyclooxygenase (COX) inhibition and beyond. J Pharm Pharm Sci 2008;11(2): 81s–110s.
6. FitzGerald GA, Patrono C. The coxibs, selective inhibitors of cyclooxygenase-2. N Engl J Med 2001;345(6):433–42.
7. Rink C, Khanna S. Significance of brain tissue oxygenation and the arachidonic acid cascade in stroke. Antioxid Redox Signal 2011;14:1889–903.
8. Mendes RT, Stanczyk CP, Sordi R, et al. Selective inhibition of cyclooxygenase-2: risks and benefits. Rev Bras Reumatol 2012;52:767–82.
9. Smyth EM, Grosser T, Wang M, et al. Prostanoids in health and disease. J Lipid Res 2009;50(Suppl):S423–8.
10. Yui K, Imataka G, Nakamura H, et al. Eicosanoids derived from arachidonic acid and their family prostaglandins and cyclooxygenase in psychiatric disorders. Curr Neuropharmacol 2015;13:776–85.
11. Harris RE, Beebe J, Alshafie GA. Reduction in cancer risk by selective and nonselective cyclooxygenase-2 (COX-2) inhibitors. J Exp Pharmacol 2012;4: 91–6.
12. Lim H, Paria BC, Das SK, et al. Multiple female reproductive failures in cyclooxygenase-2 deficient mice. Cell 1997;91:197–208.
13. Cheng HF, Wang JL, Zhang MZ, et al. Angiotensin II attenuates renal cortical cyclooxygenase-2 expression. J Clin Invest 1999;103:953–61.
14. Breder CD, DeWitt DL, Kraig RP. Characterization of inducible cyclooxygenase in rat brain. J Comp Neurol 1995;355:296–315.
15. Chandrasekharan NV, Dai H, Roos KL, et al. COX-3, a cyclooxygenase-1 variant inhibited by acetaminophen and other analgesic=antipyretic drugs: cloning, structure, and expression. Proc Natl Acad Sci U S A 2002;99:13926–31.
16. Smith WL, DeWitt DL, Garavito RM. Cyclooxygenases: structural, cellular, and molecular biology. Annu Rev Biochem 2000;69:145–82.
17. Narumiya S, FitzGerald GA. Genetic and pharmacological analysis of prostanoid receptor function. J Clin Invest 2001;108(1):25–30.

18. Samuelsson B, Morgenstern R, Jakobsson PJ. Membrane prostaglandin E synthase-1: a novel therapeutic target. Pharmacol Rev 2007;59:207–24.

19. Tanioka T, Nakatani Y, Semmyo N, et al. Molecular identification of cytosolic prostaglandin E2 synthase that is functionally coupled with cyclooxygenase 1 in immediate prostaglandin E2 biosynthesis. J Biol Chem 2000;275:32775–82.

20. Park JY, Pillinger MH, Abramson SB. Prostaglandin E2 synthesis and secretion: the role of PGE2 synthases. Clin Immunol 2006;119:229–40.

21. Trebino CE, Stock JL, Gibbons CP, et al. Impaired inflammatory and pain responses in mice lacking an inducible prostaglandin E synthase. Proc Natl Acad Sci U S A 2003;100:9044–9.

22. Sugimoto Y, Narumiya S. Prostaglandin E receptors. J Biol Chem 2007;282: 11613–7.

23. Kawabe J, Ushikubi F, Hasebe N. Prostacyclin in vascular diseases. Circ J 2010; 74:836–43.

24. Wu KK, Liou JY. Cellular and molecular biology of prostacyclin synthase. Biochem Biophys Res Commun 2005;338:45–52.

25. Noda M, Kariura Y, Pannasch U, et al. Neuroprotective role of bradykinin because of the attenuation of pro-inflammatory cytokine release from activated microglia. J Neurochem 2007;101:397–410.

26. Félétou M, Verbeuren TJ, Vanhoutte PM. Endothelium-dependent contractions in SHR: a tale of prostanoid TP and IP receptors. Br J Pharmacol 2009;156:563–74.

27. Nakahata N. The thromboxane/endoperoxide receptor (TP): the common villain. Thromboxane A2: physiology/pathophysiology, cellular signal transduction and pharmacology. Pharmacol Ther 2008;118:18–35.

28. Herlong JL, Scott TR. Positioning prostanoids of the D and J series in the immunopathogenic scheme. Immunol Lett 2006;102:121–31.

29. Rudic RD, Brinster D, Cheng Y. COX-2-derived prostacyclin modulates vascular remodeling. Circ Res 2005;96:1240–7.

30. Heymann MA, Berman W Jr, Rudolph AM, et al. Dilatation of the ductus arteriosus by prostaglandin E1 in aortic arch abnormalities. Circulation 1979;59:169–73.

31. Smith CE, Soti S, Jones TA, et al. Non-steroidal anti-inflammatory drugs are caspase inhibitors. Cell Chem Biol 2017;24:281–92.

32. Varvarigou A, Bardin CL, Beharry K, et al. Early ibuprofen administration to prevent patent ductus arteriosus in premature newborn infants. JAMA 1996;275: 539–44.

33. Van Overmeire B, Allegaert K, Casaer A, et al. Prophylactic ibuprofen in premature infants: a multicentre, randomised, double-blind, placebo-controlled trial. Lancet 2004;364(9449):1945–9.

34. Gournay V, Roze JC, Kuster A, et al. Prophylactic ibuprofen versus placebo in very premature infants: a randomised, double-blind, placebo-controlled trial. Lancet 2004;364(9449):1939–44.

35. Aranda JV, Thomas R. Systematic review: intravenous ibuprofen in preterm newborns. Semin Perinatol 2006;30:114–20.

36. Ohlsson A, Walia R, Shah SS. Ibuprofen for the treatment of patent ductus arteriosus in preterm or low birth weight (or both) infants. Cochrane Database Syst Rev 2015;(2):CD003481.

37. Aranda JV, Varvarigou A, Beharry K, et al. Pharmacokinetics and protein binding of intravenous ibuprofen in the premature newborn infant. Acta Paediatr 1997;86: 289–93.

38. Brocks DR, Jamali F. The pharmacokinetics of ibuprofen in humans and animals. Chapter 4. In: Rainsford KD, editor. Ibuprofen a critical bibliographic review. Boca Ratal (FL): CRC Press. Taylor & Francis Group; 1999. p. 87–142.

39. Durrmeyer X, Hovhannisyan S, Medard Y, et al. Are cytochrome P450 CYP2C8 and CYP2C9 polymorphisms associated with ibuprofen response in very preterm infants? PLoS One 2010;5(8):e12329.

40. Gregoire N, Desfrere L, Roze JC, et al. Population pharmacokinetic analysis of Ibuprofen enantiomers in preterm newborn infants. J Clin Pharmacol 2008;48: 1460–8.

41. Barzilay B, Youngster I, Batash D, et al. Pharmacokinetics of oral ibuprofen for patent ductus arteriosus closure in preterm infants. Arch Dis Child Fetal Neonatal Ed 2012;97:F116–9.

42. Demir N, Peker E, Ece İ, et al. Efficacy and safety of rectal ibuprofen for patent ductus arteriosus closure in very low birth weight preterm infants. J Matern Fetal Neonatal Med 2017;25:1–10.

43. Desfrere L, Zohar S, Morville P, et al. Dose-finding study of ibuprofen in patent ductus arteriosus using the continual reassessment method. J Clin Pharm Ther 2005;30:121–32.

44. Graham GG, Davies MJ, Day RO, et al. The modern pharmacology of paracetamol: therapeutic actions, mechanism of action, metabolism, toxicity and recent pharmacological findings. Inflammopharmacology 2013;21:201–32.

45. Karthein R, Dietz R, Wolfgang-Nastainczyk W, et al. Higher oxidation states of prostaglandin H synthase EPR study of a transient tyrosyl radical in the enzyme during the peroxidase reaction. Eur J Biochem 1988;171:313–20.

46. Aronoff DM, Oates JA, Boutaud O. New insights into the mechanism of action of acetaminophen: its clinical pharmacologic characteristics reflect its inhibition of the two prostaglandin H2 synthases. Clin Pharmacol Ther 2006;79:9–19.

47. Howard CR, Howard FM, Weitzman ML. Acetaminophen analgesia in neonatal circumcision: the effect on pain. Pediatrics 1994;93:641–6.

48. van Lingen RA, Quak CM, Deinum HT, et al. Effects of rectally administered paracetamol on infants delivered by vacuum extraction. Eur J Obstet Gynecol Reprod Biol 2001;94:73–8.

49. Ohlsson A, Shah PS. Paracetamol (acetaminophen) for prevention or treatment of pain in newborns. Cochrane Database Syst Rev 2016;(10):CD011219.

50. Hammerman C, Bin-Nun A, Markovitch E, et al. Ductal closure with paracetamol: a surprising new approach to patent ductus arteriosus treatment. Pediatrics 2011;128:e1618–21.

51. Terrin G, Conte F, Oncel MY, et al. Paracetamol for the treatment of patent ductus arteriosus in preterm neonates: a systematic review and meta-analysis. Arch Dis Child Fetal Neonatal Ed 2016;101:F127–36.

52. Dang D, Wang D, Zhang C, et al. Comparison of oral paracetamol versus ibuprofen in premature infants with patent ductus arteriosus: a randomized controlled trial. PLoS One 2013;8:e77888.

53. Oncel MY, Yurttutan S, Erdeve O, et al. Oral paracetamol versus oral ibuprofen in the management of patent ductus arteriosus in preterm infants: a randomized controlled trial. J Pediatr 2014;164(3):510–4.e1.

54. Acetaminophen pathway. Available at: https://www.pharmgkb.org/pathway/PA165986279. Accessed April 15, 2017.

55. Krekels EH, van Ham S, Allegaert K, et al. Developmental changes rather than repeated administration drive paracetamol glucuronidation in neonates and infants. Eur J Clin Pharmacol 2015;71:1075–82.

56. Beringer RM, Thompson JP, Parry S, et al. Intravenous paracetamol overdose: two case reports and a change to national treatment guidelines. Arch Dis Child 2011;96:307 8.
57. Walls L, Baker CF, Sarkar S. Acetaminophen-induced hepatic failure with encephalopathy in a newborn. J Perinatol 2007;27:133–5.
58. Allegaert K, Van der Marel CD, Debeer A, et al. Pharmacokinetics of single dose intravenous propacetamol in neonates: effect of gestational age. Arch Dis Child Fetal Neonatal Ed 2004;89:F25–8.
59. Palmer GM, Atkins M, Anderson BJ, et al. I.V. acetaminophen pharmacokinetics in neonates after multiple doses. Br J Anaesth 2008;101:523–30.
60. Cook SF, Roberts JK, Samiee-Zafarghandy S, et al. Population pharmacokinetics of intravenous paracetamol (acetaminophen) in preterm and term neonates: model development and external evaluation. Clin Pharmacokinet 2016;55: 107–19.
61. Veyckemans F, Anderson BJ, Wolf AR, et al. Intravenous paracetamol dosage in the neonate and small infant. Br J Anaesth 2014;112(2):380–1.
62. van Lingen RA, Deinum JT, Quak JM, et al. Pharmacokinetics and metabolism of rectally administered paracetamol in preterm neonates. Arch Dis Child Fetal Neonatal Ed 1999;80:F59–63.
63. Hansen TG, O'Brien K, Morton NS, et al. Plasma paracetamol concentrations and pharmacokinetics following rectal administration in neonates and young infants. Acta Anaesthesiol Scand 1999;43:855–9.
64. Lin YC, Sussman HH, Benitz WE. Plasma concentrations after rectal administration of acetaminophen in preterm neonates. Paediatr Anaesth 1997;7:457–9.
65. van Lingen RA, Deinum HT, Quak CM, et al. Multiple-dose pharmacokinetics of rectally administered acetaminophen in term infants. Clin Pharmacol Ther 1999; 66:509–15.
66. Friedman WF, Hirschklau MJ, Printz MP, et al. Pharmacologic closure of patent ductus arteriosus in the premature infant. N Engl J Med 1976;295:526–9.
67. Gersony WM, Peckham GJ, Ellison RC, et al. Effects of indomethacin in premature infants with patent ductus arteriosus: results of a national collaborative study. J Pediatr 1983;102:895–906.
68. Schmidt B, Davis P, Moddemann D, et al, Trial of Indomethacin Prophylaxis in Preterms Investigators. Long-term effects of indomethacin prophylaxis in extremely-low-birth-weight infants. N Engl J Med 2001;344:1966–72.
69. Ment LR, Oh W, Ehrenkranz RA, et al. Low-dose indomethacin and prevention of intraventricular hemorrhage: a multicenter randomized trial. Pediatrics 1994;93: 543–50.
70. Ment LR, Duncan CC, Ehrenkranz RA, et al. Randomized indomethacin trial for prevention of intraventricular hemorrhage in very low birth weight infants. J Pediatr 1985;107:937–43.
71. Fowlie PW, Davis PG, McGuire W. Prophylactic intravenous indomethacin for preventing mortality and morbidity in preterm infants. Cochrane Database Syst Rev 2010;(7):CD000174.
72. Evans M, Bhat R, Vidyasagar D, et al. A comparison of oral and intravenous indomethacin dispositions in the premature infant with patent ductus arteriosus. Pediatr Pharmacol 1981;1:251–8.
73. Bhat R, Vidyasagar D, Vadapalli M, et al. Disposition of indomethacin in preterm infants. J Pediatr 1979;95:313–6.
74. Duggan DE, Hogans AF, Kwan KC, et al. The metabolism of indomethacin in man. J Pharmacol Exp Ther 1972;181:563–75.

75. Friedman CA, Temple DM, Wender DF, et al. Metabolism and disposition of indomothaoin in protorm infanto. Dov Pharmacol Ther 1991;17:1–7.
76. Wiest DB, Pinson JB, Gal PS, et al. Population pharmacokinetics of intravenous indomethacin in neonates with symptomatic patent ductus arteriosus. Clin Pharmacol Ther 1991;49:550–7.
77. Yaffe SJ, Friedman WF, Rogers D, et al. The disposition of indomethacin in preterm babies. J Pediatr 1980;97:1001–6.
78. Bhat R, Vidyasagar D, Fisher E, et al. Pharmacokinetics of oral and intravenous indomethacin in preterm infants. Dev Pharmacol Ther 1980;1:101–10.
79. Thalji AA, Carr I, Yeh TF, et al. Pharmacokinetics of intravenously administered indomethacin in premature infants. J Pediatr 1980;97:995–1000.
80. Sperandio M, Beedgen B, Feneberg R, et al. Effectiveness and side effects of an escalating, stepwise approach to indomethacin treatment for symptomatic patent ductus arteriosus in premature infants below 33 weeks of gestation. Pediatrics 2005;116:1361–6.
81. Jegatheesan P, Ianus V, Buchh B, et al. Increased indomethacin dosing for persistent patent ductus arteriosus in preterm infants: a multicenter, randomized, controlled trial. J Pediatr 2008;153:183–9.
82. Gupta A, Daggett C, Drant S, et al. Prospective randomized trial of ketorolac after congenital heart surgery. J Cardiothorac Vasc Anesth 2004;18:454–7.
83. Dawkins TN, Barclay CA, Gardiner RL, et al. Safety of intravenous use of ketorolac in infants following cardiothoracic surgery. Cardiol Young 2009;19:105–8.
84. Aldrink JH, Ma M, Wang W, et al. Safety of ketorolac in surgical neonates and infants 0 to 3 months old. J Pediatr Surg 2011;46:1081–5.
85. Avila-Vazquez M, Maffrand R, Sosa M, et al. Treatment of retinopathy of prematurity with topical ketorolac tromethamine: a preliminary study. BMC Pediatr 2004;4:15.
86. Giannantonio C, Papacci P, Purcaro V, et al. Effectiveness of ketorolac tromethamine in prevention of severe retinopathy of prematurity. J Pediatr Ophthalmol Strabismus 2011;48:247–51.
87. Aranda JV, Cai CL, Ahmad T, et al. Pharmacologic synergism of ocular ketorolac and systemic caffeine citrate in rat oxygen-induced retinopathy. Pediatr Res 2016;80:554–65.
88. Zuppa AF, Mondick JT, Davis L, et al. Population pharmacokinetics of ketorolac in neonates and young infants. Am J Ther 2009;16:143–6.
89. Olkkola KT, Maunuksela EL. The pharmacokinetics of postoperative intravenous ketorolac tromethamine in children. Br J Clin Pharmacol 1991;31:182–4.
90. Brocks DR, Jamali F. Clinical pharmacokinetics of ketorolac tromethamine. Clin Pharmacokinet 1992;23:415–27.
91. Mroszczak EJ, Jung D, Yee J, et al. Ketorolac tromethamine pharmacokinetics and metabolism after intravenous, intramuscular, and oral administration in humans and animals. Pharmacotherapy 1990;10(6 Pt 2):33S–9S.
92. Hayball PJ, Wrobel J, Tamblyn JG, et al. The pharmacokinetics of ketorolac enantiomers following intramuscular administration of the racemate. Br J Clin Pharmacol 1994;37:75–8.
93. Kulo A, Smits A, Maleškić S, et al. Enantiomer-specific ketorolac pharmacokinetics in young women, including pregnancy and postpartum period. Bosn J Basic Med Sci 2017;17:54–60.
94. Kauffman RE, Lieh-Lai MW, Uy HG, et al. Enantiomer-selective pharmacokinetics and metabolism of ketorolac in children. Clin Pharmacol Ther 1999;65:382–8.

# Metformin Use in Children and Adolescents with Prediabetes

Aditi Khokhar, MBBS[a], Vatcharapan Umpaichitra, MD[b],
Vivian L. Chin, MD[b], Sheila Perez-Colon, MD[b],*

## KEYWORDS

- Metformin • Prediabetes • Obesity • Insulin resistance • Children • Adolescents

## KEY POINTS

- Early recognition and treatment of prediabetes may prevent development of type 2 diabetes.
- Clinicians consider pharmacologic intervention including metformin therapy for treatment of prediabetes when lifestyle interventions are not successful.
- There are few data in children regarding metformin therapy in diabetes prevention.
- The long-term effects of metformin have not been studied in the pediatric population.

## INTRODUCTION

Prediabetes is a state of higher than normal blood sugar levels that does not fall within the diabetes range. There is a strong association between prediabetes in childhood and the development of diabetes in young adulthood.[1] The prevalence of prediabetes among adolescents has increased.[2] It is important for physicians to identify prediabetes in obese youth for early introduction of lifestyle modifications and pharmacologic interventions when indicated. Metformin, a biguanide derivate, is the first line of pharmacologic treatment for type 2 diabetes mellitus (T2DM), in conjunction with lifestyle modifications.[3] Metformin therapy improves insulin sensitivity, as shown by a reduction in fasting plasma glucose and insulin concentrations.[4] This article focuses on

Support: No funding was sought or obtained for this review, and the authors had no conflict of interest or personal gain during its completion.
Financial Disclosure: None.
Conflicts of Interest: None.
[a] Division of Pediatric Endocrinology, Department of Pediatrics, SUNY Upstate Medical University, 3229 East Genesee Street, Syracuse, NY 13214, USA; [b] Division of Pediatric Endocrinology, Department of Pediatrics, SUNY Downstate Medical Center and Kings County Hospital Center, 445 Lenox Road, Box 49, Brooklyn, NY 11203, USA
* Corresponding author.
E-mail address: sheila.perez-colon@downstate.edu

the mechanism of action of metformin, including evidence supporting its clinical use, and its safety profile in obese prediabetic children and adolescents.

## SCREENING FOR DIABETES

Obesity is increasing worldwide and is a major risk factor for metabolic and cardiovascular morbidities. Data suggest that 16.9% of the youth in the United States are obese.[5] The increasing prevalence of obesity has led to an increased incidence of comorbidities like insulin resistance, hypertension, dyslipidemia, and T2DM.[6,7] The American Diabetes Association[8] recommends diabetes screening in asymptomatic overweight and obese (body mass index [BMI] >85th percentile for age and sex, weight for height >85th percentile, or weight >120% of ideal for height) children and adolescents, who have 2 of the following risk factors: (1) first- or second-degree relative with T2DM, (2) minority race/ethnicity, (3) signs of insulin resistance (acanthosis nigricans) or comorbidities (hypertension, dyslipidemia, polycystic ovarian syndrome), or (4) mother with diabetes or gestational diabetes during child's gestation.

## PREDIABETES DEFINITION

The American Diabetes Association defines prediabetes (category for increased risk of diabetes) as impaired fasting glucose, which is a fasting plasma glucose of 100 to 125 mg/dL (5.6–6.9 mmol/L), or impaired glucose tolerance, which is a 2-hour plasma glucose after 75 g of oral glucose intake of 140 to 199 mg/dL (7.8–11.0 mmol/L), or glycated hemoglobin (HbA1c) of 5.7% to 6.4% (39–46 mmol/mol).[9]

## PROGRESSION OF PREDIABETES TO DIABETES

The rate of progression of prediabetes to overt diabetes has been assessed to be 5% to 10% annually.[10] Besides being a precursor for development of diabetes, prediabetes itself has been associated with the development of microvascular and macrovascular complications.[11,12] The prevalence of microalbuminuria and polyneuropathy is slightly increased in patients with prediabetes compared with individuals with normoglycemia.[13,14] Once detected, prediabetes is managed with lifestyle modifications and, when needed, medication to prevent or aim to slow the transition to diabetes. Prediabetic individuals have been shown to revert to normoglycemia with a reduced risk of diabetes development after lifestyle and drug-based interventions.[15–17] Early identification of prediabetes can help to adequately direct the resources and interventions toward the patients at greatest risk for developing diabetes.

## HISTORY OF BIGUANIDES

Chemically, biguanides are composed of 2 guanidine groups joined together with the loss of ammonia. There is evidence of biguanide use in medieval Europe in the form of a herb *Galega officinalis*, commonly referred to as goat's-rue or French lilac.[18] Guanidine, the active component of *G officinalis*, was used to synthesize several antidiabetic compounds in the early 19th century, but was found to be toxic. Diguanides (synthalin A and synthalin B), composed of 2 guanidines connected by an alkyl chain, were used clinically for a short time, but marked toxicity was noted quite quickly. The 2 main biguanides, metformin and phenformin, were introduced into clinical practice in 1957; however, phenformin was withdrawn from several countries 2 decades later after recognizing its association with lactic acidosis.[19,20] Metformin continues to be used as a major oral antidiabetic medication all over the world given the impressive safety record of the drug.[21]

## MECHANISM OF ACTION OF METFORMIN

The mechanism of action of metformin is still not completely understood and is an area of active research. Two important drug sites of action that have been described include mitochondrial oxygen consumption reduction and adenosine monophosphate (AMP) activation.

Metformin requires transporters to cross membranes. It enters hepatocytes through the organic cation transporter-1 (OCT-1). Metformin can alter mitochondrial function by inhibiting complex I in the mitochondrial electron transport chain.[22] This results in insufficient flux of adenosine triphosphate required to drive energy-consuming hepatic gluconeogenesis.[23] The magnitude of inhibition of gluconeogenesis is correlated with the extent of inhibition of the respiratory chain.[24] This is an important mechanism described through which metformin lowers fasting plasma glucose concentrations.[4] It is not clear whether or not complex I is the only mitochondrial target of metformin. Lactic acidosis, a rare side effect of metformin, can be explained by the medication's effect on mitochondrial and respiratory chain inhibition, which results in accumulation of lactate from glycolysis. Compared with other biguanides such as phenformin and buformin, lactic acidosis is observed less commonly with metformin therapy.[25] This could be explained by the self-limiting mitochondrial inhibition with metformin because it depends on the mitochondria being active.[24]

The other proposed mechanism of action of metformin is via increased 5′ AMP-activated protein kinase activation, which increases peripheral glucose use and fatty acid oxidation in the skeletal muscle, and inhibition of lipid synthesis in the liver.[26] The 5′ AMP-activated protein kinase is a nutrient and energy sensor that maintains energy homeostasis.[27]

Metformin is not metabolized and is excreted in the urine and bile in an unmodified form. The pharmacokinetics of metformin are determined by its active transport by key transporters including plasma membrane monoamine transporter and OCT.[28,29] Plasma membrane monoamine transporter mediates its intestinal absorption, whereas OCT1 and OCT3 transport metformin into the hepatocytes. Multidrug and toxic compound extrusion 1 transports it out from hepatocytes into the bile and finally, OCT2 moves it into the renal tubular epithelial cells, and multidrug and toxic compound extrusion 2 into the renal tubule.[23]

## PREDIABETES TREATMENT

The benefits of lifestyle intervention for weight loss in obesity and for prevention of T2DM are well-established.[30,31] However, at times, lifestyle intervention alone is not successful and physicians have to consider pharmacologic strategies. Several groups of antidiabetic drugs such as biguanides, thiazolidinediones, α-glucosidase inhibitors, glucagon like peptide 1 analogues, and other categories of drugs and therapies such as antiobesity drugs and bariatric surgery have been studied in context of prediabetes in adults. Metformin is the only drug that has been evaluated in formal clinical trials in children.[32] It is approved by the US Food and Drug Administration for use in children (age 10 years and older) for the treatment of T2DM.[33] Results from large, randomized, clinical trials in the adult population support the efficacy of metformin in diabetes prevention.[17,30,34] The use of metformin in nondiabetic obese adults has been demonstrated to cause reduced food intake and weight loss, with reduction in fasting plasma glucose, cholesterol, and insulin concentrations.[35,36] Although the endpoint of the studies performed in the pediatric population was not diabetes prevention, metformin use has been shown to improve metabolic parameters such as BMI, body fat composition, fasting glucose and insulin, HbA1c, insulin resistance index

(Homeostatic Model Assessment for Insulin Resistance [HOMA-IR]), blood pressure, and lipid profile in children

Freemark and colleagues[37] were the first to conduct a 6-month double-blind randomized controlled trial of metformin in obese adolescents in 2001. Their results showed improved BMI (mean decrease of 0.5 kg/m$^2$ or <1.3% from baseline; $P$<.02 vs placebo), fasting insulin concentrations (from 31.5 ± 3.3 μU/mL at baseline to 19.2 ± 1.5 μU/mL after 6 months of treatment; $P$<.01), and fasting glucose levels (9.2 ± 3.9% lower than baseline levels in the metformin group and 8.7 ± 3.3% higher than baseline levels in the placebo group; $P$<.01). This study was followed by multiple short-term randomized controlled trials with small sample sizes that were done in different parts of the world (**Table 1**).

The MOCA trial (Metformin in Obese Children and Adolescents trial) in the UK has been the largest trial that included 151 obese children and adolescents (mean age, 13.7 ± 2.3 years) with hyperinsulinemia and/or increased glucose levels.[38] Participants were randomized to metformin or placebo for 6 months. Follow-up data were available from 124 participants at 3 months and 110 participants at 6 months. Significant improvement in the metformin group was observed for BMI at 6 months, with a mean change of −0.1 standard deviation (95% CI, -0.18 to −0.02; $P$ = .02). Fasting plasma glucose improved at 3 months only (−0.16 mmol/L; 95% CI, -0.31 to −0.00; $P$ = .047) and not at 6 months. Similarly, improvements in metabolic parameters such as alanine aminotransferase and adiponectin/leptin ratio were observed at 3 months, but were not sustained at 6 months.

McDonagh and colleagues[39] presented a systematic review of 14 randomized controlled trials of metformin in overweight and obese children without diabetes. All trials together accounted for a total of 946 children and adolescents with mean age range of 10 to 16 years and baseline BMI ranging from 26 to 41 kg/m$^2$. The majority of the trials were short term and lasted 6 months or less; only 2 lasted 1 year or more in duration. Metformin doses ranged from 1000 to 2000 mg/d divided twice daily or once daily in extended release formulations. Lifestyle interventions of some form were used in most studies; 2 studies included intensive lifestyle interventions.[40,41] The primary outcome of the study was weight reduction, and not HbA1c improvement or diabetes prevention.

BMI reduction with metformin use was seen in the pooled estimates of seven 6-month trials (mean difference in BMI change was −1.38; 95% CI, −1.93 to −0.82; $I^2$, 44%).[37,40,42–46] However, the 2 studies with a longer duration did not show statistically significant differences.[47,48] Patients with higher baseline BMI (>35 kg/m$^2$) and younger age (≤12 years) had greater BMI reduction.

The metformin group had greater weight loss than the control group based on the results of 8 clinical trials (−3.26; 95% CI, −4.23 to −2.30; $I^2$, 0%).[32,40,42,45–47,49,50] The greatest difference in weight loss was seen at 6 months (−3.77; 95% CI, −5.03 to −2.51), whereas the study with a 1-year duration found no significant difference between the 2 groups (0.70; 95% CI, −3.62–5.02; $P$ = .75).[47] The metformin group had a slightly greater decrease in total cholesterol compared with the control group (−4.65 mg/dL; 95% CI, −8.90 to −0.41; $I^2$, 0%). The authors concluded that short-term treatment with metformin along with lifestyle interventions might result in a less than 5% reduction in BMI in some obese children and adolescents.

Another systematic review of metformin use in obese nondiabetic children and adolescents comprising 11 clinical trials found a small but significant benefit of metformin in reducing weight after 6 to 12 months of treatment.[51] The authors were not able to derive conclusive data on the effect of metformin on insulin metabolism because different indices of insulin resistance and sensitivity were used in various

**Table 1**
Overview of principal metformin trials in pediatric population

| Study | Inclusion Criteria | n; Age (y) | Design/Duration | Therapy | Major Findings |
|---|---|---|---|---|---|
| Freemark and Bursey,[37] 2001 (United States) | BMI >30 kg/m²; fasting insulin >15 μU/mL and family history of T2DM | 29; 12–19 | RCT/6 mo | Metformin 500 mg twice daily vs placebo. No lifestyle modifications | Significant improvement in BMI, fasting insulin and FPG. No significant change in insulin sensitivity, HbA1c or lipid profile |
| Kay et al,[32] 2001 (United States) | BMI >30 kg/m²; Fasting glucose <120 mg/dL, HbA1c <7%, normal OGTT | 24; 15.6 ± 0.4 (metformin group), 15.7 ± 0.5 (placebo group) | RCT/8 wk | Metformin 850 mg twice daily vs placebo; low calorie diet | Reduction in body weight, body fat, fasting insulin, AUC insulin and leptin concentrations. No significant change in FPG |
| Srinivasan et al,[45] 2006 (Australia) | Obesity as defined by the International Obesity Task Force; fasting insulin (mu/L) to fasting glucose (mmol/L) ratio >4.5 or presence of acanthosis nigricans | 28; 9–18 | RCT with crossover at 6 months/12 mo | Metformin 1000 mg twice daily vs placebo. No lifestyle intervention | Significant improvements in weight, BMI, and waist circumference, abdominal subcutaneous fat, fasting insulin and FPG. No significant change in visceral fat or insulin sensitivity |
| Fu et al,[61] 2007 (China) | Weight >97th percentile, and >30% or 50% of weight for age and gender | 30; 7–16 | Observational uncontrolled study/3 mo | Metformin 500 mg twice daily with lifestyle modifications | Significant reductions in BMI, adiponectin level, HOMA-IR, cholesterol, triglyceride and 2-h plasma glucose |

(continued on next page)

**Table 1**
*(continued)*

| Study | Inclusion Criteria | n; Age (y) | Design/Duration | Therapy | Major Findings |
|---|---|---|---|---|---|
| Atabek and Pirgon,[42] 2008 (Turkey) | BMI >95th percentile | 120; 9–17 | RCT/6 mo | Metformin 500 mg twice daily with individualized diet and exercise regimen | Significant reduction in BMI, fasting insulin levels, improvement in HOMA-IR and QUICKI and insulin AUC |
| Love-Osborne et al,[44] 2008 (United States) | Fasting insulin >25 μU/mL or HOMA-IR >3.5 and 2 out of 3 factors (acanthosis nigricans, BMI >95th percentile, family history of T2DM) | 85; 12–19 | RCT/6 mo | Metformin 850 mg twice daily, goal setting for lifestyle modifications | No overall difference in weight loss between metformin and placebo group. No differences in insulin level changes in the 2 groups |
| Clarson et al,[43] 2009 (Canada) | BMI >95th percentile, HOMA-IR >3.0 | 25, 10–16 | RCT/6 mo | Metformin 1500 mg daily with lifestyle interventions | Significant reductions in BMI but no change in HOMA |
| Wiegand et al,[41] 2010 (Germany) | No success after 6 mo of lifestyle interventions in patients with BMI >97th percentile: ΔBMP <2, HOMA-IR >3 or 95th percentile | 70, 12–18 | RCT/6 mo | Metformin 500 mg twice daily with continued lifestyle intervention | No significant change in BMI or HOMA-IR, improved insulin sensitivity |
| Wilson et al,[48] 2010 (United States) | BMI >95th percentile | 77; 13–18 | RCT/12 mo | Metformin 2000 mg extended release once daily with lifestyle interventions | Small but significant improvement in BMI that persisted at 12–24 wk after cessation of medication. No significant changes in central adiposity, insulin indices, or lipid indices |

| Yanovski et al,[46] 2011 (United States) | BMI ≥95th percentile | 100; 6–12 y | RCT for 6 mo followed by 6 mo open-label metformin | Metformin 1000 mg twice daily along with lifestyle interventions | Significant reduction in weight, BMI, body fat, body circumference and skin fold thickness. Improved fasting insulin, FPG and HOMA-IR. No change in first phase insulin secretion of insulin sensitivity |
|---|---|---|---|---|---|
| Gómez-Díaz et al,[62] 2012 (Mexico) | Impaired glucose tolerance on OGTT per ADA criteria | 52; 4–17 | RCT/3 mo | Metformin 850 mg twice daily vs placebo; with consistent individualized diet and exercise regimen | Significant reductions in percentage weight change, resistin concentrations, HOMA-IR, HbA1c, AST, and ALT. After adjusting for weight loss, only HbA1c and resistin reductions were significant |
| Rynders et al,[63] 2012 (United States) | BMI >95th percentile | 16; 10–17 | Not placebo controlled/6 mo | Metformin 500 mg twice daily (<12 y), 1000 mg twice daily (≥12 y) with lifestyle intervention | No benefit on body composition or inflammatory markers |
| Mauras et al,[40] 2012 (United States) | BMI >95th percentile, CRP and/or fibrinogen >2 SD above mean | 42; 8–17 | Not placebo controlled/6 mo | Metformin 500 mg twice daily (<12 y), 1000 mg twice daily (≥12 y) with lifestyle intervention | Improved BMI and waist circumference. Inflammatory markers were improved in the lifestyle intervention only group compared with metformin and lifestyle intervention group |

(continued on next page)

**Table 1**
*(continued)*

| Study | Inclusion Criteria | n; Age (y) | Design/Duration | Therapy | Major Findings |
|---|---|---|---|---|---|
| The MOCA Trial, 2013 (UK)[38] | BMI >98th percentile; and OGTT 2-h plasma glucose ≥7.8 to ≤11.1 mmol/L (with or without impaired fasting glucose ≥6.1 to ≤7.0 mmol/L), or fasting insulin >26 mIU/L or 120-min insulin >89 mIU/L (pubertal/postpubertal children); fasting insulin >15 mIU/L or 120-min insulin >89 mIU/L (prepubertal children) | 151; 8–18 | Multicenter RCT/6 mo | Metformin 1000 mg in morning and 500 mg in evening vs placebo Not intensive lifestyle intervention | Significant improvements in BMI at 3 and 6 mo Improvements in FPG, AST, and adiponectin/leptin ratio at 3 mo No changes in adiponectin, resistin, or leptin concentrations No effect on CRP, fasting lipid, and fasting insulin levels |
| Van der Aa et al,[53] 2016 (Netherlands) | BMI SDS >2.3, HOMA-IR ≥3.4 | 42; 10–16 | Multicenter RCT/18 mo | Metformin 1000 mg twice daily with lifestyle interventions | BMI improved at 6–9 mo interval but was back to baseline at 18 mo No improvement in HOMA-IR or A1c Improvement in fat mass, no change in body fat percentage |

*Abbreviations:* ΔDA, American Diabetes Association; ALT, alanine transaminase; AST, aspartate transaminase; AUC, area under the curve; ΔBMP, change in basic metabolic profile; BMI, body mass index; CRP, C-reactive protein; FPG, fasting plasma glucose; HbA1c, glycated hemoglobin; HOMA-IR, homeostatic model assessment of insulin resistance; OGTT, oral glucose tolerance test; QUICKI, quantitative insulin sensitivity; RCT, randomized control trial; SD, standard deviation; SDS, standard deviation score; T2DM, type 2 diabetes mellitus.

trials. Improved fasting insulin levels as well as improved insulin resistance indices such as the HOMA-IR and Quantitative Insulin Sensitivity (QUICKI) with metformin use were noted in some studies.[37,42,45,46] These insulin resistance parameters are derived from fasting insulin and fasting glucose levels, and are primarily used in research settings.[52] These authors observed that metformin did not affect whole body (primarily muscle) insulin sensitivity.[37,45,46]

Recently, an 18-month multicenter, randomized, double-blinded, placebo-controlled trial was conducted in Netherlands among obese Caucasian adolescents with insulin resistance.[53] Inclusion criteria were age 10 to 16 years, BMI standard deviation score of greater than 2.3, and a HOMA-IR of 3.4 or greater. Participants were randomized to receive metformin 1000 mg twice daily or placebo. Total number of participants was 62, of which 42 were included in the final analyses. Study results showed that there was a decrease in BMI from baseline in the metformin group during the first 6 to 9 months of treatment; however, it subsequently returned to baseline at 18 months. In contrast, the BMI of the placebo group increased from baseline. After 18 months, median change in BMI compared with baseline was +0.2 (−2.9–1.3) in the metformin group versus +1.2 (−0.3–2.4) in the placebo group ($P$ = .015). No difference was observed for delta HOMA-IR after 18 months between the groups. HbA1c increased in both the groups while fat mass decreased in the metformin group with no change in body fat percentage.

## METFORMIN SAFETY PROFILE

The common side effects of metformin are gastrointestinal tract related, such as abdominal pain, nausea, metallic taste, bloating, and diarrhea, and were commonly noted in the clinical trials discussed. These side effects can be minimized by starting metformin at a low dose and increasing the dose gradually as tolerated.[54] Extended-release formulations of metformin seem to have better gastrointestinal tolerability than the immediate-release formulations.[55]

No serious adverse effects were noted even with long-term use (18 months) of metformin in the clinical trials. A rare but life-threatening side effect of metformin is lactic acidosis. The risk of lactic acidosis with metformin is known to be low when it is prescribed correctly.[21] There are reported cases of lactic acidosis in adolescents with metformin overdose.[56] In adults, lactic acidosis has been reported primarily in diabetic patients with significant renal insufficiency. When renal function is impaired, the plasma half-life of metformin is prolonged and its renal clearance is decreased in proportion to the decrease in creatinine clearance. In such patients, metformin dose should be adjusted based on the glomerular filtration rate.[57]

Metformin treatment has also been associated with clinically significant vitamin $B_{12}$ deficiency in some patients. It has been shown to be associated with an almost 3-fold risk of severe $B_{12}$ deficiency (vitamin $B_{12}$ <150 pg/mL) and a 2-fold risk of moderately low $B_{12}$ levels (150–220 pg/mL). The authors described that almost one-fifth to one-third of patients with T2DM on metformin have low $B_{12}$ levels.[58] A metaanalysis of 20 studies that included a total of 8009 patients found that metformin increased the risk of $B_{12}$ deficiency, with an odds ratio of 2.45 versus non–metformin-exposed individuals.[59] Monitoring $B_{12}$ levels, with supplementation when necessary, may be useful in all subjects receiving long-term treatment with metformin.

## DISCUSSION

The alarming increase in childhood obesity and its metabolic complications are well-described. Primary preventive measures including community- and family-based interventions are vital. Lifestyle interventions focusing on dietary modifications and increased physical activity should be the foundation of therapy for diabetes prevention in patients with prediabetes. At the same time, the clinicians taking care of young patients with insulin resistance and obesity need to be aware of treatment options that are relatively safe and effective. Pediatric clinical trials have shown beneficial effects of metformin by further decreasing BMI when added to lifestyle interventions. However, most of the trials were of short duration with small sample sizes, with the longest being 18 months. Long-term data are needed. Although some of the trials have shown improved insulin sensitivity indices, the results are not consistent. Few studies did not report any improvement in insulin sensitivity indices, body composition, or lipid profile. Moreover, diabetes prevention, which is the essential goal while treating prediabetic individuals with metformin, has not been studied so far in pediatric population. Data from adult studies demonstrate the efficacy of metformin and supports its use in adults with prediabetes.[17] Currently, the therapy for obese children and adolescents with prediabetes is individualized. The 2017 Pediatric Obesity Clinical Guidelines from The Endocrine Society recommend pediatricians to refrain from the practice of prescribing pharmacotherapy, including metformin, for only weight loss in obese children.[60] Complete clinical scenario including metabolic profile, comorbidities, and the feasibility of lifestyle interventions and access to resources should be taken into account. Metformin is a safe drug with significant proven benefits and may be considered in some cases. More research is needed to study its effects on diabetes prevention and to establish its long-term benefits in children.

## REFERENCES

1. Nguyen QM, Srinivasan SR, Xu JH, et al. Fasting plasma glucose levels within the normoglycemic range in childhood as a predictor of prediabetes and type 2 diabetes in adulthood: the Bogalusa Heart Study. Arch Pediatr Adolesc Med 2010; 164(2):124–8.
2. Li C, Ford ES, Zhao G, et al. Prevalence of pre-diabetes and its association with clustering of cardiometabolic risk factors and hyperinsulinemia among U.S. adolescents: National Health and Nutrition Examination Survey 2005-2006. Diabetes Care 2009;32(2):342–7.
3. American Diabetes Association. Standards of medical care in diabetes-2016: summary of revisions. Diabetes Care 2016;39(Suppl 1):S4–5.
4. Hermann LS, Melander A. Biguanides: basic aspects and clinical uses, vol. 1. Chichester (England): John Wiley; 1992.
5. Ogden CL, Carroll MD, Flegal KM. Prevalence of obesity in the United States. JAMA 2014;312(2):189–90.
6. Cruz ML, Shaibi GQ, Weigensberg MJ, et al. Pediatric obesity and insulin resistance: chronic disease risk and implications for treatment and prevention beyond body weight modification. Annu Rev Nutr 2005;25:435–68.
7. Weiss R, Dziura J, Burgert TS, et al. Obesity and the metabolic syndrome in children and adolescents. N Engl J Med 2004;350(23):2362–74.
8. American Diabetes Association. Standards of medical care in diabetes-2017: summary of revisions. Diabetes Care 2017;40(Suppl 1):S11–24.
9. American Diabetes Association. Standards of medical care in diabetes-2016. Diabetes Care 2016;39(Suppl 1):S1–109.
10. Gerstein HC, Santaguida P, Raina P, et al. Annual incidence and relative risk of diabetes in people with various categories of dysglycemia: a systematic overview

and meta-analysis of prospective studies. Diabetes Res Clin Pract 2007;78(3): 305–12.

11. Diabetes Prevention Program Research Group. The prevalence of retinopathy in impaired glucose tolerance and recent-onset diabetes in the Diabetes Prevention Program. Diabet Med 2007;24(2):137–44.

12. Nagi DK, Pettitt DJ, Bennett PH, et al. Diabetic retinopathy assessed by fundus photography in Pima Indians with impaired glucose tolerance and NIDDM. Diabet Med 1997;14(6):449–56.

13. Tapp RJ, Shaw JE, Zimmet PZ, et al. Albuminuria is evident in the early stages of diabetes onset: results from the Australian Diabetes, Obesity, and Lifestyle Study (AusDiab). Am J Kidney Dis 2004;44(5):792–8.

14. Ziegler D, Rathmann W, Dickhaus T, et al. Prevalence of polyneuropathy in prediabetes and diabetes is associated with abdominal obesity and macroangiopathy: the MONICA/KORA Augsburg Surveys S2 and S3. Diabetes Care 2008; 31(3):464–9.

15. Diabetes Prevention Program Research Group, Knowler WC, Fowler SE, Hamman RF, et al. 10-year follow-up of diabetes incidence and weight loss in the Diabetes Prevention Program Outcomes Study. Lancet 2009;374(9702): 1677–86.

16. Investigators DT, Gerstein HC, Yusuf S, et al. Effect of rosiglitazone on the frequency of diabetes in patients with impaired glucose tolerance or impaired fasting glucose: a randomised controlled trial. Lancet 2006;368(9541):1096–105.

17. Ramachandran A, Snehalatha C, Mary S, et al. The Indian Diabetes Prevention Programme shows that lifestyle modification and metformin prevent type 2 diabetes in Asian Indian subjects with impaired glucose tolerance (IDPP-1). Diabetologia 2006;49(2):289–97.

18. Bailey CJ, Day C. Traditional plant medicines as treatments for diabetes. Diabetes Care 1989;12(8):553–64.

19. Bailey CJ. Biguanides and NIDDM. Diabetes Care 1992;15(6):755–72.

20. Nattrass M, Alberti KG. Biguanides. Diabetologia 1978;14(2):71–4.

21. Cryer DR, Nicholas SP, Henry DH, et al. Comparative outcomes study of metformin intervention versus conventional approach the COSMIC Approach Study. Diabetes Care 2005;28(3):539–43.

22. El-Mir MY, Nogueira V, Fontaine E, et al. Dimethylbiguanide inhibits cell respiration via an indirect effect targeted on the respiratory chain complex I. J Biol Chem 2000;275(1):223–8.

23. Rena G, Pearson ER, Sakamoto K. Molecular mechanism of action of metformin: old or new insights? Diabetologia 2013;56(9):1898–906.

24. Owen MR, Doran E, Halestrap AP. Evidence that metformin exerts its anti-diabetic effects through inhibition of complex 1 of the mitochondrial respiratory chain. Biochem J 2000;348 Pt 3:607–14.

25. Salpeter SR, Greyber E, Pasternak GA, et al. Risk of fatal and nonfatal lactic acidosis with metformin use in type 2 diabetes mellitus. Cochrane Database Syst Rev 2010;(4):CD002967.

26. Zhou G, Myers R, Li Y, et al. Role of AMP-activated protein kinase in mechanism of metformin action. J Clin Invest 2001;108(8):1167–74.

27. Hardie DG, Ross FA, Hawley SA. AMPK: a nutrient and energy sensor that maintains energy homeostasis. Nat Rev Mol Cell Biol 2012;13(4):251–62.

28. Procter KL. The aetiology of childhood obesity: a review. Nutr Res Rev 2007; 20(1):29–45.

29. Koepsell H, Lips K, Volk C. Polyspecific organic cation transporters: structure, function, physiological roles, and biopharmaceutical implications. Pharm Res 2007;24(7):1227–51.

30. Knowler WC, Barrett-Connor E, Fowler SE, et al. Reduction in the incidence of type 2 diabetes with lifestyle intervention or metformin. N Engl J Med 2002; 346(6):393–403.

31. Tuomilehto J, Lindstrom J, Eriksson JG, et al. Prevention of type 2 diabetes mellitus by changes in lifestyle among subjects with impaired glucose tolerance. N Engl J Med 2001;344(18):1343–50.

32. Kay JP, Alemzadeh R, Langley G, et al. Beneficial effects of metformin in normoglycemic morbidly obese adolescents. Metabolism 2001;50(12):1457–61.

33. George MM, Copeland KC. Current treatment options for type 2 diabetes mellitus in youth: today's realities and lessons from the TODAY study. Curr Diab Rep 2013; 13(1):72–80.

34. Zinman B, Harris SB, Neuman J, et al. Low-dose combination therapy with rosiglitazone and metformin to prevent type 2 diabetes mellitus (CANOE trial): a double-blind randomised controlled study. Lancet 2010;376(9735):103–11.

35. Fontbonne A, Charles MA, Juhan-Vague I, et al. The effect of metformin on the metabolic abnormalities associated with upper-body fat distribution. BIGPRO Study Group. Diabetes Care 1996;19(9):920–6.

36. Lee A, Morley JE. Metformin decreases food consumption and induces weight loss in subjects with obesity with type II non-insulin-dependent diabetes. Obes Res 1998;6(1):47–53.

37. Freemark M, Bursey D. The effects of metformin on body mass index and glucose tolerance in obese adolescents with fasting hyperinsulinemia and a family history of type 2 diabetes. Pediatrics 2001;107(4):E55.

38. Kendall D, Vail A, Amin R, et al. Metformin in obese children and adolescents: the MOCA trial. J Clin Endocrinol Metab 2013;98(1):322–9.

39. McDonagh MS, Selph S, Ozpinar A, et al. Systematic review of the benefits and risks of metformin in treating obesity in children aged 18 years and younger. JAMA Pediatr 2014;168(2):178–84.

40. Mauras N, DelGiorno C, Hossain J, et al. Metformin use in children with obesity and normal glucose tolerance–effects on cardiovascular markers and intrahepatic fat. J Pediatr Endocrinol Metab 2012;25(1–2):33–40.

41. Wiegand S, l'Allemand D, Hubel H, et al. Metformin and placebo therapy both improve weight management and fasting insulin in obese insulin-resistant adolescents: a prospective, placebo-controlled, randomized study. Eur J Endocrinol 2010;163(4):585–92.

42. Atabek ME, Pirgon O. Use of metformin in obese adolescents with hyperinsulinemia: a 6-month, randomized, double-blind, placebo-controlled clinical trial. J Pediatr Endocrinol Metab 2008;21(4):339–48.

43. Clarson CL, Mahmud FH, Baker JE, et al. Metformin in combination with structured lifestyle intervention improved body mass index in obese adolescents, but did not improve insulin resistance. Endocrine 2009;36(1):141–6.

44. Love-Osborne K, Sheeder J, Zeitler P. Addition of metformin to a lifestyle modification program in adolescents with insulin resistance. J Pediatr 2008;152(6): 817–22.

45. Srinivasan S, Ambler GR, Baur LA, et al. Randomized, controlled trial of metformin for obesity and insulin resistance in children and adolescents: improvement in body composition and fasting insulin. J Clin Endocrinol Metab 2006;91(6): 2074–80.

46. Yanovski JA, Krakoff J, Salaita CG, et al. Effects of metformin on body weight and body composition in obese insulin-resistant children: a randomized clinical trial. Diabetes 2011;60(2):477–85.

47. Lavine JE, Schwimmer JB, Van Natta ML, et al. Effect of vitamin E or metformin for treatment of nonalcoholic fatty liver disease in children and adolescents: the TONIC randomized controlled trial. JAMA 2011;305(16):1659–68.

48. Wilson DM, Abrams SH, Aye T, et al. Metformin extended release treatment of adolescent obesity: a 48-week randomized, double-blind, placebo-controlled trial with 48-week follow-up. Arch Pediatr Adolesc Med 2010;164(2):116–23.

49. Burgert TS, Duran EJ, Goldberg-Gell R, et al. Short-term metabolic and cardiovascular effects of metformin in markedly obese adolescents with normal glucose tolerance. Pediatr Diabetes 2008;9(6):567–76.

50. Evia-Viscarra ML, Rodea-Montero ER, Apolinar-Jimenez E, et al. The effects of metformin on inflammatory mediators in obese adolescents with insulin resistance: controlled randomized clinical trial. J Pediatr Endocrinol Metab 2012; 25(1–2):41–9.

51. Brufani C, Crino A, Fintini D, et al. Systematic review of metformin use in obese nondiabetic children and adolescents. Horm Res Paediatr 2013;80(2):78–85.

52. Hrebicek J, Janout V, Malincikova J, et al. Detection of insulin resistance by simple quantitative insulin sensitivity check index QUICKI for epidemiological assessment and prevention. J Clin Endocrinol Metab 2002;87(1):144–7.

53. van der Aa MP, Elst MA, van de Garde EM, et al. Long-term treatment with metformin in obese, insulin-resistant adolescents: results of a randomized double-blinded placebo-controlled trial. Nutr Diabetes 2016;6(8):e228.

54. Scarpello JHB. Optimal dosing strategies for maximising the clinical response to metformin in type 2 diabetes. Br J Diabetes Vasc Dis 2001;1(1):28–36.

55. Feher MD, Al-Mrayat M, Brake J, et al. Tolerability of prolonged-release metformin (Glucophage) in individuals intolerant to standard metformin: results from four UK centres. Br J Diabetes Vasc Dis 2007;7(5):225–8.

56. Lacher M, Hermanns-Clausen M, Haeffner K, et al. Severe metformin intoxication with lactic acidosis in an adolescent. Eur J Pediatr 2005;164(6):362–5.

57. Lu WR, Defilippi J, Braun A. Unleash metformin: reconsideration of the contraindication in patients with renal impairment. Ann Pharmacother 2013;47(11): 1488–97.

58. Singh AK, Kumar A, Karmakar D, et al. Association of B12 deficiency and clinical neuropathy with metformin use in type 2 diabetes patients. J Postgrad Med 2013; 59(4):253–7.

59. Niafar M, Hai F, Porhomayon J, et al. The role of metformin on vitamin B12 deficiency: a meta-analysis review. Intern Emerg Med 2015;10(1):93–102.

60. Styne DMArslanian SACE, Farooqi IS, Murad MH, et al. Pediatric obesity— assessment, treatment, and prevention: an Endocrine Society Clinical Practice Guideline. J Clin Endocrinol Metab 2017;102(3):1–49.

61. Fu JF, Liang L, Zou CC, et al. Prevalence of the metabolic syndrome in Zhejiang Chinese obese children and adolescents and the effect of metformin combined with lifestyle intervention. Int J Obes (Lond) 2007;31(1):15–22.

62. Gómez-Díaz RA, Talavera JO, Pool EC, et al. Metformin decreases plasma resistin concentrations in pediatric patients with impaired glucose tolerance: a placebo-controlled randomized clinical trial. Metabolism 2012;61(9):1247–55.

63. Rynders C, Weltman A, Delgiorno C, et al. Lifestyle intervention improves fitness independent of metformin in obese adolescents. Med Sci Sports Exerc 2012; 44(5):786–92.

# Inhaled Drugs and Systemic Corticosteroids for Bronchopulmonary Dysplasia

CrossMark

Dirk Bassler, MD, MSc[a],*, John van den Anker, MD, PhD[b,c]

## KEYWORDS

- Bronchopulmonary dysplasia • Inhaled corticosteroids • Inhaled bronchodilators
- Systemic corticosteroids • Dexamethasone • Hydrocortisone • Pharmacology

## KEY POINTS

- A contemporary definition of bronchopulmonary dysplasia (BPD) that correlates with neurodevelopment and respiratory morbidity in childhood is desirable.
- Despite some positive effects on BPD, more information about the long-term effects of early inhaled corticosteroids is required to assess the overall efficacy and associated risks.
- Clinicians should balance the risks of neurodevelopmental impairment owing to systemic corticosteroids against those of BPD itself.
- Too little evidence is currently available to show positive or negative effects of bronchodilators for BPD.
- Future research focusing on the design of appropriate aerosol delivery systems and on the pharmacokinetics of inhaled drugs and systemic corticosteroids is needed.

## DEFINING BRONCHOPULMONARY DYSPLASIA

In 1967, Northway and colleagues[1] described a previously unrecorded abnormality of the lung after hyaline membrane disease in preterm infants that were relatively mature and coined the term bronchopulmonary dysplasia (BPD). In their view, the disease seemed to be a prolongation of the healing phase of respiratory distress syndrome combined with an injury triggered by mechanical ventilation and oxygen. They characterized BPD by its clinical course, radiographic findings, and histopathology. Twelve

Disclosure Statement: D. Bassler is principal investigator and J. van den Anker member of the steering committee of the Neonatal European Study of Inhaled Steroids (NEUROSIS). Other than this, the authors have nothing to disclose.
[a] University of Zurich, University Hospital Zurich, Department of Neonatology, Frauenklinikstrasse 10, Zurich 8091, Switzerland; [b] Division of Paediatric Pharmacology and Pharmacometrics, University of Basel Children's Hospital, Spitalstrasse 33, 4056 Basel, Switzerland; [c] Division of Clinical Pharmacology, Children's National Medical Center, 111 Michigan Avenue NorthWest, Washington, DC 20010, USA
* Corresponding author.
E-mail address: dirk.bassler@usz.ch

http://dx.doi.org/10.1016/j.pcl.2017.08.012
0031-3955/17/© 2017 Elsevier Inc. All rights reserved.

years later, Tooley[2] introduced a functional definition and suggested that oxygen use at 28 days of age might better identify preterm infants with BPD. The emphasis on the functional abnormality was reinforced by Shennan and colleagues,[3] who aimed for a definition that could separate those who would be normal from abnormal in the long term. They proposed, in 1988, that the best predictor of abnormal pulmonary outcomes at 2 years of age among very preterm infants was the clinical use of oxygen at 36 weeks postmenstrual age (PMA) with a corresponding accuracy of 85%. To address the problem of a definition that treats BPD as a dichotomous "yes" or "no" diagnosis, the National Institute of Child Health and Human Development proposed a consensus definition that includes 3 levels of severity (mild, moderate, and severe) based on an assessment at 36 weeks PMA.[4] This is preceded by an assessment that included the use of oxygen for at least 28 days (not necessarily consecutive). To control for the variable clinical use of targeted oxygen saturations, Walsh and colleagues[5] suggested an alternative definition, the so-called physiologic definition. They defined BPD as the requirement for positive pressure support, the requirement for supplemental oxygen at a fraction of inspired oxygen exceeding 0.3, or, in infants receiving low amounts of oxygen, an inability to maintain an oxygen saturation value of greater than 90% during a structured, short period of saturation monitoring coupled with gradual weaning from oxygen to ambient air (the oxygen reduction test).

All of these definitions have their limitations and shortcomings. Recently, Isayama and colleagues[6] conducted a retrospective cohort study in the Canadian Neonatal Network with the objective to identify the optimal definition of BPD that best predicts respiratory and neurodevelopmental outcomes in preterm infants. They concluded that defining BPD by the use of oxygen alone is inadequate and suggested a combined criterion of oxygen and/or positive pressure respiratory support. Furthermore, they proposed to apply this criterion at 40 weeks PMA rather than at 36 weeks PMA because of a better ability to predict serious respiratory morbidity and neurosensory morbidity at 18 to 21 months. This finding was confirmed by another study that assessed the contribution of the prevalence (mild, moderate, or severe) and the time of diagnosis of BPD in the prediction of neurodevelopmental impairment at the corrected age of 2 years in a single-center, retrospective analysis of 754 children with a gestational age (GA) of less than 30 weeks who were born between 2000 and 2013. (Malavolti AM, Bassler D, Arlettaz-Mieth R, et al. Severe bronchopulmonary dysplasia is a better predictor of neurological impairment in very preterm infants when diagnosed at 40 compared to 36 postmenstrual weeks. Submitted for publication.) Additionally, this group found that severe BPD was a better independent predictor of neurodevelopmental impairment at the age of 2 years than mild or moderate BPD.

## SHORTCOMINGS OF CURRENTLY AVAILABLE BRONCHOPULMONARY DYSPLASIA DEFINITIONS

The use of different definitions for BPD has been an ongoing challenge. In addition, contemporary changes in management of infants such as high-flow nasal cannula pose further challenges and limit application of existing definitions, which may result in misclassifications. In a scoping review, Hines and colleagues[7] found that the incidence of BPD ranged from 6% to 57%, depending on the definition chosen and that studies that investigated correlations with long-term pulmonary and/or neurosensory outcomes reported moderate-to-low predictive values regardless of the BPD criteria. In their review, these authors concluded that a comprehensive and evidence-based definition for BPD is needed for benchmarking and prognostic use. Poindexter and colleagues[8] applied 3 commonly used definitions of BPD to surviving infants at 36 weeks PMA in a prospective, multicenter, observational cohort of extremely preterm infants. They found large differences between existing definitions with respect to ease of data collection and number of unclassifiable cases. Similarly to Hines and colleagues,[7] Poindexter and colleagues[8] concluded that a contemporary definition of BPD that correlates with respiratory morbidity in childhood is urgently needed. In 2017, members of the NeoVitaAStudy Group came up with a suggestion to harmonize the definition of BPD.[9] They proposed a definition that was adapted from the National Institute of Child Health and Human Development network definition. It incorporates aspects that evolve over time, such as the use of high-flow nasal cannulas, and takes into account differences between clinical centers, including different target oxygen saturations. The suggested definition covers the aspect of evolving BPD measured in days, and of the assessment of definite BPD at a PMA of 36 weeks. Currently, the International Neonatal Consortium of the Critical Path Institute—a global collaboration formed to forge a predictable regulatory path for evaluating the safety and effectiveness of therapies for neonates that unites stakeholders from research institutions, drug developers, regulatory agencies, patient advocacy, and other organizations (available: https://c-path.org/programs/inc/)—is dedicating an ongoing project to BPD with the aim of drafting a new definition that allows for a better standardization of endpoints addressing the needs of patients, parents, clinical trialists, drug developers, and regulators.

## INHALED DRUGS FOR THE PREVENTION OR TREATMENT OF BRONCHOPULMONARY DYSPLASIA

Many pharmacologic interventions are currently used to prevent or treat BPD in preterm infants, among them inhaled medications such as bronchodilators and corticosteroids.

### Bronchodilators

The rationale for using bronchodilators in BPD patients comes from their potential effect of dilating small airways that have muscular hypertrophy and the association of BPD with an increased airway resistance, decreased dynamic compliance, and wheezing. Increased compliance and tidal volume and decreased pulmonary resistance have been documented when bronchodilators were used in short-term studies of pulmonary mechanics in infants with BPD.

### High-level evidence

There are numerous studies on bronchodilator use in BPD patients and an updated systematic review from the Cochrane Collaboration from 2016,[10] including systemic[11] and inhaled[12] bronchodilators. This review includes only 1 study investigating the role of inhaled bronchodilators (salbutamol).[12] This study enrolled 173 infants and aimed at the prevention of BPD.[12] According to GRADE (available http://www.gradeworkinggroup.org/), the quality of the evidence was moderate. Prophylaxis with salbutamol led to no statistically significant differences in mortality (relative risk [RR] 1.08; 95% CI, 0.50–2.31) or in BPD (RR, 1.03; 95% CI, 0.78–1.37). Results showed no differences in other complications associated with BPD or preterm birth. Investigators in this study did not comment on side effects owing to salbutamol. The authors of the systematic review from the Cochrane Collaboration found no eligible trial that studied the use of bronchodilator therapy for treatment of individuals with established BPD. They concluded that there is too little evidence to show positive or negative effects of bronchodilators for the prevention or treatment of BPD in preterm infants.

*Pharmacologic considerations (inhaled and systemic)*
Most studies in infants with BPD investigated the effect of inhaled bronchodilators, but there were also studies using the intravenous or the oral route of administration. Based on their mechanism of action, $\beta_2$-agonists lead to an increase in heart rate, which can be problematic in hemodynamically unstable young infants.

The pharmacokinetics and effects of intravenously administered salbutamol (albuterol) on respiratory mechanics was investigated in 6 infants with BPD (GA, 24–28 weeks; postnatal age, 54–105 days; body weight, 1.1–3.2 kg).[13] Salbutamol, which was administered at a dose of 30 µg/kg over 30 minutes, caused improvement in total respiratory system compliance and in airflow resistance, but a correlation between salbutamol serum concentration and pulmonary function could not be established. Clearance was 7.5 ± 2.6 (standard error of the mean in mL/min/kg), volume of distribution was 1291 ± 397 mL/kg and elimination half-life was 118 ± 13.9 minutes. Salbutamol's area under the curve correlated inversely with the change in heart rate (r = 0.92) and also a significant correlation between the apparent volume of distribution and heart rate change was found (r = 0.87). The authors concluded that preterm infants have measurable activity of bronchiolar β-2 receptor responsive to salbutamol.

Steady-state serum theophylline concentrations after equal doses of intravenous aminophylline and oral theophylline were comparable in 30 preterm infants with a GA of 29.2 ± 2.9 weeks (8.2 ± 2.2 µg/mL vs 8.4 ± 1.9 µg/mL; $P$ = .483).[14]

The pharmacokinetics of aminophylline was assessed in 7 preterm Korean infants (birth weight, 1190 ± 253 g; GA, 31.5 ± 1.99 weeks).[15] The mean theophylline maintenance dosage was 1.28 ± 0.15 mg/kg (standard error of the mean), given as equivalent aminophylline solution every 6 hours. The mean volume of distribution, 0.937 ± 0.232 L/kg, elimination rate constant, 0.0249 ± 0.0095/h, elimination half-life, 32.1 ± 12.1 h, and total body clearance, 21.7 ± 6.18 mL/h/kg, of theophylline were comparable with the values of neonates in other countries.

Two aminophylline loading doses, 8 and 6 mg/kg, were compared in 61 preterm infants weighing less than 1500 g.[16] After the loading dose of the 8 mg/kg, the recommended serum theophylline levels (7–12 µg/mL) were more frequently achieved than in the 6 mg/kg group (39% vs 3%; $P$ = .002). Subsequent levels were similar between the groups. There were no increases in side effects with the higher loading dose.

## Corticosteroids

Because inflammation seems to be a primary mediator of injury in the pathogenesis of BPD, antiinflammatory agents such as corticosteroids have long been the focus of preventive research activities. However, systemic corticosteroids, although reducing BPD, have frequently been linked to adverse neurodevelopmental outcomes and these considerations may have contributed to the recently reported widespread use of inhaled corticosteroids in neonatal units in North America, Europe, and Asia.[17–22] Theoretically, the administration of inhaled corticosteroids may allow for beneficial effects on the pulmonary system of infants with evolving or established BPD with a lower risk of undesirable side effects compared with systemic corticosteroids.

### High-level evidence
Systematic reviews from the Cochrane Collaboration have attempted to separate studies of prevention and treatment of BPD. Shah and colleagues[23] reported a metaanalysis of studies of "early" postnatal inhaled corticosteroids, defined as administration that was started before the age of 2 weeks. Onland and colleagues[24] conducted a metaanalysis of "late" studies defined as treatment started after 7 days of age. A recent systematic review that was conducted outside the Cochrane

Collaboration did not distinguish between "early" and "late" administration and pooled all studies in which inhaled corticosteroids were compared with placebo for the prevention or treatment of BPD in preterm infants.[25,26]

In an updated version from 2017 that includes 10 studies and 1644 patients, the Cochrane authors focusing on early administration found that there is increasing evidence that early administration of inhaled steroids to very low birth weight neonates is effective in reducing the incidence of death or BPD at 36 weeks of PMA among, either all randomized infants or among survivors. Even though there is statistical significance, the authors of the review questioned the clinical relevance as the upper CI limit for the outcome of death or BPD at 36 weeks of PMA is infinity.

The Cochrane review focusing on the "late" administration includes 8 trials and 232 preterm infants. Inhaled corticosteroids did not reduce the separate or combined outcomes of death or BPD. Furthermore, inhaled steroids did not impact short-term respiratory outcomes, such as failure to extubate and total duration of mechanical ventilation or oxygen dependency.

The metaanalysis combining both approaches, prevention and treatment, and including preterm infants from birth onward includes 16 trials. Overall, the 16 studies include 1596 infants, 804 in the active intervention groups and 792 in the control groups. Inhaled corticosteroids were associated with a significant reduction in death or BPD at 36 weeks of PMA (RR, 0.86; 95% CI, 0.75–0.99; 6 trials; $n = 1285$). BPD was significantly reduced (RR, 0.77; 95% CI, 0.65–0.91; 7 trials; $n = 1168$) and there was no effect on death (RR, 0.97; 95% CI, 0.42–2.2; 7 trials; n = 1270). No difference was found for death or BPD at 28 days of PMA. The use of systemic corticosteroids was significantly reduced in treated infants (13 trials; $n = 1537$; RR, 0.87; 95% CI, 0.76–0.98).

All 3 systematic reviews concluded that more information about the long-term effects of inhaled corticosteroids for the prevention or treatment of BPD is needed before firm clinical recommendations can be made. Unfortunately, even today, hardly any information is available. Among the 10 qualifying trials that were included in the Cochrane systematic review of the administration of inhaled corticosteroids within 2 weeks after birth, only 2 trials report long-term outcomes. Nakamura and colleagues[27] assessed death or neurodevelopmental impairment at 18 months of PMA in 187 infants available at follow-up. There was no difference between the 2 groups (RR 1.09; 95% CI, 0.70–1.70). At 3 years of age the authors report 2 additional composite outcomes. For 179 infants, death or neurodevelopmental impairment was not significantly different between the 2 groups (RR 1.03; 95% CI, 0.68–1.56), nor was death or cerebral palsy in 190 infants available at follow-up (RR 1.12; 95% CI, 0.64–1.96). Jangaard and colleagues[28] report long-term outcomes for 56 patients at the age of 3 years. There was no difference in the incidence of cerebral palsy among survivors (RR 1.33; 95% CI, 0.33–5.42) or in the incidence of mean developmental index on Bayley II Scales of Infant Development less than 2 standard deviations of the mean among survivors (RR, 1.25; 95% CI, 0.37–4.17). More information about the long-term effects of inhaled corticosteroids from the NEUROSIS study (Neonatal European Study of Inhaled Steroids) is expected to be published in 2017. NEUROSIS is a placebo-controlled, double-blind randomized controlled trial conducted in 40 centers in 9 countries including 863 preterm infants with a GA of 23 weeks 0 days to 27 weeks 6 days.[29,30] Infants were enrolled before an age of 12 hours and were either mechanically ventilated or on nasal respiratory support. Infants with major congenital anomalies or multiple births other than the second-born infant were excluded. Budesonide (200 µg/puff by metered dose inhaler via mini-Aerochamber: 2 puffs 2 times a day for 2 weeks then 1 puff 2 times a day) was administered until 32 weeks or off oxygen or ventilation. The primary outcome, a composite of BPD or death at 36 weeks of

PMA, was of borderline statistical significance (RR, 0.86; 95% CI, 0.75–1.00; $P$ = .05). The incidence of BPD was 27.8% in the budesonide group versus 38.0% in the placebo group (RR, 0.74; 95% CI, 0.60–0.91; $P$ = .004); death occurred in 16.9% and 13.6% of the patients, respectively (RR, 1.24; 95% CI, 0.91–1.69; $P$ = .17). The prespecified secondary long-term outcome, neurodevelopmental disability, was defined as a composite of cerebral palsy, cognitive delay (defined as a Mental Developmental Index score of <85 on the Bayley Scales of Infants Development), deafness, or blindness at a corrected age of 18 to 22 months.

### Pharmacologic considerations
In addition to the paucity of data on the long-term effects of inhaled steroids, there is also very limited pharmacologic information concerning the use of inhaled corticosteroids such as beclomethasone, fluticasone, and budesonide in infants with BPD.

At present, there is no evidence of adrenal insufficiency during beclomethasone therapy, but it was associated with a small decrease in basal cortisol levels in preterm infants less than 33 weeks of GA and with a body weight of less than 1250 g. However, there was no difference in cortisol response to stimulation tests in the beclomethasone versus the control group.[31] Another study also found no adverse reactions to inhaled beclomethasone, especially no evidence of hypothalamic–pituitary–adrenal axis suppression.[32] No immediate adverse effects were seen in 116 very low birth weight infants after early postnatal exposure to budesonide, but in the largest multicenter trial to date in 863 preterm infants with GAs between 23 and 28 weeks the advantage of a lower incidence of BPD might have been gained at the expense of an increased mortality.[30,33]

### LIMITATIONS OF INHALATION IN PRETERM INFANTS

Compared with children and adults, infants have a low tidal volume, vital capacity, and functional residual capacity, and short respiratory cycles. These anatomic and physiologic characteristics lead to a low residence time for aerosol particles.[34] Infants with BPD have an even lower tidal volume in addition to reduced lung compliance and increased airway resistance.[1,35] Therefore, when using inhaled drugs for the prevention or treatment of BPD, the mode of administration is an important factor to consider. The response to inhaled therapies depends the amount of aerosol delivered to the peripheral airways. There are numerous factors known to affect aerosol efficiency, such as the principle of aerosol generation, particle size, gas flow, and location within the ventilator circuit. Different principles of aerosol generation have been used for ventilated infants, among them metered dose inhalers, jet, vibrating mesh, and ultrasonic.[36] Despite their widespread use, aerosol delivery systems have not been systematically evaluated for use in mechanically ventilated infants or in infants receiving continuous positive airway pressure. Unfortunately, direct estimation of lung deposition of inhaled drugs in infants with BPD is a methodologic challenge. Most studies used indirect methods, in vitro filters, or animal lung models. All of these methods have important limitations leading to an inaccurate estimation of lung deposition in neonates. Direct estimation of lung deposition in neonates using radiotracers provides more accurate estimates of the actual pulmonary dose and drug distribution, but radiolabeled aerosols are no longer used. In the only study that measured radiolabeled aerosol (albuterol) lung deposition in preterm infants with BPD, 10 ventilated and 13 nonventilated low birth weight infants were randomly assigned to either inhalation using a jet nebulizer or a metered dose inhaler in a crossover sequence.[37] Although both methods resulted in a low pulmonary dose and the study also reported marked intersubject variability in lung deposition, the metered dose inhaler was associated with a significantly higher pulmonary deposition relative to the jet nebulizer when results were expressed as a percentage of initial nebulizer reservoir activity, both in the nonventilated and in the ventilated group.

In recent years, in vitro and in vivo study methods that do not depend on radiolabeling have overcome some of the methodologic challenges, and future research focusing on the design of appropriate aerosol delivery systems for ventilated infants and neonates on continuous positive airway pressure that efficiently transport aerosols without impairment of ventilator support is needed.

## SYSTEMIC CORTICOSTEROIDS FOR THE PREVENTION OR TREATMENT OF BRONCHOPULMONARY DYSPLASIA

Dexamethasone and hydrocortisone are the most studied systemic corticosteroids for the prevention or treatment of BPD, but they behave differently. In the brain, hydrocortisone binds to both mineralocorticoid receptors and glucocorticoid receptors; dexamethasone binds only to glucocorticoid receptors and suppresses native cortisol production, which promotes apoptosis and results in adverse outcomes in animal models.

### Dexamethasone

Dexamethasone is a synthetic corticosteroid with potent glucocorticoid effects. In the 1980s, the first randomized, controlled trials in infants with BPD were conducted that demonstrated short-term benefits such as earlier weaning from respiratory support and higher success rates of endotracheal extubation. After these findings were published, dexamethasone became widely used in the 1990s for the prevention and treatment of BPD,[38] often with prolonged courses and high doses.[39] In 2002, a collective statement of the American Academy of Pediatrics and the Canadian Pediatric Society was published suggesting a causal link between dexamethasone and cerebral palsy, concluding that routine dexamethasone therapy for the prevention or treatment of BPD could not be recommended and that alternative corticosteroids should undergo further study.[40] At present, the neonatal community is left with the difficult task of weighing the potential risks and benefits of dexamethasone in infants at high risk of BPD.

### High-level evidence

Two systematic reviews from the Cochrane Collaboration showed that dexamethasone reduces the rate of BPD in mechanically ventilated extremely preterm infants, regardless of initiation of therapy during or after the first week of life.[41] Despite this clear benefit, the authors of the review concluded that the lower risk of BPD "may not outweigh" the actual or potential adverse effects of dexamethasone. Early (<8 days of life) dexamethasone increases the risks of gastrointestinal perforation and hypertrophic cardiomyopathy.[42] Cerebral palsy was increased with early dexamethasone (RR, 1.75; 95% CI, 1.20–2.55; 7 studies and 1452 infants), as was major neurosensory disability. However, it remains uncertain if late (>7 days of life) dexamethasone results in similar long-term harm. Short-term adverse effects of late dexamethasone include hyperglycemia, glycosuria, and hypertension. Late dexamethasone may also increase the risk of severe retinopathy of prematurity. The risk of cerebral palsy at 1 to 3 years of age was not increased among surviving infants treated with late dexamethasone (60 of 322; 18.6%) compared with controls (53 of 309; 17.2%; RR, 1.05; 95% CI, 0.75–1.47).

In addition to the time point of initiation ("early" vs "late"), the cumulative dose may also play a role in safety and efficacy. Onland and colleagues[43] evaluated the effects of different dosing regimens on rates of BPD and long-term neurodevelopment in another systematic review from the Cochrane Collaboration. They concluded that although some of the included studies reported a modulating effect of treatment regimens in favor of higher dosage regimens on the incidence of BPD and neurodevelopmental impairment, recommendations on the optimal type of corticosteroid, the optimal dosage, or the optimal timing of initiation for the prevention of BPD in preterm infants cannot be made based on current level of evidence.

An alternative way to interpret the available clinical trial data was suggested by Doyle at al[44,45] in an innovative metaregression originally published in 2005 and updated in 2014. The authors suggested to plot net benefit or net harm (death or cerebral palsy at 2 years) against baseline BPD event rate (in control groups of infants) in randomized, controlled trials then published. An excess risk associated with steroid use when there is a low control group event rate of BPD shifts to a net benefit when started at a higher event rate. This study emphasizes the important fact that one needs to carefully balance the risks of neurodevelopmental impairment owing to corticosteroids against those of BPD itself. Thus, future studies should focus on infants with a very high risk of developing BPD.

### Pharmacologic considerations

The pharmacokinetics of intravenously administered dexamethasone was studied in 9 premature neonates with a mean GA of 27.3 weeks and a postnatal age of 21.8 days.[46] A strong correlation between clearance (4.96 mL/min/kg) and GA (r = 0.884) could be established. Mean clearance in infants with a GA of less than 27 weeks was 1.69 mL/min/kg and in infants with a GA of more than 27 weeks was 7.57 mL/min/kg. The mean distribution volume in groups I and II was 1.26 L/kg (<27 weeks GA) and 2.19 L/kg (>27 weeks GA), respectively. No significant relationships were noted between pharmacokinetics and ventilator requirements or adverse effects.

The dosage and duration of early corticosteroids given to small premature infants influences the risk of the side effects and the early outcome.[47] The 2 most relevant side effects are growth restriction and suppression of the hypothalamic–pituitary–adrenal axis. Short-term growth of premature infants treated with dexamethasone, assessed by miniknemometry, showed that lower doses seemed to have an equivalent effect without long-term effect on lower leg length. In higher doses, the growth was suppressed for more than 24 hours.[48] Significant suppression of the hypothalamic–pituitary–adrenal axis was seen after 7 days of a dexamethasone treatment regimen.[49]

### Hydrocortisone

Hydrocortisone may have fewer or no adverse effects on neurosensory development in preterm infants and it has been the focus of recent clinical research activity.

#### High-level evidence

**Evidence from systematic reviews** Currently available data from systematic reviews do not support the use of hydrocortisone for the prevention of BPD, because there is little evidence about this benefit when used in the first week of life.[42] A systematic review, published in 2010, did not identify randomized studies to substantiate the use of hydrocortisone in chronically ventilator-dependent infants with established or evolving BPD.[50]

**Recent randomized, controlled trials** In 2016, Baud and colleagues[51] published the primary outcome results of the French PREMILOC study (Trial to Prevent Bronchopulmonary Dysplasia in Very Preterm Neonates) of low-dose hydrocortisone. This study was a double-blind, randomized, placebo-controlled, parallel-group clinical trial with a sequential design. The study team enrolled extremely preterm neonates within the first 24 postnatal hours. Infants were eligible if they were inborn and delivered between $24^{+0}$ and $27^{+6}$ weeks of gestation. Infants received equal volumes of either intravenous placebo or hydrocortisone hemisuccinate, 1 mg/kg per day divided into 2 doses per day for 7 days, followed by one dose of 0.5 mg/kg per day for 3 days. The primary outcome was survival without BPD at 36 weeks of PMA. The trial was stopped early owing to "financial and technical support limitations." One hundred fifty-three (60%) of 255 infants assigned to receive hydrocortisone, and 136 (51%) of 266 infants assigned to placebo survived without BPD. The result was just statistically significant (odds ratio, 1.48; 95% CI, 1.02–2.16; $P$ = .04). The long-term neurodevelopmental outcomes have been published in April 2017.[52] Four hundred six infants survived until 2 years of age, when neurologic assessment has been done using clinical staging and the Revised Brunet-Lezine scale for cognitive and motor assessment. In total, 194 of the 207 surviving children (94%) treated by hydrocortisone and 185 of the 199 children (93%) assigned to the placebo group had a neurologic assessment at 2 years. The distribution of patients without neurodevelopmental impairment (73% in the hydrocortisone group vs 70% in the placebo group), with mild neurodevelopmental impairment (20% in the hydrocortisone group vs 18% in the placebo group), or with moderate to severe neurodevelopmental impairment (7% in the hydrocortisone group vs 11% in the placebo group) was not statistically significantly different between the groups ($P$ = .33). The incidence of cerebral palsy or other major neurologic impairments did not differ significantly between the 2 groups.

**Ongoing randomized, controlled trials**
   **The National Institute of Child Health and Human Development neonatal research network trial** The National Institute of Child Health and Human Development Neonatal Research Network is currently recruiting patients for a study that will test the safety and efficacy of a 10-day course of hydrocortisone for infants who have an estimated GA of less than 30 weeks and are intubated at 14 to 28 days of life. Infants will be randomized to receive hydrocortisone or placebo. This study will determine if hydrocortisone improves infants' survival without moderate or severe BPD and if it will be associated with improvement in survival without moderate or severe neurodevelopmental impairment at 22 to 26 months of corrected age (clinicaltrials. gov NCT01353313).

   **The STOP-BPD trial** The STOP-BPD trial (Systemic Hydrocortisone To Prevent Bronchopulmonary Dysplasia in preterm infants) from the Netherlands and Belgium is a randomized, double-blind, placebo-controlled, multicenter study including 400 very low birth weight infants (available: www.neonatologiestudies.nl/stopbpd).[53] It aims to investigate if hydrocortisone is safe and effective in reducing the incidence of the combined outcome death or BPD at 36 weeks PMA in chronically ventilated preterm infants, as compared with placebo. This study does not aim to successfully extubate ventilator-dependent preterm infants with the lowest possible use of corticosteroids (ie, hydrocortisone), but to use corticosteroids as an early intervention (7–14 d after birth) to reduce the risk of death or BPD in these ventilator-dependent preterm infants.

*Pharmacologic considerations*
No adverse effects of hydrocortisone were observed in infants with a birthweight of less than 1000 g receiving low-dose hydrocortisone. Hydrocortisone had no effect on regional brain volumes or pulmonary outcomes before neonatal intensive care unit discharge.[54]

An increase in spontaneous gastrointestinal perforations in the hydrocortisone-treated group lead to premature termination of a study investigating the effect of prophylactic hydrocortisone administration on early adrenal insufficiency to prevent BPD.[55]

Finally, low-dose hydrocortisone therapy did not suppress adrenal function or compromise short-term growth.

## SUMMARY

Since the term BPD was first coined by William Northway and colleagues in 1967, several definitions of this frequent morbidity of prematurity have been suggested in the neonatal literature. All of these definitions have limitations and a new definition is desirable. This new definition should facilitate future clinical trials, benchmarking and prognostic prediction of respiratory and neurologic development of extremely preterm infants in later life. Neonatal pharmacologic therapies are an important tool to reduce the burden of BPD among very immature infants and different inhaled and systemic drugs are currently used to prevent or treat BPD. When using inhaled drugs, the mode of administration is an important factor to consider. The response to inhaled therapies depends on the amount of aerosol delivered to the peripheral airways and there is currently insufficient information available about appropriate aerosol delivery systems for ventilated infants and neonates on continuous positive airway pressure. However, it has been convincingly shown in a large randomized, controlled trial and confirmed by several metaanalyses that early inhaled budesonide reduces BPD. However, more information about the effects of inhaled corticosteroids is required to assess overall efficacy and associated risks. The information currently available to show positive or negative effects of inhaled bronchodilators for BPD is insufficient, and future and large well-designed studies are needed. Today, dexamethasone and hydrocortisone are the most studied systemic corticosteroids for the prevention or treatment of BPD. Dexamethasone is a synthetic corticosteroid with potent glucocorticoid effects that is associated with cerebral palsy if given in the first week of life. Hydrocortisone may have fewer or no adverse effects on neurosensory development in preterm infants. As with inhaled corticosteroids, more information about the long-term effects of hydrocortisone is required to assess overall efficacy and associated risks. Until such information becomes available, neonatologists need to carefully balance the risks of neurodevelopmental impairment owing to systemic corticosteroids against those of BPD itself. Future studies should, therefore, focus on infants with a very high risk of developing BPD and include pharmacokinetics and long-term developmental outcomes.

## REFERENCES

1. Northway WH Jr, Rosan RC, Porter DY. Pulmonary disease following respirator therapy of hyaline-membrane disease. Bronchopulmonary dysplasia. N Engl J Med 1967;276:357–68.
2. Tooley WH. Epidemiology of bronchopulmonary dysplasia. J Pediatr 1979;95: 851–8.
3. Shennan AT, Dunn MS, Ohlsson A, et al. Abnormal pulmonary outcomes in premature infants: prediction from oxygen requirement in the neonatal period. Pediatrics 1988;82:527–32.
4. Jobe AH, Bancalari E. Bronchopulmonary dysplasia. Am J Respir Crit Care Med 2001;163:1723–9.
5. Walsh MC, Wilson-Costello D, Zadell A, et al. Safety, reliability, and validity of a physiologic definition of bronchopulmonary dysplasia. J Perinatol 2003;23:451–6.

6. Isayama T, Lee SK, Yang J, et al, Canadian Neonatal Network and Canadian Neonatal Follow-Up Network Investigators. Revisiting the definition of broncho-pulmonary dysplasia: effect of changing panoply of respiratory support for pre-term neonates. JAMA Pediatr 2017;171:271–9.

7. Hines D, Modi N, Lee SK, et al, International Network for Evaluating Outcomes (iNeo) of Neonates. Scoping review shows wide variation in the definitions of bronchopulmonary dysplasia in preterm infants and calls for a consensus. Acta Paediatr 2017;106(3):366–74.

8. Poindexter BB, Feng R, Schmidt B, et al, Prematurity and Respiratory Outcomes Program. Comparisons and limitations of current definitions of bronchopulmonary dysplasia for the prematurity and respiratory outcomes program. Ann Am Thorac Soc 2015;12:1822–30.

9. Meyer S, Franz AR, Bay J, et al, NeoVitaA Study Group. Developing a better and practical definition of bronchopulmonary dysplasia. Acta Paediatr 2017;106(5): 842.

10. Ng G, da Silva O, Ohlsson A. Bronchodilators for the prevention and treatment of chronic lung disease in preterm infants. Cochrane Database Syst Rev 2016;(12):CD003214.

11. Armanian AM, Badiee Z, Afghari R, et al. Reducing the incidence of chronic lung disease in very premature infants with aminophylline. Int J Prev Med 2014;5: 569–76.

12. Denjean A, Paris-Llado J, Zupan V, et al. Inhaled salbutamol and beclometha-sone for preventing bronchopulmonary dysplasia: a randomised double-blind study. Eur J Pediatr 1998;157:926–31.

13. Kirpalani H, Koren G, Schmidt B, et al. Respiratory response and pharmacoki-netics of intravenous salbutamol in infants with BPD. Crit Care Med 1990;18: 1374–7.

14. Al-Omran A, al-Alaiyari S. Theophylline concentrations following equal doses of intravenous doses of aminophylline and oral theophylline in preterm infants. Am J Perinatol 1997;14:147–9.

15. Ahn H, Shin W, Park K, et al. Pharmacokinetics of theophylline and caffeine after intravenous administration of aminophylline to premature neonates in Korea. Res Commun Mol Pathol Pharmacol 1999;105:105–13.

16. Hochwald C, Kennedy K, Chang J, et al. A randomized, controlled, double blind trial comparing two loading doses of aminophylline. J Perinatol 2002;22:275–8.

17. Bassler D. Inhaled budesonide for the prevention of bronchopulmonary dysplasia. J Matern Fetal Neonatal Med 2017;30(19):2372–4.

18. Bassler D. Inhalation or instillation of steroids for the prevention of bronchopulmo-nary dysplasia. Neonatology 2015;107(4):358–9.

19. Maas C, Poets CF, Bassler D. Survey of practices regarding utilization of inhaled steroids in 223 German neonatal units. Neonatology 2010;98:404–8.

20. Job S, Clare P. Current UK practices in steroid treatment of chronic lung disease. Arch Dis Child Fetal Neonatal Ed 2015;100(4):F371.

21. Slaughter JL, Stenger MR, Reagan PB, et al. Utilization of inhaled corticosteroids for infants with bronchopulmonary dysplasia. PLoS One 2014;9:e106838.

22. Ogawa R, Mori R, Sako M, et al. Drug treatment for bronchopulmonary dysplasia in Japan: questionnaire survey. Pediatr Int 2015;57:189–92.

23. Shah VS, Ohlsson A, Halliday HL, et al. Early administration of inhaled corticoste-roids for preventing chronic lung disease in ventilated very low birth weight pre-term neonates. Cochrane Database Syst Rev 2017;(1):CD001969.

24. Onland W, Offringa M, van Kaam A. Late (> 7 days) inhalation corticosteroids to reduce bronchopulmonary dysplasia in preterm infants [review]. Cochrane Database Syst Rev 2012;(4):CD002311.

25. Shinwell ES, Portnov I, Meerpohl J, et al. Use of inhaled corticosteroids for the prevention and/or treatment of bronchopulmonary dysplasia in preterm infants: a systematic review protocol. Syst Rev 2015;4:127.

26. Shinwell ES, Portnov I, Meerpohl JJ, et al. Inhaled corticosteroids for bronchopulmonary dysplasia: a meta-analysis. Pediatrics 2016;138(6) [pii:e20162511].

27. Nakamura T, Yonemoto N, Nakayama M, et al. Early inhaled steroid use in extremely low birthweight infants: a randomised controlled trial. Arch Dis Child Fetal Neonatal Ed 2016;10:F1–5.

28. Jangaard KA, Stinson DA, Allen AC, et al. Early prophylactic inhaled beclomethasone in infants less than 1250 g for the prevention of chronic lung disease. Paediatr Child Health 2002;7:13–9.

29. Bassler D, Halliday HL, Plavka R, et al. The Neonatal European Study of Inhaled Steroids (NEUROSIS): an EU-funded international randomised controlled trial in preterm infants. Neonatology 2010;97:52–5.

30. Bassler D, Plavka R, Shinwell ES, et al. Early Inhaled budesonide for the prevention of bronchopulmonary dysplasia. N Engl J Med 2015;373:1497–506.

31. Cole C, Shah B, Abbas S, et al. Adrenal function in premature infants during inhaled beclomethasone therapy. J Pediatr 1999;135:65–70.

32. Zimmerman J, Gabbert D, Shivpuri C, et al. Meter-dosed, inhaled beclomethasone attenuates bronchoalveolar oxyradical inflammation in premature infants at risk for bronchopulmonary dysplasia. Am J Perinatol 1998;15:567–76.

33. Yeh T, Lin H, Chang C, et al. Early intratracheal instillation of budesonide using surfactant as a vehicle to prevent CLD in preterm infants: a pilot study. Pediatrics 2008;121:e1310–8.

34. Fink JB. Aerosol delivery to ventilated infant and pediatric patients. Respir Care 2004;49:653–65.

35. Bancalari E, Abdenour GE, Feller R, et al. Bronchopulmonary dysplasia: clinical presentation. J Pediatr 1979;95:819–23.

36. Mazela J, Polin RA. Aerosol delivery to ventilated newborn infants: historical challenges and new directions. Eur J Pediatr 2011;170:433–44.

37. Fok TF, Monkman S, Dolovich M, et al. Efficiency of aerosol medication delivery from a metered dose inhaler versus jet nebulizer in infants with bronchopulmonary dysplasia. Crit Care Med 1997;25:140–4.

38. Watterberg K. Evidence-based neonatal pharmacotherapy: postnatal corticosteroids. Clin Perinatol 2012;39:47–59.

39. Demauro SB, Dysart K, Kirpalani H. Stopping the swinging pendulum of postnatal corticosteroid use. J Pediatr 2014;164:9–11.

40. American Academy of Pediatrics, Committee on Fetus and Newborn, Canadian Paediatric Society, Fetus and Newborn Committee. Postnatal corticosteroids to treat or prevent chronic lung disease in preterm infants. Pediatrics 2002;109:330–8.

41. Doyle LW, Ehrenkranz RA, Halliday HL. Late (> 7 days) postnatal corticosteroids for chronic lung disease in preterm infants. Cochrane Database Syst Rev 2014;(5):CD001145.

42. Doyle LW, Ehrenkranz RA, Halliday HL. Early (< 8 days) postnatal corticosteroids for preventing chronic lung disease in preterm infants. Cochrane Database Syst Rev 2014;(5):CD001146.

43. Onland W, De Jaegere AP, Offringa M, et al. Systemic corticosteroid regimens for prevention of bronchopulmonary dysplasia in preterm infants. Cochrane Database Syst Rev 2017;(1):CD010941.

44. Doyle LW, Halliday HL, Ehrenkranz RA, et al. Impact of postnatal systemic corticosteroids on mortality and cerebral palsy in preterm infants: effect modification by risk for chronic lung disease. Pediatrics 2005;115:655–61.

45. Doyle LW, Halliday HL, Ehrenkranz RA, et al. An update on the impact of postnatal systemic corticosteroids on mortality and cerebral palsy in preterm infants: effect modification by risk of bronchopulmonary dysplasia. J Pediatr 2014;165: 1258–60.

46. Lugo R, Nahata M, Menke J, et al. Pharmacokinetics of dexamethasone in premature neonates. Eur J Clin Pharmacol 1996;49:477–83.

47. Anttila E, Peltoniemi O, Haumont D, et al. Early neonatal dexamethasone treatment for prevention of bronchopulmonary dysplasia. Randomised trial and meta-analysis evaluating the duration of dexamethasone therapy. Eur J Pediatr 2005;164:472–81.

48. Keller A, Keller E, Hermanussen M, et al. Short-term growth of premature infants treated with dexamethasone assessed by mini-knemometry. Ann Hum Biol 2004; 31:389–97.

49. Rivzi Z, Aniol H, Myers T, et al. Effects of dexamethasone on the hypothalamic-pituitary-adrenal axis in preterm infants. J Pediatr 1992;120:961–5.

50. Doyle LW, Ehrenkranz RA, Halliday HL. Postnatal hydrocortisone for preventing or treating bronchopulmonary dysplasia in preterm infants: a systematic review. Neonatology 2010;98:111–7.

51. Baud O, Maury L, Lebail F, et al. Effect of early low-dose hydrocortisone on survival without bronchopulmonary dysplasia in extremely preterm infants (PREMILOC): a double-blind, placebo-controlled, multicentre, randomised trial. Lancet 2016;387:1827–36.

52. Baud O, Trousson C, Biran V, et al. Association between early low-dose hydrocortisone therapy in extremely preterm neonates and neurodevelopmental outcomes at 2 years of age. JAMA 2017;317:1329–37.

53. Onland W, Offringa M, Cools F, et al. Systemic hydrocortisone to prevent bronchopulmonary dysplasia in preterm infants (the SToP-BPD study); a multicenter randomized placebo controlled trial. BMC Pediatr 2011;11:102.

54. Parikh N, Kennedy K, Lasky R, et al. Pilot randomized trial of hydrocortisone in ventilator-dependent extremely preterm infants: effects on regional brain volumes. J Pediatr 2013;162:685–90.

55. Watterberg K, Gerdes J, Cole C, et al. Prophylaxis of early adrenal insufficiency to prevent bronchopulmonary dysplasia: a multicenter trial. Pediatrics 2004;114: 1649–55.

# New Antimicrobial Agents for the Treatment of Staphylococcal Infections in Children

 CrossMark

Roopali Sharma, PharmD[a,b], Densley Francois, PharmD[c,d],
Margaret R. Hammerschlag, MD[d,e],*

## KEYWORDS

- *Staphylococcus aureus* • MRSA • Vancomycin • Ceftaroline • Daptomycin
- Dalbavancin • Telavancin • Tedizolid

## KEY POINTS

- Decreased susceptibility of methicillin-resistant *Staphylococcus aureus* (MRSA) to vancomycin is increasing and associated with treatment failure, even when MRSA strains are fully susceptible to vancomycin.
- Treatment with vancomycin requires careful monitoring of drug levels because there is a potential for nephrotoxicity.
- In the last few years several new antimicrobial agents—daptomycin, ceftaroline, telavancin, dalbavancin, and tedizolid—have been approved for treatment staphylococcal infections, including MRSA, in adults.
- Ceftaroline and daptomycin have been approved for use in children.
- Ceftaroline, the first beta-lactam antibiotic with activity against MRSA, has been approved for treatment of community-acquired bacterial pneumonia and complicated skin and skin structure infections.

---

Disclosure: The authors do not have any commercial or financial conflicts of interest and any funding sources to disclose.

[a] Department of Pharmacy Practice, Touro College of Pharmacy, 230 West 125th Street, New York, NY 10027, USA; [b] Department of Medicine, SUNY Downstate Medical Center, 450 Clarkson Avenue, Brooklyn, NY 11203, USA; [c] Department of Pharmacy, SUNY Downstate Medical Center, 450 Clarkson Avenue, Brooklyn, NY 11203, USA; [d] Department of Pediatrics, SUNY Downstate Medical Center, 450 Clarkson Avenue, Brooklyn, NY 11203, USA; [e] Division of Pediatric Infectious Diseases, SUNY Downstate Medical Center, 450 Clarkson Avenue, Brooklyn, NY 11203, USA
* Corresponding author. SUNY Downstate Medical Center, 450 Clarkson Avenue, Brooklyn, NY 11203.
E-mail address: mhammerschlag@downstate.edu

Pediatr Clin N Am 64 (2017) 1369–1387
http://dx.doi.org/10.1016/j.pcl.2017.08.005

pediatric.theclinics.com

## INTRODUCTION

Staphylococcus aureus was first identified as bacterial pathogens in the 19th century. Penicillins were considered the drug of choice until S aureus developed penicillin resistance by production of beta-lactamase. This led to discovery of semisynthetic penicillins such as dicloxacillin and nafcillin but quickly methicillin-resistant S aureus (MRSA) emerged owing to the acquisition of genes that have decreased affinity for beta-lactams, including antistaphylococcal penicillins, cephalosporins, and carbapenems.[1] In the last 50 years, vancomycin has been the agent of choice to treat MRSA infections, although other agents such as clindamycin, tetracyclines, and cotrimoxazole have also been used. However, vancomycin treatment failure is not uncommon, even when MRSA strains are fully susceptible to vancomycin (minimum inhibitory concentration [MIC] $\leq 2$ mg/mL).[2] Treatment with vancomycin requires careful monitoring of drug levels because there is a potential for nephrotoxicity. In addition, resistance to clindamycin is not infrequent, which also limits therapeutic options for treating infections owing to MRSA in children. In the last few years, tedizolid, daptomycin, telavancin, dalbavancin, and ceftaroline have been approved for the treatment of staphylococcal infections, including MRSA, in adults. Ceftaroline and daptomycin have been approved by the US Food and Drug Administration (FDA) for use in children. Ceftaroline, daptomycin, dalbavancin, telavancin, and tedizolid offer a number of advantages over currently available drugs to treat staphylococcal and other Gram-positive infections, especially vancomycin, including improved antimicrobial activity; superior pharmacokinetics, pharmacodynamics, tolerability, and dosing, including once-daily and weekly regimens; and less need for monitoring drug levels.

## CEFTAROLINE
### Chemistry and Pharmacology

Cephalosporins are beta-lactam antibiotics derived from the fungus *Cephalosporium* (now called *Acremonium*). There are numerous agents in this class, each containing a beta-lactam ring fused to a 6-member dihydrothiazine ring, and 2 side chains that can be modified to affect antibacterial activity and pharmacokinetic properties.[3] Ceftaroline fosamil is water soluble, an *N*-phosphono type prodrug of a cephalosporin class of beta-lactam antibacterial drugs, rapidly converted to the active form, ceftaroline.[4] Ceftaroline was synthesized with specific manipulations of the side chains to provide enhanced activity against MRSA and multidrug-resistant *Streptococcus pneumoniae* isolates, making it the first available beta-lactam with this ability.[5] One of the mechanisms of resistance to beta-lactam agents is through mutations of the penicillin-binding proteins (PBP). MRSA and penicillin-resistant *S pneumoniae* produce PBP2a and PBP-2x variants, respectively.[6]

Similar to other cephalosporins, ceftaroline binds to PBPs, inhibiting transpeptidation. This interaction blocks the final stage of peptidoglycan synthesis and inhibits bacterial cell wall synthesis, ceftaroline binds to PBP 1 to 4 and has a high affinity to PBP2a, the protein responsible for conferring methicillin resistance in *S aureus*.[6] Ceftaroline also has activity against penicillin-resistant *S pneumoniae* owing to binding affinity to PBP2x.[6]

### Pharmacokinetics and Pharmacodynamics

Limited pharmacokinetic studies on ceftaroline exist for pediatric patients. In a phase I open-label, noncomparative study, a single dose was examined for pharmacokinetics in 9 subjects aged 12 to 17 years.[7] A single 1-hour infusion of ceftaroline 8 mg/kg was administered to hospitalized patients for suspected infection who weighed less than 75 kg or 600 mg for subjects who weighed 75 kg or more. Patients were excluded if they were allergic to beta-lactam agents, have a history of seizures, or were critically ill. The peak plasma concentration ($C_{max}$) reported in these patients was 15 ± 6 μg/mL, which is comparable with what is reported in adults.[7] This study did not include patients who were obese or critically ill. A pharmacokinetic study of ceftaroline was conducted in 53 children less than 12 years of age who were hospitalized with an infection.[8] It was open-label, single-dose, phase IV study. Patients were excluded from the study if they had hypersensitivity to beta-lactam agents, renal insufficiency, or a history of seizures. The patients received various doses of ceftaroline based on their age. The results of this study are not published. In this study, some patients received a ceftaroline dose of 15 mg/kg, which is more than the FDA recommended dose of 8 to 12 mg/kg for this age group. Riccobene and colleagues[9] conducted a population pharmacokinetic modeling and target simulations by combining the results of 5 pediatric studies that included 305 children from birth to age 18 years to investigate the dosing of ceftaroline in patients that had acute bacterial skin and skin structure infections (ABSSSI) and community-acquired pneumonia (CAP). The studies used dosing of 8 mg/kg every 8 hours for children aged 2 months or less and less than 2 years. Children older than 2 years received a dose of 12 mg/kg every 8 hours up to a weight of 33 kg. Older children weighing more than 33 kg received 400 mg every 8 hours or an adult dose of 600 mg every 12 hours. The objective of the study was to estimate ceftaroline exposures and percentage of time that free drug concentrations of ceftaroline were above the MIC (%$fT$ > MIC) for pediatric dose regimens. The various dosing regimens in pediatric patients maintained a concentration greater than a MIC of 1 μg/mL more than 75% of the time.[9] More than 90% of children were predicted to achieve a target of 36% $fT$ of greater than MIC at an MIC of 2 μg/mL, and more than 97% were predicted to achieve 44% $fT$ of greater than MIC at an MIC of 1 μg/mL. The 12-hour dosing alternative for older children maintained concentrations above the MIC of 1 μg/mL 44% of the time in 97% of children and above MIC of 2 mg/mL for 36% of the time in more than 90% of children. Other pharmacokinetic parameters are summarized in **Table 1**. The

**Table 1**
**Pharmacokinetic parameters of ceftaroline by age based on simulations for children with normal renal function following doses used in the pediatric ABSSSI and CABP studies**

| Age Range | Dose[a] | Weight, kg | $C_{max,ss}$, μg/mL | $AUC_{0-24h,ss}$, μg.h/mL |
|---|---|---|---|---|
| 12 to <18 y | 12 mg/kg q8h | 52.9 (36.8, 75.3) | 19.7 (11.0, 34.2) | 122 (72.7, 201) |
| 6 to <12 y | 12 mg/kg q8h | 28.5 (19.3, 46.5) | 27.6 (16.4, 43.3) | 157 (99.7, 245) |
| 2 to <6 y | 12 mg/kg q8h | 15.8 (11.8, 22.2) | 27.1 (16.8, 41.8) | 144 (92.6, 225) |
| 18 to <24 mo | 12 mg/kg q8h | 11.7 (9.81, 14.1) | 28.3 (17.6, 43.4) | 160 (104, 247) |
| 12 to <18 mo | 12 mg/kg q8h | 10.4 (8.60, 12.7) | 28.7 (17.9, 44.0) | 168 (109, 260) |
| 6 to <12 mo | 12 mg/kg q8h | 8.43 (6.55, 10.7) | 29.3 (18.2, 45.1) | 182 (116, 282) |
| 2 to <6 mo | 8 mg/kg q8h | 5.75 (4.12, 7.66) | 19.2 (12.1, 29.7) | 134 (86.6, 208) |
| Adults | 600 mg q12h | 77.6 (52.5, 105) | 21.0 (11.9, 36.5) | 97.3 (59.1, 164) |

Abbreviations: ABSSSI, acute bacterial skin and skin structure infection; $AUC_{0-24h,ss}$, area under the plasma concentration–time curve from time 0 to 24 hours at steady state, assuming q8h dosing; CABP, community-acquired bacterial pneumonia; $C_{max,ss}$, maximum plasma drug concentration at steady state.

[a] All doses administered as 1-hour infusions. All pediatric doses were up to a maximum of 400 mg based on weight.

Adapted from Riccobene T, Khariton T, Knebel W, et al. Population PK modeling and target attainment simulations to support dosing of ceftaroline fosamil in pediatric patients with acute bacterial skin and skin structure infections and community-acquired bacterial pneumonia. J Clin Pharmacol 2017;57(3):345–55.

elimination half-life was not calculated for the pediatric patients. The authors of this study concluded that the tested dosing regimen would produce similar drug exposures to adult dosing. One of the limitations of this study was that the authors did not study the impact of renal function on dosing of ceftaroline.

Pharmacokinetic data are lacking in special populations of children, such as patients with cystic fibrosis (CF), burn patients, or pediatric patients with central nervous system infections. There is 1 case report published by Molloy and colleagues[10] that describes pharmacokinetic dosing in a 6-year-old male patient with CF and MRSA infection. The MRSA isolate had a ceftaroline MIC of 1 μg/mL and the dose given to this patient was 200 mg every 8 hours (32.4 mg/kg/d). Serum ceftaroline concentrations remained greater than the MIC for only 21% of the dosage interval; however, the patient improved clinically.[10] Ceftaroline, like most other beta-lactam agents is a time-dependent (concentration-dependent) antibiotic. The pharmacodynamic parameter that best predicts ceftaroline efficacy is a $f$%T of greater than MIC.[11] A Monte Carlo simulation of ceftaroline 600 mg every 12 hours given to healthy adults predicted $f$T% of greater than MIC of 71% and 51% for organisms with MICs of 1 and 2 μg/mL, respectively. The probability of target attainment of 40% $f$T of greater than MIC was 100% at an MIC of 1 μg/mL and 90% at an MIC of 2 μg/mL.[12,13]

### Adverse Events and Drug Interactions

Ceftaroline was approved in May of 2016 for the treatment of ABSSSI and community-acquired bacterial pneumonia (CABP) in children less than 2 months of age based on 3 studies.[14–16] To date, the safety of ceftaroline has been evaluated in 3 active control studies and 2 single-dose pharmacokinetic studies in a total of 319 pediatric subjects.[7,8,14–16] These 2 randomized, controlled studies evaluated the safety of ceftaroline in children.[15,16] Adverse events in both studies were similar between ceftaroline and comparative agents (22% vs 23% in the ABSSSI and 45% vs 46% in the CABP studies, respectively). The most common side effects experienced in these patients were diarrhea, rash, nausea, vomiting, and fever. Ceftaroline should be used with caution in patients with a previous history of hypersensitivity to beta-lactam antibiotics and is contraindicated in patients where anaphylaxis has occurred. Direct Coombs' test seroconversion is a known side effect of ceftaroline and is listed in the warning section of the package insert for adult patients.[17] In pediatric subjects, the ceftaroline arm experienced a higher incidence of direct Coombs' seroconversion as compared with comparators.[15,16] Hemolytic anemia or hemolysis was not documented in any of the patients receiving ceftaroline. This warning is also added for the pediatric patients. Ceftaroline is hydrolyzed into its inactive metabolite, ceftaroline M-1. It undergoes little hepatic metabolism and is not a substrate, inhibitor, or inducer of the cytochrome P 450 enzyme system and therefore is not likely to cause cytochrome P 450-related drug–drug interactions.[18]

### Dosing and Administration

Dosing of ceftaroline is based on both age and weight (**Table 2**). According to the package insert, children between the ages of 2 months and less than 2 years should receive a lower dose at 8 mg/kg every 8 hours. Patients aged 2 years or more should be given 12 mg/kg every 8 hours with a maximum dose of 400 mg per dose in patients weighing more than 33 kg.[17] Alternatively, a 600-mg dose may be given every 12 hours. The duration of therapy of ceftaroline depends on the type of infection being treated. The typical duration is 5 to 14 days. Ceftaroline is excreted by the kidneys and the elimination of ceftaroline is altered in patients with renal insufficiency. Dosing

**Table 2**
**Ceftaroline dosing in children**

| Age | FDA-Approved Dose for CABP and ABSSSI | Suggested[a] cCABP, CF, MRSA Bacteremia/Endocarditis |
|---|---|---|
| 2 mo <2 y | 8 mg/kg every q8h | Age <6 mo: 10 mg/kg q8h<br>Age 6 mo to <2 y: 15 mg/kg q8h |
| ≥2 y[a] | 12 mg/kg q8h<br>Maximum 1200 mg/d, divided q8-12h | 15 mg/kg q8h<br>Maximum 1800 mg/d, divided q8h |

*Abbreviations:* ABSSSI, acute bacterial skin and skin structure infection; CABP, community-acquired bacterial pneumonia; cCABP, complicated community-acquired bacterial pneumonia; CF, cystic fibrosis; FDA, US Food and Drug Administration; MRSA, methicillin-resistant *Staphylococcus aureus.*

[a] Limited data, not prospectively evaluated for safety outside of cCABP.

*Data from* Teflaro® (ceftaroline fosamil) [package insert]. St Louis, MO: Forest Pharmaceuticals, Inc; 2016; and Corey A, So T-Y. Current clinical trials on the use of ceftaroline in the pediatric population. Clin Drug Investig 2017. http://dx.doi.org/10.1007/s40261-017-0523-2.

adjustments are recommended in adult patients with a creatinine clearance of less than 50 mL/min and who are on hemodialysis. Intermittent hemodialysis removes approximately 21% of ceftaroline.[19] Dosing recommendations in pediatric patients with renal insufficiency or hemodialysis are lacking; therefore, children should not receive ceftaroline until further studies are conducted to ensure an optimal dosing regimen.

Ceftaroline is only available as an intravenous (IV) agent. Ceftaroline should be reconstituted to be used within 6 hours at room temperature and within 24 hours if refrigerated. The IV infusion time has been approved between 5 and 60 minutes; because ceftaroline is a time-dependent antibiotic it is best to administer the agent over 60 minutes.[17]

## DAPTOMYCIN
### Chemistry and Pharmacology

Daptomycin, a fermentation product derived from *Streptomyces roseosporus*, is the first member of a novel class of antibiotics called the cyclic lipopeptides and presents an attractive option for the treatment of invasive infections owing to Gram-positive organisms. The mechanism of daptomycin is calcium dependent because, to exert its antimicrobial effect, it must first bind to calcium forming micelles that enhance its affinity for the bacterial cytoplasmic membrane.[20,21] The daptomycin–calcium complex then inserts deep into the membrane, causing rapid depolarization of the membrane potential, arrest of DNA and RNA synthesis, and cell death without lysis and release of inflammatory mediators.[21]

As a result of its unique mechanism of action in targeting the cell membrane, daptomycin has several advantageous microbiological characteristics, including efficacy against a majority of Gram-positive organisms, including *Staphylococcus* and *Enterococcus* species resistant to vancomycin, linezolid, and quinupristin/dalopristin; rapid bactericidal activity; and antimicrobial effect at all growth phases of the bacterial cell.[22,23] One limitation to daptomycin use is its interaction with pulmonary surfactant, which inactivates daptomycin and reduces its efficacy in the treatment of alveolar pneumonia.[23] Daptomycin is currently FDA approved in adults for the treatment of complicated skin and soft tissue infections, *S aureus* bacteremia, and right-sided endocarditis associated with *S aureus* bacteremia. It was approved for treatment of ABSSSI in children in 2017.

### Pharmacokinetics and Pharmacodynamics

Daptomyoin is a concentration-dependent, bactericidal agent that follows first-order linear pharmacokinetics. In adults, it is 90% protein bound, distributes into the extracellular fluid, and is eliminated renally as intact drug with an average half-life of about 8 hours. An adult given a dose of 4 to 6 mg/kg given IV daily yields the pharmacokinetic parameters that are associated with efficacy: $C_{max}$ 50 to 90 μg/mL and an area under the curve (AUC) of 400 to 600 mg·L/h.[23–26] Children have several developmental pharmacokinetic differences compared with adults, including greater total body water content with an increased extracellular fluid proportion and decreased protein binding. Renal function is impaired at birth with improvement up to and beyond adult values throughout childhood. Such pharmacokinetic changes would theoretically result in an increased volume of distribution, lower peak concentrations, and more rapid clearance of daptomycin.[23] Several small cases series have been conducted evaluating the pharmacokinetics of daptomycin in newborns to adolescents. Pharmacokinetic parameters and corresponding current dosing recommendations from these studies are detailed in **Table 2**.

### Pharmacokinetic and Pharmacodynamic Data in Children 2 to 17 Years Old

In 2008, Abdel-Rahman and colleagues[24] conducted a single dose pharmacokinetic study in 2- to 17-year-old children receiving daptomycin at a dose of 4 mg/kg daily for proven or suspected gram-positive infections. Pharmacokinetic analyses resulted in suboptimal daptomycin AUC and $C_{max}$ levels compared with adults in children less than 12 years old with appropriate levels in those greater than 12 years old.[26] Abdel-Rahman and colleagues[27] then conducted a second study specifically in children 2 to 6 years old, stratifying the patient population into 2 dosing groups, namely, 8 and 10 mg/kg daily. Pharmacokinetic parameters achieved in this study were similar to those targeted in adults. The average half-life was between 5 and 7 hours in both studies. Current recommended dosing is detailed in **Table 3**.

**Table 3**
**Pharmacokinetic and pharmacodynamic data and associated dosing recommendations in children**

| Author, Year | Age, n | Daily Dose | In-Study Evaluations | AUC (mg·L/h) | $t_{1/2}$ (h) | Current Recommended Dosing |
|---|---|---|---|---|---|---|
| Children 2–17 y old | | | | | | |
| Abdel-Rahman et al,[24] 2008 | 2–17 y, n = 22 | 4 mg/kg | 12–17 y | 374 | 6.7 | >12 y: 4-6 mg/kg daily |
| | | | 7–11 y | 271[a] | 5.6 | |
| | | | 2–6 y | 215[a] | 5.3 | 6–11 y: 7 mg/kg |
| Abdel-Rahman, et al,[27] 2011 | 2–6 y, n = 12 | 8 mg/kg, 10 mg/kg | 8 mg/kg | 429.1 | 5.4 | daily |
| | | | 10 mg/kg | 549.1 | 5.7 | 2–5 y: 10 mg/kg daily |
| Children <2 y old | | | | | | |
| Cohen-Wolowiez et al,[28] 2012 | <120 d, n = 20 | 6 mg/kg | n/a | 262.4[a] | 6.2 | <2 y: 10 mg/kg/d Neonates: 6 mg/kg |
| Bradley et al,[29] 2014 | 3–24 mo n = 23 | 4 mg/kg 6mg/kg | 2–12 mo | 217[a] | NR | q12h |
| | | | 13–24 mo | 281[a] | NR | |

*Abbreviations:* AUC, area under the curve; n/a, not applicable; NR, not reported; $t_{1/2}$, half-life.
[a] Suboptimal AUC based on levels of 400 to 600 mg·L/h normally achieved in adults.[4–6]
*Data from* Refs.[23–25]

*Pharmacokinetic and Pharmacodynamic Data in Children less than 2 Years Old*

Cohen-Wolkowiez and colleagues[28] conducted a single dose pharmacokinetic study in children less than 120 days old receiving daptomycin at a dose of 6 mg/kg for a suspected systemic infection. The AUC and $C_{max}$ values were reportedly lower than target adult exposure values. Therefore, young infants seem to require a higher dose requirement, similar to children 2 to 6 years old to achieve typical adult pharmacokinetic parameters. The second study was performed in children 3 to 24 months old with children 2 to 12 months old receiving 4 mg/kg and children 13 to 24 months old receiving 6 mg/kg. Pharmacokinetic parameters were proportionally higher in the children receiving 6 mg/kg compared with 4 mg/kg.[29] The average half-life was between 5 and 7 hours in both studies. Three published case reports describing 4 neonates with gram positive bacteremia used a dosing regimen of 6 mg/kg per dose given every 12 hours and attained pharmacokinetic parameters similar to those associated with efficacy in adults.[30–33]

*Drug Interactions*

Owing to the potential for creatine phosphokinase (CPK) elevations with daptomycin, theoretically there is a concern for the use of 3-hydroxy-3-methyl-glutaryl-coenzyme A reductase inhibitors with daptomycin and the development of myopathy. Current experience with concomitant therapy is limited; however, in a study evaluating daptomycin use for *S aureus* endocarditis, 4 of the 11 patients who experienced increases in CPK were also on a 3-hydroxy-3-methyl-glutaryl-coenzyme A reductase inhibitor.[34] There have also been reports for daptomycin causing a significant concentration-dependent false elevation of the prothrombin time and International Normalized Ratio. This interaction potential can be reduced by drawing these levels at the time of daptomycin trough concentrations. Last, increased daptomycin and decreased tobramycin concentrations have been reported with concomitant use, although this interaction has not been evaluated clinically.[25]

*Adverse Drug Reactions in Adults*

In a phase III clinical trial performed in adults receiving 4 mg/kg of daptomycin for ABSSSI, 2.8% of patients were reported to have a drug-related CPK elevation. The side effects reported in more than 2% of patients included diarrhea (5.2%), headache (5.4%), dizziness, rash, abnormal liver function tests, urinary tract infections, hypotension, and dyspnea (all occurring in <5% of patients). All side effects were comparable with the vancomycin comparator group.[26] In the a trial evaluating daptomycin for *S aureus* bacteremia/endocarditis in adults, daptomycin was given at a dose of 6 mg/kg and 9.3% of patient experienced CPK elevations; however, this proportion was not significantly different than the comparator group.[34]

*Adverse Reactions Reported in Children*

The limited studies in children report similar side effects to adults. A large, retrospective review of hospitalized children over a 9-year period evaluated 1035 different hospitalizations with a least 1 administration of daptomycin in 794 children. About one-half of the children (47.3%) were less than 10 years of age. Adverse events were reported in 8 children, 7 had rhabdomyolysis and 1 had pulmonary eosinophilia.[35] In a systematic review of 29 studies performed in children, 10 studies reported no side effects and 93% of the reported adverse effects were considered unrelated to daptomycin. The most common side effects related to daptomycin included increased liver function tests, headache, phlebitis, and infusion site reactions, with 1 serious side effect of anaphylaxis reported.[36]

## DALBAVANCIN

Although dalbavancin is not yet approved for use in children, its unique pharmacology deserves to be examined.

### Chemistry and Pharmacology

Dalbavancin is a semisynthetic lipoglycopeptide derived from a teicoplanin-like glyco-peptide agent by derivatization and modification of the functional groups and removal or substitution of sugar moieties while preserving the binding site required for antimi-crobial activity.[37,38] Similar to teicloplanin, dalbavancin has a long lipophilic acyl moi-ety in an amide linkage to glucosamine component. This lipophilic side chain is useful in improving the activity by anchoring the molecule to the bacterial cell membrane, which prolongs the interaction of the agent with the bacteria.[37]

Dalbavancin inhibits cell wall synthesis by binding to the D-alanyl-D-alanine of the growing peptidoglycan chains, interfering with cross-linking and polymerization. Dal-bavancin is more potent against staphylococci than vancomycin is, and this property may be due to an additional mechanism.[38,39] In addition to inhibiting peptidoglycan synthesis, dalbavancin may inhibit transglycosylation by direct interaction with en-zymes involved in the final stages of peptidoglycan synthesis.[38]

### Pharmacokinetics and Pharmacodynamics

Dalbavancin has interesting pharmacokinetic characteristics, including a long half-life and good tissue distribution mainly owing to its highly reversible protein binding to serum albumin.[39] Dalbavancin has renal and nonrenal clearance via feces. Approxi-mately 30% of dalbavancin is excreted unchanged via the kidney. Hepatic metabolism does not seem to affect dalbavancin clearance and dose modifications may not be needed in patients with hepatic impairment, although data are limited in patients with moderate to severe hepatic impairment.[39,40]

The disposition of dalbavancin in children has been published in 2 phase I, open-label, multicenter studies.[41,42] Bradley and colleagues[41] studied the pharmacokinetics of IV dalbavancin in children 12 to 17 years of age. A single dose of 1000 mg of dal-bavancin was administered to children weighing 60 kg or greater and 15 mg/kg for children weighing less than 60 kg. Pharmacokinetic parameters were determined us-ing noncompartmental analysis. There were total of 10 subjects, 5 in the dalbavancin 1000 mg and 5 in the dalbavancin 15 mg/kg groups. The $C_{max}$ and AUC in either 1000 mg for those who weighed greater than 60 kg or 15 mg/kg for those weighing less than 60 kg was similar. The terminal half-life was approximately 9 days in both dosing groups, compared with 15 days in adult patients in published studies, high-lighting that this pharmacokinetic difference in half-life may be owing to age.[41] In this study, the AUC was 30% less than those documented in adult studies, which probably can be explained by enhanced hepatic and renal clearance in healthy ado-lescents compared with adults. Nine of the 10 subjects had detectable plasma levels of dalbavancin 55 days after administration.

The second pediatric study examined the pharmacokinetics of IV dalbavancin after the administration of a single dose in hospitalized pediatric patients 3 months to 11 years of age.[42] The authors of this study used published data from the study of Bradley and colleagues[41] to further categorize disposition characteristics of dalbavan-cin in pediatric subjects aged greater than 3 months and to perform a population pharmacokinetics analysis to identify optimal dalbavancin dosing in children.[42] Three hundred eleven dalbavancin serum concentrations from 43 subjects were analyzed. Thirty-one patients were males, the median age and weight from the pooled data were 5.9 years (range, 0.3–16.9) and 18.9 kg (range, 5.7–105.2), respectively. The median dose in both studies was 15 mg/kg (range, 9.5–25.7). The optimal pediatric age-dependent dosing of dalbavancin based on the population pharmacokinetics model was as follows: age 6 to less than 18 years, 12 mg/kg (1000 mg maximum) on day 1, and 6 mg/kg (500 mg maximum) on day 8; and age 3 months to less than 6 years, 15 mg/kg (1000 mg maximum) on day 1, and 7.5 mg/kg (500 mg maximum) on day 8. This dosing regimen in children would achieve similar dalbavancin exposure compared with that in adults administered a 2-dose regimen (1000 mg on day 1 plus 500 mg on day 8). Similarly, the following age-dependent regimen was found to match adult exposure after a single-dose (1500 mg): age 6 to less than 18 years, 18 mg/kg (1500 mg maximum) on day 1; and age 3 months to less than 6 years, 22.5 mg/kg (1500 mg maximum) on day 1. The data on pharmacokinetics in children are limited to these 2 studies. There is no dosage defined for neonates and further studies are needed to define an optimum dose of dalbavancin for maximum efficacy and limited toxicity in pediatric population.

The pharmacodynamic parameters of dalbavancin have not been established in children. Based on in vitro and in animal studies, the 24-hour AUC/MIC parameter and the $C_{max}$/MIC is highly associated with in vivo activity.[39] These pharmacodynamic parameters endorse the infrequent administration of large doses and the pharmacodynamic parameter most likely to predict efficacy of dalbavancin is AUC/MIC. In adults, a regimen of 1500 mg given on day 1 and then again on day 8 is expected to achieve an AUC similar to that for a 1000-mg initial dose, followed by 4 subsequent 500-mg weekly doses. Although the same total AUC should provide similar outcomes, experimental data suggest that the efficacy of drugs with a long half-life, such as dalbavancin, is enhanced by providing higher doses earlier in the course of therapy. This finding has been observed in animal studies with dalbavancin in which better outcomes were observed when the same total dose was delivered in larger amounts earlier and less frequently.

### Adverse Events and Drug Interactions

Dalbavancin seems to be well-tolerated, with most of the adverse events being mild. Studies conducted in adult patients with dalbavancin using an IV 2-dose scheme of 1000 mg on day 1 followed by 500 mg 1 week later or a 1-time 1100-mg dose have consistently demonstrated that the drug is well-tolerated, with no dose-limiting toxicities or relevant laboratory values alterations.[39] One study in adult patients using a similar dosing strategy reported patients having oral candidiasis, diarrhea, constipation, and fever; however, no patients required discontinuation of the drug.[39] Safety data from phase II and III studies of dalbavancin in adults revealed 52% of patients had at least 1 adverse event, which was comparable with 56.9% in the comparator arms of these studies. Approximately 3.5% of patients in the dalbavancin group discontinued the study medication compared with 3.8% in the comparator arm.[39,43]

A single dose of dalbavancin seems to be well-tolerated in children. No severe or serious adverse events have been related to this agent, including ototoxicity, nephrotoxicity, and hepatotoxicity. Despite the lack of reported toxicities, additional data are necessary to confirm the safety of dalbavancin in the pediatric population.[44]

It is interesting that anaphylactoid reactions, such as flushing, hypotension, and rash, which are commonly seen with other glycopeptides, have not been reported with dalbavancin. Dalbavancin has not been widely used in children and the maximum tolerated dose of dalbavancin has not been established. Given the pharmacokinetic profile of dalbavancin, which has a prolonged half-life, if an adverse event did occur, reversing the adverse event may take an extended period of time, which is an important consideration.[39] Dalbavancin does not have significant drug–drug interactions because it is not a substrate, inhibitor, or inducer of the cytochrome P450 system.[39]

## SPECTRUM OF ACTIVITY
### Ceftaroline

The comparative activities of ceftaroline and daptomycin against selected Gram-positive bacteria are shown in **Table 4**. Ceftaroline is the first cephalosporin approved for use in children that has activity against MRSA. Its overall spectrum of activity is similar to ceftriaxone; in addition to activity against S aureus (MSSA and MRSA), it has excellent activity against Haemophilus influenzae and Escherichia coli.[45,46] Ceftaroline is more active against S pneumoniae; 99.9% of isolates were found to be sensitive to ceftaroline compared with 92.2% sensitive to ceftriaxone.[45] Pfaller and colleagues,[45] in a study of 1460 bacterial isolates from children with skin and soft tissue infections and CAP from US hospitals from 2012 to 2014, found ceftaroline to be 4 times more active than ceftriaxone against MSSA. Of interest, they reported that 16% of MSSA and 13.1% of MRSA tested were resistant clindamycin. However, a multicenter study from China published in 2015 found that only 66.5% of MRSA isolates from patients with skin and soft tissue infection were susceptible to ceftaroline, 33.5% were intermediate, and none were fully resistant.[47] However, emergence of resistance of MRSA to ceftaroline has been described during therapy.[48] Cannavino and colleagues[14] reported isolating a ceftaroline resistant MRSA from a 4-year-old girl with CF after 22 courses of the antibiotic, the MIC increase from 0.5 to 4.0 μg/mL. They identified an alteration in the PBP 2 that seemed to be responsible for the resistance. Children with CF eliminate beta-lactam antibiotics faster than normal children. These data are concerning and suggest that we need continued surveillance of MRSA isolates in the United States.

**Table 4**
**In vitro activity of ceftaroline and daptomycin against selected bacteria**

| Bacteria | Ceftaroline | | Daptomycin | |
|---|---|---|---|---|
| | $MIC_{50/90}$ (μg/mL) | MIC Range | $MIC_{50/90}$ (μg/mL) | MIC Range |
| *Staphylococcus aureus* | | | | |
| MSSA | 0.12/0.25 | 0.06–1.0 | 0.25/0.25 | 0.25 |
| MRSA | 0.5/2.0 | <0.06–4.0 | 0.25/0.5 | 0.06–2.0 |
| Coagulase-negative *S aureus* | | | | |
| MS | 0.25/0.5 | <0.06–0.5 | 0.25/1.0 | 0.06–4.0 |
| MR | 0.25/0.5 | <0.06–2.0 | 0.5/0.5 | 0.06–2.0 |
| *S pneumoniae* | | | | |
| PCN sensitive | ≤0.015/0.12 | ≤0.015–1.0 | — | — |
| PCN resistant | 0.12/0.25 | 0.06–1.0 | — | — |
| CTX resistant | 0.25/0.5 | 0.25–1.0 | — | — |

*Abbreviations:* CTX, ceftriaxone; $MIC_{50/90}$, minimum inhibitory concentration for 50% and 90% of isolates; MR, methicillin resistant; MRSA, methicillin-resistant *S aureus*; MS, methicillin sensitive; MSSA, methicillin-sensitive *S aureus*; PCN, penicillin.
    *Data from Refs.*[45–47]

## Daptomycin

Daptomycin is active against all clinically significant Gram-positive bacteria, including MSSA, MRSA, and coagulase-negative staphylococci, streptococci and enterococci, including vancomycin-resistant enterococcus,[49–52] as shown in **Table 3**. Although daptomycin is active against S pneumoniae, the drug cannot be used to treat pneumonia because it is inactivated by surfactant. Resistance to daptomycin developing during treatment of infections owing to MRSA in patients with endocarditis and osteomyelitis has been well-documented in adults.[21,25,50] Many of these patients received prior treatment with vancomycin.[52] The occurrence of vancomycin MIC creep can influence not only susceptibility to vancomycin, but to daptomycin.[52,53] Reduced susceptibility to vancomycin in vancomycin-intermediate S aureus isolates is due to the synthesis of an unusually thickened cell wall containing dipeptides (D-Ala-D-Ala) capable of binding vancomycin, thereby reducing the availability of the drug for intracellular target molecules.[54,55] The altered cell wall results in a reduced diffusion coefficient of vancomycin and sequestration of vancomycin within the cell wall by these false targets. S aureus strains with higher vancomycin MICs also tend to have higher daptomycin MICs.[21,53,54] Daptomycin resistance in these strains has been linked to polymorphisms in the mprF gene, leading to altered membrane phospholipid profiles and cell wall thickening. Jacobson and colleagues[52] reported on a 15-year-old boy with MRSA bacteremia after sustaining 90% body surface area flame burns, where the MRSA became resistant to daptomycin within 5 days of the initiation of therapy. The patient had not received prior vancomycin. The daptomycin MIC, by E-test, increased from 1 to 4 μg/mL. It was also confirmed as nonsusceptible by broth microdilution with an MIC of 2 μg/mL. The patient was switched to vancomycin and, although the initial MRSA isolate had a vancomycin MIC of 1 μg/mL, the MIC on day 5 had increased to 2 μg/mL, also by microdilution. Although the isolate was at the breakpoint and technically susceptible, many patients with invasive MRSA infections with vancomycin MICs of 1.5 to 2.0 μg/mL do not do well on vancomycin.[2]

## Dalbavancin and Telavancin

Both dalbavancin and telavancin have similar spectrum of activity against Gram-positive bacteria as vancomycin.[48,49,55–57] Gram-negative bacteria are intrinsically resistant to lipoglycopeptides. As shown in **Table 5**, both drugs are almost 17 times more active than vancomycin against S aureus, including MRSA, with MIC$_{90}$s of 0.06 μg/mL compared with 1 μg/mL for vancomycin.[56,57] They are also more active than vancomycin against enterococci, including vancomycin-resistant enterococcus. There are few data on activity against MRSA strains with high vancomycin MICs. It has been pointed out that it took more than 30 years for resistance to vancomycin to emerge.[56] Because these semisynthetic lipoglycopeptides have multiple mechanisms of action, it is expected that the frequency of resistance will be lower.[55] Telavancin-resistant strains of MRSA have been selected in vitro after serial passage, but there are no reports of resistance developing during therapy.[55] Similar results have been reported for dalbavancin.[55]

## Tedizolid

Tedizolid is an expanded oxazolidinone antibiotic, similar to linezolid. It has been approved for treatment of ABSSSIs in adults, and phase III pediatric studies are currently underway. Tedizolid acts by inhibiting protein synthesis by interacting with the 23S ribosomal RNA component of the 50S ribosomal subunit.[56] The spectrum of activity of tedizolid is essentially the same as linezolid, with excellent activity against

**Table 5**
**In vitro activity of vancomycin and linezolid compared with new antibiotics against MSSA and MRSA**

| Antibiotic | MSSA MIC Range (μg/mL) | MRSA MIC Range (μg/mL) |
|---|---|---|
| Vancomycin | 0.5–1.0 | 0.5–2.0 |
| Dalbavancin | 0.03–0.06 | 0.03–0.06 |
| Telavancin | 0.03–0.06 | 0.03–0.12 |
| Linezolid | 0.12–2.0 | 2.0–4.0 |
| Tedizolid | 0.25–0.5 | 0.25–0.5 |

Abbreviations: $MIC_{50/90}$, minimum inhibitory concentration for 50% and 90% of isolates; MRSA, methicillin-resistant Staphylococcus aureus MSSA, methicillin-sensitive S aureus.
Data from Refs.[37,48,49,51,56,57]

S aureus, including MRSA, streptococci, and enterococci (see **Table 5**). It has activity against linezolid-resistant S aureus and MRSA.[56] Tedizolid is approximately 4- to 16-fold more active than linezolid against MSSA and MRSA. There are no commercially available testing methods available for tedizolid at the time of this writing. As seen with linezolid, mutations of the 23 ribosomal RNA gene can occur and have been associated with increases of the MIC to greater than 4 μg/mL.[56]

## CLINICAL DATA

Only ceftaroline and daptomycin have FDA approval for use in children. Although there are studies of the pharmacology of dalbavancin, telavancin, and tedizolid in children, and phase III studies are currently being conducted, there are no published clinical data on the use of these drugs in children.

### Ceftaroline

Ceftaroline was approved by the FDA in May 2016 for treatment of ABSSSI and CABP in children 2 months of age and older. Approval was based on 2 randomized, controlled, observer-blinded studies.[14,15] Currently approved FDA dosage regimens for treatment of CAP and ABSSSI are 8 to 12 mg/kg every 8 hours in children 6 months to 2 years of age, and 12 mg/kg every 8 hours in children 2 to less than 18 years of age, to a divided maximum dose of 1200 mg/d 8 to 12 over hours. Increased doses of up to 10 mg/kg in children less than 6 months of age and 15 mg/kg in children greater than 6 months, to a maximum of 1800 mg/d for complicated CABP, patients with CF, and MRSA bacteremia/endocarditis may be given. The CAP study found that ceftaroline was comparable with ceftriaxone with clinical cure rates of 88% and 89%, respectively.[14] Patients with suspected MRSA infection were excluded.

The ABSSSI trial used the same dosing as the CABP study. Patients were randomized to receive ceftaroline or vancomycin or cefazolin with or without aztreonam.[15] Patients with bone and joint infections, burns, bite wounds, and necrotizing infections (ie, necrotizing fasciitis) were excluded. As seen with the CABP study, initial clinical cure rates were similar—94% for the ceftaroline group compared with 87% in patients who received the comparator. The incidences of adverse events were similar in both studies, with no differences between ceftaroline and the comparators. One exception was seroconversion to a positive direct Coombs test was seen more frequently in the patients who were treated with ceftaroline in the CABP study (17% vs 3% of patients who received ceftriaxone). Similar results were seen in the ABSSI study. There is an additional pediatric study of complicated CABP that compared monotherapy with ceftaroline to ceftriaxone plus vancomycin.[58] Patients with empyema, pleural effusion requiring a chest tube, and admission to an intensive care unit were excluded. Higher doses of ceftaroline were used: 10 mg/kg per dose every 8 hours in children less than 6 months and 15 mg/kg per dose in children greater than 6 months and older up to a maximum of 600 mg per dose. Clinical cure was observed in 90% of children (26 of 29) in the ceftaroline group compared with 100% (9 of 9) in the ceftriaxone plus vancomycin group. Of note, the incidence of adverse events was twice as frequent in the ceftriaxone plus vancomycin group (80% vs 40% in those who were treated with ceftaroline). Another study currently underway is an open trial of ceftaroline plus or minus gentamicin for treatment of late-onset sepsis in infants 34 weeks of gestation or older. No data have been presented so far.

### Daptomycin

Daptomycin was approved for treatment of ABSSSI in children 1 year of age and older in March 2017. It has been approved for use in adults since 2003. Safety and effectiveness in pediatric patients younger than the age of 1 year have not been established. Use of daptomycin in pediatric patients younger than 1 year of age should be avoided owing to the risk of potential effects on muscular, neuromuscular, and/or nervous systems observed in neonatal dogs.[25] Daptomycin is not indicated in pediatric patients with renal impairment because a dosage has not been established in these patients.[25] Overall, the safety profile in pediatric patients was similar to that observed in adult patients. There are a number of case reports, and retrospective and prospective phase I studies of use of daptomycin in children published since 2008.[35,36,59–63] Conditions included cellulitis and abscesses, bacteremia (MSSA, MRSA, enterococci), catheter-related bloodstream infections (coagulase-negative staphylococci, enterococcus, MSSA, MRSA), endocarditis (MRSA), osteomyelitis, and septic arthritis (MRSA) and ventricular peritoneal shunt infection (vancomycin intermediate S hemolyticus, vancomycin-resistant enterococcus). Overall response rates in terms of clinical cure and bacterial eradication were excellent. Side effects were also similar to those reported in adults. Increases in CPK were less than 5%. As of this writing, there is only 1 published, randomized, controlled trial in children 1 to 17 years of age for the treatment of ABSSSI, which compared daptomycin with local standard of care for skin and soft tissue infections.[64] Local standard of care included IV vancomycin, clindamycin, or a semisynthetic penicillin. A total of 257 patients received daptomycin and 132 received standard of care, which was primarily clindamycin or vancomycin. Thirty-five percent of the patients had confirmed MRSA infection. The overall therapeutic success rate was comparable in both groups: 97% for those patients who were treated with daptomycin compared with 98.7% of those who received standard of care. The use of daptomycin was not associated with increased muscular or neurologic toxicity. There were also no instances of emergence of resistance to daptomycin during therapy.

### Dalbavancin

Dalbavancin was approved by the FDA for treatment of ABSSSI in adults in 2014. Studies in adults have demonstrated that a single, weekly dose of dalbavancin, as a single 1500-mg infusion, was as effective as a 2-dose regimen (1000 mg on day 1 followed by 500 mg 1 week later).[65] Clinical outcomes were similar in both groups, including those patients with confirmed MRSA infection.

The potential advantages of use of dalbavancin in children include possibility of fewer doses owing to a long half-life. These characteristics of an antibiotic are particularly important, especially for pediatric population, owing to decreased durations of stay and decreased need for central venous access. This factor may lead to significant cost savings, with the possibility to save beds and reduce hospital duration of stay. Pharmacoeconomic studies on dalbavancin use in comparison with other antibiotics with similar antimicrobial spectrum are needed. Possible indications for this drug in the pediatric age group include neonatal sepsis, central line-associated bloodstream infection, acute hematogenous osteomyelitis, and severe skin and soft tissue infections. However, dalbavancin should only be used when there is a confirmed staphylococcal infection. It probably should not be used for presumptive treatment in the absence of a specific microbiologic diagnosis, because the drug persists in the body for several weeks; the terminal half-life of dalbavancin is approximately 14 days.[56] This factor can be important for patients who may have an adverse reaction.

### Tedizolid

Tedizolid was approved in adults for treatment of ABSSSI owing to susceptible Gram-positive organisms including *S aureus* (MSSA and MRSA), *S pyogenes, S agalactaie, S anginous* group, and *E faecalis* in 2014. Tedizolid has the advantage of being available in an oral as well as an IV formulation. Although there are no published data on the clinical use of tedizolid in children, a study of the pharmacokinetics, safety, and tolerability of single 200-mg oral or IV dose in adolescents (12–17 years old) was published in 2016.[66] The overall results were similar to those in adults. There was excellent bioavailability after oral dosing. Clinical trials of tedizolid for treatment of ABSSSI and other indications (osteomyelitis) in adolescents, using a 200-mg single daily dose, and younger children are currently ongoing. Unlike the other new antistaphylococcal drugs covered herein, tedizolid offers the option of an early IV to oral switch. Once-a-day dosing and increased antimicrobial activity offers a number of advantages over linezolid.

## THE FUTURE

Ceftaroline and daptomycin are currently approved for use in children. It is expected that the approved indications will continue to expand beyond ABSSSI for both and for CAPB for ceftaroline. Dalbavancin, telavancin, and tedizolid are currently in phase III trials in children in the United States. FDA approval is anticipated within 2 to 3 years. As described in this review, these drugs offer significant advantages over vancomycin for the treatment of MRSA infections in children. Ceftaroline is a beta-lactam antibiotic with expanded coverage, not only for *S aureus* and MRSA, but also for other Gram-positive bacteria, including *S pneumoniae.* Ceftaroline has an excellent safety profile and does not require monitoring of serum levels. Daptomycin has once daily dosing, making it suitable for outpatient IV therapy against a wide range of potentially resistant Gram-positive infections. One major drawback is that it cannot be used for pulmonary infections. Prolonged therapy with daptomycin has also been associated with the emergence of resistance, especially if the patient has received prior vancomycin. The emergence of daptomycin resistance may be avoided by using combination therapy with a beta-lactam antibiotic, which seems to also be synergistic. Although dalbavancin and telavancin are not yet approved, they offer superior antimicrobial activity, safety, and ease of dosing to vancomycin. Tedizolid is the only new antistaphylococcal agent that is also available in an oral formulation. This strength, plus once-a-day, dosing offers major advantages over linezolid, although cost will be an issue, especially because linezolid will shortly be available generically. The use of these drugs has the potential to shorten hospitalization and significantly reduce costs for pediatric care. Stay tuned.

## REFERENCES

1. Stewart GT, Holt RJ. Evolution of natural resistance to the newer penicillins. Br Med J 1963;1:308–11.

2. Arun A, Swamy S, Jacob K, et al. Evaluation of clinical outcome in children and adolescents receiving vancomycin for invasive infections due to methicillin-resistant *Staphylococcus aureus*: impact of increasing vancomycin MICs. Minerva Pediatr 2016. [Epub ahead of print].

3. Ghamrawi RJ, Neuner E. Ceftaroline fosamil: a super-cephalosporin? Cleve Clin J Med 2015;82(7):437–44.

4. Ishikawa T, Matsunaga N, Tawada H, et al. TAK-599, a novel N-phosphono type prodrug of anti-MRSA cephalosporin T-91825: synthesis, physicochemical and pharmacological properties. Bioorg Med Chem 2003;11:2427–37.

5. Ikeda Y, Ban J, Ishikawa T, et al. Stability and stabilization studies of TAK-599 (ceftaroline fosamil), a novel-N-phosphono type prodrug of anti-methicillin resistant *Staphylococcus aureus* cephalosporin T-91825. Chem Pharm Bull 2008;56: 1406–11.

6. Kosowska-Shick K, McGhee PL, Appelbaum PC. Affinity of ceftaroline (CPT) and other β-lactams for penicillin-binding proteins (PBPs) from *Staphylococcus aureus* and *Streptococcus pneumoniae*. Antimicrob Agents Chemother 2010; 54(5):1670–7.

7. Forest Laboratories. Pharmacokinetics of ceftaroline in subjects 12–17 years of age. In: ClinicalTrials.gov. [Internet]. Bethesda, (MD): National Library of Medicine (US). 2000. NLM Identifier: NCT00633126. Available at: https://clinicaltrials.gov/ct2/study/NCT00633126. Accessed April 28, 2017.

8. Forest Laboratories. Study of blood levels of ceftaroline fosamil in children who are receiving antibiotic therapy in hospital. In: ClinicalTrials.gov. [Internet]. Bethesda, (MD): National Library of Medicine (US). 2000. NLM Identifier: NCT01298843. Available at: https://clinicaltrials.gov/show/NCT01298843. Accessed April 28, 2017.

9. Riccobene T, Khariton T, Knebel W, et al. Population PK modeling and target attainment simulations to support dosing of ceftaroline fosamil in pediatric patients with acute bacterial skin and skin structure infections and community-acquired bacterial pneumonia. J Clin Pharmacol 2017;57(3):345–55.

10. Molloy L, Snyder AH, Srivastava R, et al. Ceftaroline fosamil for methicillin-resistant *Staphylococcus aureus* pulmonary exacerbation in a pediatric cystic fibrosis patient. J Pediatr Pharmacol Ther 2014;19(2):135–40.

11. Andes D, Craig WA. Pharmacodynamics of a new cephalosporin, PPI- 0903 (TAK-599), activity against methicillin-resistant *Staphylococcus aureus* in murine thigh and lung infection models: identification of an in vivo pharmacokinetic-pharmacodynamic target. Antimicrob Agents Chemother 2006;50:1376–83.

12. Ge Y, Liao S, Thye DA, et al. Ceftaroline (CPT) dose adjustment recommendations for subjects with mild or moderate renal impairment (RI). Abstracts of the 47th Interscience Conference on Antimicrobial Agents and Chemotherapy.

Chicago (IL), Washington, DC: American Society for Microbiology. Abstract, Abstract A-35. September 17-20, 2007.

13. Ge Y, Liao S, Talbot GH. Population pharmacokinetics (PK) analysis of ceftaroline (CPT) in volunteers and patients with complicated skin and skin structure infection (cSSSI). Abstracts of the 47th Interscience Conference on Antimicrobial Agents and Chemotherapy. Chicago (IL). Washington, DC: American Society for Microbiology. Abstract A-34. September 17-20, 2007.

14. Cannavino C, Nemeth A, Korczowski B, et al. A randomized, prospective study of pediatric patients with community-acquired pneumonia treated with ceftaroline versus ceftriaxone. Pediatr Infect Dis J 2016;35:752–9.

15. Blumer J, Ghonghadze T, Cannavino C, et al. A multicenter, randomized, observer-blinded, active-controlled study evaluating the safety and effectiveness of ceftaroline compared with ceftriaxone plus vancomycin in pediatric patients with complicated community-acquired bacterial pneumonia. Pediatr Infect Dis J 2016;35:760–6.

16. Korczowski B, Antadze T, Giorgobiani M, et al. A multicenter, randomized, observer-blinded, active-controlled study to evaluate the safety and efficacy of ceftaroline versus comparator in pediatric patients with acute bacterial skin and skin structure infection. Pediatr Infect Dis J 2016;35:e239–47.

17. Teflaro® (ceftaroline fosamil) [package insert]. St Louis, MO: Forest Pharmaceuticals, Inc; 2016.

18. Riccobene TA, Rekeda L, Rank D, et al. Evaluation of the effect of a supratherapeutic dose of intravenous ceftaroline fosamil on the corrected QT interval. Antimicrob Agents Chemother 2013;57(4):1777–83.

19. Shirley D, Heil E, Johnson J. Ceftaroline fosamil: a brief clinical review. Infect Dis Ther 2013;2:95–110.

20. Hancock RE. Mechanisms of action of newer antibiotics for gram-positive pathogens. Lancet Infect Dis 2005;5(4):209–18.

21. Miller WR, Bayer AS, Arias CA, et al. Mechanism of action and resistance to daptomycin in Staphylococcus aureus and Enterococci. Cold Spring Harb Perspect Med 2016;6:a026997.

22. Sader HS, Farrell DJ, Flamm RK, et al. Daptomycin activity tested against 164457 bacterial isolates from hospitalised patients: summary of 8 years of a Worldwide Surveillance Programme (2005–2012). Int J Antimicrob Agents 2014;43:465–9.

23. Principi N, Caironi M, Venturini F, et al. Daptomycin in paediatrics: current knowledge and the need for future research. J Antimicrob Chemother 2015;70(3):643–8.

24. Abdel-Rahman SM, Benziger DP, Jacobs RF, et al. Single-dose pharmacokinetics of daptomycin in children with suspected or proved gram-positive infections. Pediatr Infect Dis J 2008;27(4):330–4.

25. Daptomycin for injection. Full prescribing reference. Monograph: cubicin. Lexington (MA): Cubist Pharmaceuticals; 2011.

26. Arbeit RD, Maki D, Tally FP, et al. The safety and efficacy of daptomycin for the treatment of complicated skin and skin-structure infections. Clin Infect Dis 2004;38(12):1673–81.

27. Abdel-Rahman SM, Chandorkar G, Akins RL, et al. Single-dose pharmacokinetics and tolerability of daptomycin 8 to 10 mg/kg in children aged 2 to 6 years with suspected or proved Gram-positive infections. Pediatr Infect Dis J 2011; 30(8):712–4.

28. Cohen-Wolkowiez M, Watt KM, Hornik CP, et al. Pharmacokinetics and tolerability of single-dose daptomycin in young infants. Pediatr Infect Dis J 2012;31(9): 935–7.

29. Bradley JS, Benziger D, Bokesch P, et al. Single-dose pharmacokinetics of daptomycin in pediatric patients 3-24 months of age. Pediatr Infect Dis J 2014;33(9): 936–9.

30. Sarafidis K, Iosifidis E, Gikas E, et al. Daptomycin use in a neonate: serum level monitoring and outcome. Am J Perinatol 2010;27(5):421–4.

31. Cohen-Wolkowiez M, Smith PB, Benjamin DK Jr, et al. Daptomycin use in infants: report of two cases with peak and trough drug concentrations. J Perinatol 2008; 28(3):233–4.

32. Gawronski KM. Successful use of daptomycin in a preterm neonate with persistent methicillin-resistant *Staphylococcus epidermidis* bacteremia. J Pediatr Pharmacol Ther 2015;20(1):61–5.

33. Bradley JS, Nelson JD, Barnett E, et al. Nelson's pediatric antimicrobial therapy. 22nd edition. Illinois: American Academy of Pediatrics; 2016.

34. Fowler VG Jr, Boucher HW, Corey GR, et al. Daptomycin versus standard therapy for bacteremia and endocarditis caused by *Staphylococcus aureus*. N Engl J Med 2006;355(7):653–65.

35. Larru B, Cowden CL, Zaoutis TE, et al. Daptomycin use in United States children's hospitals. J Pediatric Infect Dis Soc 2015;4(1):60–2.

36. Karageorgos SA, Miligkos M, Dakoutrou M, et al. Clinical effectiveness, safety profile, and pharmacokinetics of daptomycin in pediatric patients: a systematic review. J Pediatric Infect Dis Soc 2016;5(4):446–57.

37. Malabarba A, Goldstein BP. Origin, structure, and activity in vitro and in vivo of dalbavancin. J Antimicrob Chemother 2005;55:ii15–20.

38. Leimkuhler C, Chen L, Barrett D, et al. Differential inhibition of *Staphylococcus aureus* PBP2 by glycopeptide antibiotics. J Am Chem Soc 2005;127:3250–1.

39. Billeter M, Zervos MJ, Chen AY, et al. Dalbavancin: a novel once-weekly lipoglycopeptide antibiotic. Clin Infect Dis 2008;46(4):577–83.

40. Klinker K, Borgert S. Beyond vancomycin: the tail of the lipoglycopeptides. Clin Ther 2015;37(12):2619–36.

41. Bradley JS, Puttagunta S, Rubino C. Pharmacokinetics, safety and tolerability of single dose dalbavancin in children 121-7 years of age. Pediatr Infect Dis J 2015; 34:748–52.

42. Gonzalez D, Bradley J, Blumer J. Dalbavancin pharmacokinetics and safety in children 3 months to 11 years of age. Pediatr Infect Dis J 2017;36(7):645–53.

43. Andes D, Craig WA. In vivo pharmacodynamics activity of the glycopeptide dalbavancin. Antimicrob Agents Chemother 2007;51(5):1633–42.

44. Esposito S, Bianchini S. Dalbavancin for the treatment of paediatric infectious diseases. Eur J Clin Microbiol Infect Dis 2016;35:1895–901.

45. Pfaller MA, Mendes RE, Castanheira M, et al. Ceftaroline activity tested against bacterial isolates causing community-acquired respiratory tract infections and skin and skin structure infections in pediatric patients from United States Hospitals: 2012-2014. Pediatr Infect Dis J 2017;36(5):486–90.

46. Rolston KVI, Jamal MA, Nesher L, et al. In vitro activity of ceftaroline and comparator agents against gram-positive and gram-negative clinical isolates from cancer patients. Int J Antimicrob Agents 2017;49:416–21.

47. Zhang H, Xiao M, Kon F, et al. A multicentre study of methicillin-resistant *Staphylococcus aureus* in acute bacterial skin and skin structure infections in China:

susceptibility to ceftaroline and molecular epidemiology. Int J Antimicrob Agents 2015;45:347–50.

48. Sweeny D, Shinabarger DL, Arhin FF, et al. Comparative in vitro activity of orita-vancin and other agents against methicillin-susceptible and methicillin-resistant *Staphylococcus aureus*. Diagn Microbiol Infect Dis 2017;87:121–8.

49. Huband MD, Castanheira M, Farrell DJ, et al. In vitro activity of dalbavancin against multidrug-resistant Staphylococcus aureus and streptococci from pa-tients with documented infections in Europe and surrounding regions (2011-2013). Int J Antimicrob Agents 2016;47:495–9.

50. Gonzalez-Ruiz A, Seaton RA, Hamed K. Daptomycin: an evidence-based review of its role in the treatment of Gram-positive infections. Infect Drug Resist 2016;9: 47–58.

51. Atkas G, Derbentli S. *In vitro* activity of daptomycin combined with dalbavancin and linezolid and dalbavancin with linezolid against MRSA strains. J Antimicrob Chemother 2017;72:441–3.

52. Jacobson LM, Milstone AM, Zenilman J, et al. Daptomycin therapy failure in an adolescent with methicillin-resistant *Staphylococcus aureus* bacteremia. Pediatr Infect Dis J 2009;28(5):445–7.

53. Sakoulas G, Alder J, Thauvin-Eliopoulos C, et al. Induction of daptomycin hetero-geneous susceptibility in *Staphylococcus aureus* by exposure to vancomycin. Antimicrob Agents Chemother 2006;50:1581–5.

54. Sieradzki K, Tomasz A. Alterations of cell wall structure and metabolism accom-pany reduced susceptibility to vancomycin in an isogenic series of clinical iso-lates of *Staphylococcus aureus*. J Bacteriol 2003;185:7103–10.

55. Zeng D, Debabov D, Hartsell TL, et al. Approved glycopeptides antibacterial drugs: mechanism of action and resistance. Cold Spring Harb Perspect Med 2016;6:a026989.

56. Crotty MP, Krekel T, Burnham CAD, et al. New gram-positive agents: the next generation of oxazolidinones and lipoglycopeptides. J Clin Microbiol 2016; 54(9):2225–32.

57. Jones RN, Flamm RK, Castanheira M, et al. Activity of telavancin against Gram-positive pathogens isolated from bone and joint infections in North American, Latin American, European and Asia-Pacific nations. Diagn Microbiol Infect Dis 2017. http://dx.doi.org/10.1016/j.diagmicrobio.2017.03.003.

58. Corey A, So T-Y. Current clinical trials on the use of ceftaroline in the pediatric pop-ulation. Clin Drug Investig 2017. http://dx.doi.org/10.1007/s40261-017-0523-2.

59. Namtu KC, Crain JC, Messina AF, et al. Clinical experience with daptomycin in pediatrics. Pharmacotherapy 2017;3(1):105–8.

60. Tedeschi S, Tumietto F, Conti M, et al. Use of daptomycin in critically ill children with bloodstream infections and complicated skin and soft-tissue infections. Pe-diatr Infect Dis J 2016;35(2):180–2.

61. Syriopoulou V, Dailiana Z, Dmitriy N, et al. Clinical experience with daptomycin for the treatment of gram-positive infections in children and adolescents. Pediatr Infect Dis J 2016;35(5):511–6.

62. Garazzino S, Castagnola E, Di Gangi M, et al. Daptomycin for children in clinical practice experience. Pediatr Infect Dis J 2016;35(6):639–41.

63. Ardura MI, Mejías A, Katz KS, et al. Daptomycin therapy for invasive gram-positive bacterial infections in children. Pediatr Infect Dis J 2007;26(12):1128–32.

64. Bradley J, Glasser C, Patino H, et al. Daptomycin for complicated skin infections: a randomized trial. Pediatrics 2017;139(3):e20162477.

65. Dunne MW, Puttagunta S, Giordano P, et al. A randomized clinical trial of single-dose versus weekly dalbavancin for treatment of acute bacterial skin and skin structure infection. Clin Infect Dis 2016;62(5):545–51.
66. Bradley JS, Flanagan SD, Arrieta AC, et al. Pharmacokinetics, safety, tolerability of single oral or intravenous administration of 200 mg tedizolid phosphate in adolescents. Pediatr Infect Dis J 2016;35(6):628–33.

# Antifungal Drugs in Newborns and Children

 CrossMark

Mihai Puia-Dumitrescu, MD, MPH[a,b], P. Brian Smith, MD, MPH, MHS[a,b],*

## KEYWORDS

- Antifungal agents • Newborns • Children • Immunocompromised hosts

## KEY POINTS

- Many studies of antifungals in children are small, dosing studies.
- There are minimal safety/ efficacy data, needed to support labeling.
- Dosing for infants and children with invasive fungal infections cannot be extrapolated from adults.

## INTRODUCTION AND BACKGROUND

Invasive fungal infections continue to be a significant cause of morbidity and mortality in infants and children. The most common fungi affecting children and neonates are *Candida* and *Aspergillus*. Candidemia is the fourth most common cause of nosocomial bloodstream infections in the United States and much of the developed world.[1] *Candida* spp are the third most common pathogens in nosocomial blood stream infections among premature infants[2–4] and commonly isolated in hospitalized older pediatric patients.[5,6] Invasive *Candida* infections are associated with high mortality—34% in very low-birth-weight infants (<1500 g birth weight)[7,8] and 16% to 28% in older children.[9,10] Invasive infections caused by *Aspergillus* are common in severely immunocompromised children and associated with mortality as high as 50%.[11]

Invasive fungal infections are of increasing importance as physicians care for a growing number of immunocompromised infants and children. The options for treatment are evolving and therapeutic alternatives are more available as more is learned about the dosing of antifungals in infant and children.[12–14] Appropriate use of antifungals in this vulnerable population is important for both prevention and treatment of infection. Successful identification and treatment of invasive fungal infections are required to maximize the antifungal activity of the agents and minimize toxicity.

[a] Department of Pediatrics, Division of Neonatal Medicine, Duke University Medical Center, 2424 Erwin Road, Suite 504, Durham, NC 27705, USA; [b] Department of Pediatrics, Duke Clinical Research Institute, P.O. Box 17969, Durham, NC 27715, USA
* Corresponding author. Division of Neonatal-Perinatal Medicine, Duke University Medical Center, Duke Clinical Research Institute, Durham, NC.
*E-mail address:* brian.smith@duke.edu

Pediatr Clin N Am 64 (2017) 1389–1402
http://dx.doi.org/10.1016/j.pcl.2017.08.013
0031-3955/17/© 2017 Elsevier Inc. All rights reserved.

Currently, there are 4 widely used classes of drugs in the treatment of invasive fungal infections in children and infants, including the polyenes, pyrimidine analogues, azoles, and echinocandins (**Table 1**).

## POLYENES

The class of polyene macrolides is the oldest antifungal class. Included in this class are amphotericin B deoxycholate (AmB) and the later developed lipid-based formulations: amphotericin B liposomal complex (ABLC), amphotericin B colloidal dispersion (ABCD), and liposomal amphotericin B (L-AmB). Lipid formulations of amphotericin are associated with less nephrotoxicity.[15–17]

### Amphotericin B Deoxycholate

For the past 6 decades, AmB has been one of the most used antifungals in infants and children. The mechanism of action is characterized by binding to fungal membrane ergosterols, which increases cell permeability and ultimately cell death.[18] With broad-spectrum coverage, AmB remained one of the most used antifungals for treatment of invasive infections, including *Candida* spp (excluding *Candida lusitaniae*), *Aspergillus* spp, and *Zygomycetes*. AmB is used for the treatment of *Candida* meningoencephalitis due to penetration of central nervous system (CNS) (but not the cerebrospinal fluid).[19]

Despite the lack of specific Food and Drug Administration (FDA) guidance in infants, AmB is frequently used to treat invasive candidiasis in this age group.[20,21] Safety and effectiveness have not been established in pediatrics. In infants, the risk of toxicity is low, with data suggesting transient elevation of creatinine and hypokalemia.[22] Infusion-related toxicities (fever and chills/rigors), nephrotoxicity, and electrolyte disturbances have been reported in older children.[23]

Most phamacokinetic (PK) studies in children suggest a dose of 1 mg/kg/d.[23,24] The recommended dose in infants is 1 mg/kg/d.[25]

### Lipid-Based Amphotericin B Preparations

ABCD, ABLC, and L-AmB are FDA approved in infants and children aged 1 month to 16 years for neutropenic patients with persistent fever despite broad-spectrum antibiotic therapy and patients with invasive fungal infections who are refractory to or intolerant of conventional AmB therapy. Compared with AmB, they require higher doses for equivalent antifungal efficacy in vitro and in animals models, but these lipid formulations have the same mechanism of action and antifungal spectrum. Dosing recommendations for ABCD are 3 mg/kg/d to 5 mg/kg/d,[26] for ABLC 2.5 mg/kg/d to 5 mg/kg/d,[27] and for L-AmB 3 mg/kg/d to 5 mg/kg/d.[26,28]

## PYRIMIDINE ANALOGUES

Flucytosine is a fluorinated pyrimidine analogue that interferes with fungal nucleic acid synthesis.[29] Flucytosine has been shown to be active against *Candida* spp and *Cryptococcus neoformans*. Given the rapid development of resistance, it should be used in combination with other antifungal agents.[25] The combination therapy with AmB is supported by well-designed, randomized clinical trials for the treatment of cryptococcal meningitis.[30] Other than PK data included in the FDA label, flucytosine is not approved for use in neonates.[31]

Flucytosine is rarely used in children, and PK studies are limited in this population.[24,32] Given the limited PK, safety, and efficacy data in children and infants and the lack of safe target plasma concentrations, flucytosine use is discouraged.[33]

**Table 1**
Summary of antifungals in infants and children

| Drug | Neonatal | Pediatric | Food and Drug Administration Approved in Children | Food and Drug Administration Indication |
|------|----------|-----------|---------------------------------------------------|-----------------------------------------|
| Polyenes | | | | |
| AmB | 1 mg/kg/d | 1 mg/kg/d | No | Potentially life-threatening fungal infections: aspergillosis, cryptococcosis (torulosis), North American blastomycosis, systemic candidiasis, coccidioidomycosis, histoplasmosis, zygomycosis, including mucormycosis due to susceptible species of the genera *Absidia*, *Mucor*, and *Rhizopus*, and infections due to related susceptible species of *Conidiobolus* and *Basidiobolus*, and sporotrichosis |
| L-AmB | 3 mg/kg/d | 3–5 mg/kg/d | 1 mo to 16 y | Empirical therapy for presumed fungal infection in febrile, neutropenic patients; treatment of *Cryptococcus* meningitis in HIV-infected patients; treatment of patients with *Aspergillus* spp, *Candida* spp, and/or *Cryptococcus* spp infections refractory to AmB or in patients where renal impairment or unacceptable toxicity precludes the use of AmB; treatment of visceral leishmaniasis |

*(continued on next page)*

**Table 1**
*(continued)*

| Drug | Neonatal | Pediatric | Food and Drug Administration Approved in Children | Food and Drug Administration Indication |
|------|----------|-----------|---------------------------------------------------|------------------------------------------|
| ABLC | 5 mg/kg/d | 2.5–5 mg/kg/d | <16 y | Invasive fungal infections in patients who are refractory to or intolerant of conventional amphotericin B therapy |
| ABCD | No data | 3–5 mg/kg/d | <16 y | Invasive aspergillosis in patients where renal impairment or unacceptable toxicity precludes the use of AmB in effective doses and in patients with invasive aspergillosis where prior AmB therapy has failed |
| **Pyrimidine analogues** | | | | |
| Flucytosine | 25–100 mg/kg/d divided q8h–q24h | 100–150 mg/kg/d divided q6h | No | Serious infections caused by susceptible strains of *Candida* and/or *Cryptococcus* |
| **Azoles** | | | | |
| Fluconazole | Loading dose: 25 mg/kg Maintenance: 12 mg/kg q24h (3–6 mg/kg twice weekly for prophylaxis) | 6–12 mg/kg q24h (3 mg/kg q24h for prophylaxis) | >6 mo | Oropharyngeal candidiasis, esophageal candidiasis, systemic candidiasis, cryptococcal meningitis, and prophylaxis of invasive candidiasis in immunocompromised children |
| Itraconazole | No data | 2.5–5 mg/kg q12h (2.5 mg/kg q24h for prophylaxis) | No | Oropharyngeal and esophageal candidiasis |

| Drug | | Dose | Age | Indications |
|---|---|---|---|---|
| Voriconazole | No data | Loading dose: 9 mg/kg q12h for 2 doses<br>Maintenance: 8 mg/kg q12h<br>Maximum daily dose: 700 mg | >12 y | Invasive aspergillosis, candidemia in non-neutropenic patients, esophageal candidiasis, serious fungal infections caused by *Scedosporium apiospermum* and *Fusarium* spp, including *Fusarium solani*, in patients intolerant of, or refractory to, other therapy |
| Posaconazole | No data | 800 mg/d divided q6–12h (>12 years old) | 13–17 y | Prophylaxis of invasive *Aspergillus* and *Candida* infections and treatment of oropharyngeal candidiasis, including oropharyngeal candidiasis refractory to itraconazole and/or fluconazole |
| Isavuconazole | No data | No data | No | Treatment of invasive aspergillosis and mucormycosis |
| Echinocandins | | | | |
| Caspofungin | 25 mg/m² q24h | Initial: 70 mg/m² once<br>Maintenance: 50 mg/m² q24h<br>Maximum daily dose: 70 mg/m² | >3 mo | Empirical therapy for presumed fungal infections in febrile, neutropenic patients; treatment of candidemia and the following *Candida* infections: intra-abdominal abscesses, peritonitis and pleural space infections; treatment of esophageal candidiasis; and treatment of invasive aspergillosis in patients who are refractory to or intolerant of other therapies |

(continued on next page)

**Table 1**
*(continued)*

| Drug | Neonatal | Pediatric | Food and Drug Administration Approved in Children | Food and Drug Administration Indication |
|------|----------|-----------|---------------------------------------------------|------------------------------------------|
| Micafungin | 10 mg/kg q24h | 2–4 mg/kg/d (1 mg/kg for prophylaxis) Maximum daily dose: 100 mg | >4 mo | Candidemia, acute disseminated candidiasis, *Candida* peritonitis and abscesses; treatment of patients with esophageal candidiasis; prophylaxis for patients undergoing hematopoietic stem cell transplantation |
| Anidulafungin | Initial: 3 mg/kg once followed by 1.5 mg/kg q24h | Initial: 3 mg/kg once followed by 1.5 mg/kg/d | No | Candidemia and other forms of *Candida* infections (intra-abdominal abscess and peritonitis), esophageal candidiasis |

The currently recommended dose in children greater than 1 month of age is 100 mg/kg to 150 mg/kg in 4 divided dosages.[25,26] Flucytosine can be used for infants with disseminated candidiasis and involvement of the CNS and/or urinary tract, and a dose of 25 mg/kg to 100 mg/kg daily in 1 to 3 divided dosages is recommended.[32]

## AZOLES

The mechanism of action for triazole agents involves interfering with the fungal cytochrome P450–dependent enzyme lanosterol 14$\alpha$-demethylase required for sterol synthesis, causing accumulation of aberrant and toxic sterols in the cell membrane.[34–36] The triazoles provided for orally bioavailable alternatives to the polyenes and echinocandins. The most commonly prescribed agents include first-generation fluconazole and itraconazole as well as second-generation voriconazole, posaconazole, and ravuconazole. The first-generation agents are available as oral and parenteral formulations. Fluconazole is commonly used against multiple *Candida* spp.[12] Itraconazole, voriconazole, posaconazole, and ravuconazole are active against both *Candida* spp and *Aspergillus* spp.

### Fluconazole

Fluconazole is a triazole that was approved by the FDA for treatment of cryptococcosis and *Candida* infections and is the most used antifungal in the neonatal period[37] for prophylaxis against invasive fungal disease in high-risk infants. Fluconazole undergoes minimal metabolism and is primarily excreted unchanged in the urine.[38] Fluconazole has been used for treatment of candidiasis due to its effective penetration into the CNS and the urinary tract, both important sites of invasive *Candida* infection in infants.[39] Fluconazole has been used for the treatment of invasive candidiasis in infants.[40] Fluconazole is used extensively for older children for the prevention and treatment of disseminated candidiasis. Fluconazole is indicated for use in children for the treatment of oropharyngeal candidiasis, esophageal candidiasis, systemic candidiasis, cryptococcal meningitis, and prophylaxis of invasive candidiasis in immunocompromised children. The safety profile of fluconazole in children ages 1 day to 17 years has been studied, whereas efficacy has not been established in infants less than 6 months of age.[41]

In recent years the resistance to fluconazole has been increasing. There are reports of resistance among *Candida* isolates as high as 8%, mostly among non-albicans species.[42] *Candida krusei* is generally considered inherently resistant to fluconazole and 20% to 50% of *Candida glabrata* isolates are resistant.[42,43]

The fungistatic activity of fluconazole is time dependent; optimal dosing requires that the area under the curve be maintained above the minimum inhibitory concentration for longer periods of time.[12] Given fluconazole's action on a fungal-specific enzymatic pathway, its toxicity is limited, even in premature infants.

The recommended dose in infants 12 mg/kg/d, with the potential need of a loading dose of 25 mg/kg to achieve rapid steady state concentrations, achieves surrogate pharmacodynamic targets.[44,45] Fluconazole is effective as a prophylactic agent for invasive *Candida* infection in premature infants.[12] Most neonatal units use doses of 6 mg/kg twice weekly for prophylaxis in high-risk infants.[46] Prophylaxis is recommended for use in extremely low-birth-weight infants (<1000 g) in units with high incidence of invasive fungal infections, but the criteria used to determine which infants are at high risk for invasive fungal infection vary by center.[33]

## Itraconazole

Itraconazole use is approved for the treatment of oropharyngeal and esophageal candidiasis in adult HIV patients or other immunocompromised patients by the FDA[47] but is not labeled for pediatric populations. Itraconazole is extensively metabolized in the liver, primarily by cytochrome P450 3A4[48] and variable oral absorption. The clinical use of itraconazole is primarily limited to treatment of fungi that do not cause CNS disease.[49] There are no large studies in infants, but case reports of candidiasis show itraconazole effective and well-tolerated.[50,51]

Routine drug monitoring should be considered. The use of itraconazole in infants is still not recommended due to lack of efficacy and safety data.[12,33] The bioavailability of itraconazole is dose dependent, and a dose of 2.5 mg/kg to 5 mg/kg twice daily is preferred to achieve levels comparable to adults.[52,53]

## Voriconazole

Voriconazole is a second-generation triazole engineered to extend the antifungal spectrum of fluconazole to *Aspergillus* spp.[29] Voriconazole is available in both intravenous (IV) and oral formulations with approximately 90% oral bioavailability. Voriconazole is metabolized by the liver. Similar to fluconazole, it has excellent CNS penetration. Voriconazole is FDA approved for treatment of mucocutaneous and systemic candidiasis. It is FDA indicated in children greater than 12 years of age with invasive candidiasis or aspergillosis.[54] Voriconazole is commonly used for prophylaxis against yeast and mold infections in high-risk patients, such as bone marrow transplantation candidates.[55] The use of voriconazole in infants is not recommended due to lack of PK efficacy and safety data.[12,33]

A dosing regimen of 9 mg/kg every 12 hours for 2 doses followed by 8 mg/kg every 12 hours has been suggested by pharmacokinetic models and clinical studies in older children.[56] Therapeutic drug monitoring is recommended because trough levels less than 1 mg/L have been associated with increased mortality in older patients.[57] Serum levels necessary for treatment success have not been determined in infants.

## Posaconazole

Posaconazole is a broad-spectrum antifungal, active against fluconazole-susceptible isolates of *Candida, Cryptococcus*, dimorphic fungi, and *Aspergillus*. In addition, posaconazole is active against many *Zygomycetes*.[49,58] Posaconazole can be used for prophylaxis of systemic fungal infections[59] but does not penetrate the cerebrospinal fluid well.[58] Posaconazole is available orally and in 2014 the FDA approved an IV formulation well tolerated in adult patients at risk for invasive fungal infections.[60] The safety and effectiveness of posaconazole have been established in children 13 years to 17 years of age.[61] There are few studies evaluating the dosing in children less than 13 years and the results regarding a correct dosing regimen in this group are inconclusive given highly variable trough concentration.[62] The recommended dose based on data from children 8 years to 17 years with proved or probable invasive fungal infections is 800 mg/d divided every 6 hours to 12 hours to have median serum concentrations that are comparable with adults.[63]

## Isavuconazole

Isavuconazole is FDA approved for the treatment of invasive aspergillosis and invasive mucormycosis for patients 18 years and older.[64] Isavuconazonium sulfate, a water-soluble prodrug is available as a capsule or for IV administration. Isavuconazonium sulfate was found similarly effective to voriconazole for the treatment of patients with proved or probable invasive fungal disease caused by filamentous fungi, including *Aspergillus*.[49] In open-label trials involving adults with proved, probable, or possible invasive fungal disease, mortality among patients receiving isavuconazole was similar to those who received AmB or posaconazole.[65] Isavuconazole use in children is not recommended because there are no studies evaluating the PK/pharmacodynamic, efficacy, and safety in the pediatric population, and the clinical experience knowledge is mostly limited for adults.[12,33]

## ECHINOCANDINS

The echinocandins are the newest class of antifungals, with caspofungin, micafungin, and anidulafungin approved by the FDA for IV administration.[49,66] The mechanism of action is characterized by inhibition of the $\beta$-(1,3)-D-glucan synthase complex, which disrupts cell membrane permeability. Given this unique pathway, they are considered the safest antifungals at this time. Similar to the polyenes, these agents do not penetrate cerebrospinal fluid but can penetrate brain parenchyma.[33] The echinocandins have a broad spectrum of coverage consisting of fungicidal activity against most *Candida* spp, including fluconazole-resistant species,[67] low toxicity, and minimal drug interactions.[12,67] In the 2016 Infectious Diseases Society of America candidiasis guidelines, echinocandins are the primary drugs of choice for invasive candidiasis.[26] Echinocandins are not active against *Cryptococcus*, dimorphic fungi, or *Zygomycetes*.

### Caspofungin

Caspofungin is a fungicidal agent against *Candida* spp with a concentration-dependent effect and up to 12 hours' postantifungal effect.[68] It was approved by the FDA for children greater than 3 months of age for treatment of candidemia, empirical therapy in febrile neutropenic patients, and invasive aspergillosis refractory to other antifungals.[69] Caspofungin has linear PK and hepatic metabolism, with a terminal half-life of approximately 10 hours.[70,71] The recommended dose is a single 70-mg/m$^2$ loading dose on day 1, followed by 50 mg/m$^2$ once daily thereafter. The efficacy of caspofungin for invasive candidiasis in infants less than 3 months of age is limited and a dose of 25 mg/m$^2$/d has been shown to achieve exposures similar to adults.[72] There are safety studies done in children but not in neonates. Caspofungin is well tolerated in this age group and the most common adverse effects include fever, hypokalemia, and elevated liver enzymes.[73]

### Micafungin

Micafungin is fungicidal against *Candida* spp and fungistatic in vitro against *Aspergillus*. Micafungin has a half-life of approximately 12 hours and it exhibits linear PK with the highest drug concentrations detected in the lung, liver, spleen, and kidney. Infants demonstrate greater clearance of micafungin compared with older children and adults. Due to differences in pharmacokinetic parameters, infants needed a higher dosing compared with adults to achieve similar drug exposures.[74] For infants, a daily dose of 10 mg/kg[7,12] has been used for treating *Candida* infections, including meningoencephalitis.[75] Based on an open-label study, infants have been shown to tolerate 15 mg/kg and, given concern for CNS involvement, 10 mg/kg is now recommended.[76] Safety and effectiveness in pediatric patients less than 4 months of age have not been established.[77] Micafungin is approved by FDA for the treatment of invasive candidiasis,[78] with a dose of 2 mg/kg daily.

## Anidulafungin

Anidulafungin has a fungicidal effect against *Candida* spp. It has linear PK and has a longer half-life than other echinocandins (20 hours).[79] An anidulafungin loading dose of 3 mg/kg, followed by daily 1.5 mg/kg, was suggested in infants and children.[80] Despite available PK data in children, clinical experience remains insufficient for supporting the use of anidulafungin. The safety and effectiveness of anidulafungin in children less than or equal to 16 years of age have not been established.[81]

## SUMMARY

Over the past decade, new antifungals have been developed and approved for use in newborns and children and offered physicians more options when faced with severe invasive infections. Optimization of the dosing for older antifungals in this population is needed. With the development of new agents, pharmacokinetic properties, clinical implications, and toxicity studies are expected, including safety and efficacy data specific for this vulnerable population. Combination therapy and new classes of antifungals are being developed and evaluated as potential strategies for combating drug-resistance and adverse effects.

## REFERENCES

1. Wisplinghoff H, Bischoff T, Tallent SM, et al. Nosocomial bloodstream infections in US hospitals: analysis of 24,179 cases from a prospective nationwide surveillance study. Clin Infect Dis 2004;39(3):309–17.
2. Benjamin DK, DeLong E, Cotten CM, et al. Mortality following blood culture in premature infants: increased with gram-negative bacteremia and candidemia, but not gram-positive bacteremia. J Perinatol 2004;24(3):175–80.
3. Kaufman D. Strategies for prevention of neonatal invasive candidiasis. Semin Perinatol 2003;27(5):414–24.
4. Stoll BJ, Gordon T, Korones SB, et al. Late-onset sepsis in very low birth weight neonates: a report from the National Institute of Child Health and Human Development Neonatal Research Network. J Pediatr 1996;129(1):63–71.
5. Grohskopf LA, Sinkowitz-Cochran RL, Garrett DO, et al. A national point-prevalence survey of pediatric intensive care unit-acquired infections in the United States. J Pediatr 2002;140(4):432–8.
6. Wisplinghoff H, Seifert H, Tallent SM, et al. Nosocomial bloodstream infections in pediatric patients in United States hospitals: epidemiology, clinical features and susceptibilities. Pediatr Infect Dis J 2003;22(8):686–91.
7. Benjamin DK Jr, Stoll BJ, Gantz MG, et al, Eunice Kennedy Shriver National Institute of Child Health and Human Development Neonatal Research Network. Neonatal candidiasis: epidemiology, risk factors, and clinical judgment. Pediatrics 2010;126(4):e865–73.
8. Stoll BJ, Hansen N, Fanaroff AA, et al. Late-onset sepsis in very low birth weight neonates: the experience of the NICHD Neonatal Research Network. Pediatrics 2002;110(2 Pt 1):285–91.
9. Singhi SC, Reddy TC, Chakrabarti A. Candidemia in a pediatric intensive care unit. Pediatr Crit Care Med 2004;5(4):369–74.
10. Young GA, Bosly A, Gibbs DL, et al. A double-blind comparison of fluconazole and nystatin in the prevention of candidiasis in patients with leukaemia. Antifungal Prophylaxis Study Group. Eur J Cancer 1999;35(8):1208–13.

11. Burgos A, Zaoutis TE, Dvorak CC, et al. Pediatric invasive aspergillosis: a multi-center retrospective analysis of 139 contemporary cases. Pediatrics 2008;121(5): e1286–94.

12. Autmizguine J, Guptill JT, Cohen-Wolkowiez M, et al. Pharmacokinetics and pharmacodynamics of antifungals in children: clinical implications. Drugs 2014;74(8): 891–909.

13. Stockmann C, Constance JE, Roberts JK, et al. Pharmacokinetics and pharmacodynamics of antifungals in children and their clinical implications. Clin Pharmacokinet 2014;53(5):429–54.

14. Watt K, Benjamin DK Jr, Cohen-Wolkowiez M. Pharmacokinetics of antifungal agents in children. Early Hum Dev 2011;87(Suppl 1):S61–5.

15. Al Arishi H, Frayha HH, Kalloghlian A, et al. Liposomal amphotericin B in neonates with invasive candidiasis. Am J Perinatol 1998;15(11):643–8.

16. Sandler ES, Mustafa MM, Tkaczewski I, et al. Use of amphotericin B colloidal dispersion in children. J Pediatr Hematol Oncol 2000;22(3):242–6.

17. Walsh TJ, Hiemenz JW, Seibel NL, et al. Amphotericin B lipid complex for invasive fungal infections: analysis of safety and efficacy in 556 cases. Clin Infect Dis 1998;26(6):1383–96.

18. Cohen-Wolkowiez M, Moran C, Benjamin DK Jr, et al. Pediatric antifungal agents. Curr Opin Infect Dis 2009;22(6):553–8.

19. Kethireddy S, Andes D. CNS pharmacokinetics of antifungal agents. Expert Opin Drug Metab Toxicol 2007;3(4):573–81.

20. Jeon GW, Koo SH, Lee JH, et al. A comparison of AmBisome to amphotericin B for treatment of systemic candidiasis in very low birth weight infants. Yonsei Med J 2007;48(4):619–26.

21. Linder N, Klinger G, Shalit I, et al. Treatment of candidaemia in premature infants: comparison of three amphotericin B preparations. J Antimicrob Chemother 2003; 52(4):663–7.

22. Le J, Adler-Shohet FC, Nguyen C, et al. Nephrotoxicity associated with amphotericin B deoxycholate in neonates. Pediatr Infect Dis J 2009;28(12):1061–3.

23. Koren G, Lau A, Klein J, et al. Pharmacokinetics and adverse effects of amphotericin B in infants and children. J Pediatr 1988;113(3):559–63.

24. Baley JE, Meyers C, Kliegman RM, et al. Pharmacokinetics, outcome of treatment, and toxic effects of amphotericin B and 5-fluorocytosine in neonates. J Pediatr 1990;116(5):791–7.

25. Lestner JM, Smith PB, Cohen-Wolkowiez M, et al. Antifungal agents and therapy for infants and children with invasive fungal infections: a pharmacological perspective. Br J Clin Pharmacol 2013;75(6):1381–95.

26. Pappas PG, Kauffman CA, Andes DR, et al. Clinical practice guideline for the management of Candidiasis: 2016 update by the Infectious Diseases Society of America. Clin Infect Dis 2016;62(4):e1–50.

27. Andes D, Pascual A, Marchetti O. Antifungal therapeutic drug monitoring: established and emerging indications. Antimicrob Agents Chemother 2009;53(1): 24–34.

28. Juster-Reicher A, Flidel-Rimon O, Amitay M, et al. High-dose liposomal amphotericin B in the therapy of systemic candidiasis in neonates. Eur J Clin Microbiol Infect Dis 2003;22(10):603–7.

29. Denning DW, Hope WW. Therapy for fungal diseases: opportunities and priorities. Trends Microbiol 2010;18(5):195–204.

30. Dismukes WE, Cloud G, Gallis HA, et al. Treatment of cryptococcal meningitis with combination amphotericin B and flucytosine for four as compared with six weeks. N Engl J Med 1987;317(6):334–41.

31. Valeant. Flucytosine. Available at. https://dailymed.nlm.nih.gov/dailymed/drugInfo.cfm?setid=aea0df00-a88c-4a16-abcf-750f3ff2004e. Accessed March 3, 2017.

32. Soltani M, Tobin CM, Bowker KE, et al. Evidence of excessive concentrations of 5-flucytosine in children aged below 12 years: a 12-year review of serum concentrations from a UK clinical assay reference laboratory. Int J Antimicrob Agents 2006;28(6):574–7.

33. Botero-Calderon L, Benjamin DK Jr, Cohen-Wolkowiez M. Advances in the treatment of invasive neonatal candidiasis. Expert Opin Pharmacother 2015;16(7): 1035–48.

34. Frattarelli DA, Reed MD, Giacoia GP, et al. Antifungals in systemic neonatal candidiasis. Drugs 2004;64(9):949–68.

35. Watt K, Manzoni P, Cohen-Wolkowiez M, et al. Triazole use in the nursery: fluconazole, voriconazole, posaconazole, and ravuconazole. Curr Drug Metab 2013; 14(2):193–202.

36. Odds FC, Brown AJ, Gow NA. Antifungal agents: mechanisms of action. Trends Microbiol 2003;11(6):272–9.

37. Hsieh EM, Hornik CP, Clark RH, et al, Best Pharmaceuticals for Children Act-Pediatric Trials Network. Medication use in the neonatal intensive care unit. Am J Perinatol 2014;31(9):811–21.

38. Blum RA, D'Andrea DT, Florentino BM, et al. Increased gastric pH and the bioavailability of fluconazole and ketoconazole. Ann Intern Med 1991;114(9): 755–7.

39. Benjamin DK Jr, Poole C, Steinbach WJ, et al. Neonatal candidemia and end-organ damage: a critical appraisal of the literature using meta-analytic techniques. Pediatrics 2003;112(3 Pt 1):634–40.

40. Schwarze R, Penk A, Pittrow L. Treatment of candidal infections with fluconazole in neonates and infants. Eur J Med Res 2000;5(5):203–8.

41. Physicians Total Care Inc. Fluconazole. Available at: https://dailymed.nlm.nih.gov/dailymed/drugInfo.cfm?setid=926100a4-98b2-40ec-8592-56f86fa0cf22. Accessed March 1, 2017.

42. Cleveland AA, Farley MM, Harrison LH, et al. Changes in incidence and antifungal drug resistance in candidemia: results from population-based laboratory surveillance in Atlanta and Baltimore, 2008-2011. Clin Infect Dis 2012;55(10): 1352–61.

43. Pfaller MA, Messer SA, Boyken L, et al. Variation in susceptibility of bloodstream isolates of Candida glabrata to fluconazole according to patient age and geographic location. J Clin Microbiol 2003;41(5):2176–9.

44. Turner K, Manzoni P, Benjamin DK, et al. Fluconazole pharmacokinetics and safety in premature infants. Curr Med Chem 2012;19(27):4617–20.

45. Wade KC, Wu D, Kaufman DA, et al, National Institute of Child Health and Development Pediatric Pharmacology Research Unit Network. Population pharmacokinetics of fluconazole in young infants. Antimicrob Agents Chemother 2008; 52(11):4043–9.

46. Benjamin DK Jr, Hudak ML, Duara S, et al, Fluconazole Prophylaxis Study Team. Effect of fluconazole prophylaxis on candidiasis and mortality in premature infants: a randomized clinical trial. JAMA 2014;311(17):1742–9.

47. Janssen Pharmaceuticals Inc. Itraconazole. Available at: https://dailymed.nlm. nih.gov/dailymed/drugInfo.cfm?setid=a4d555fa-787c-40fb-bb7d-b0d4f7318fd0. Accessed March 2, 2017.

48. Heykants J, Van Peer A, Van de Velde V, et al. The clinical pharmacokinetics of itraconazole: an overview. Mycoses 1989;32(Suppl 1):67–87.

49. Chang YL, Yu SJ, Heitman J, et al. New facets of antifungal therapy. Virulence 2017;8(2):222–36.

50. Bhandari V, Narang A, Kumar B, et al. Itraconazole therapy for disseminated candidiasis in a very low birthweight neonate. J Paediatr Child Health 1992; 28(4):323–4.

51. Sciacca A, Betta P, Cilauro S, et al. Oral administration of itraconazole in a case of neonatal hepatic candidiasis. Pediatr Med Chir 1995;17(2):173–5 [in Italian].

52. Groll AH, Wood L, Roden M, et al. Safety, pharmacokinetics, and pharmacodynamics of cyclodextrin itraconazole in pediatric patients with oropharyngeal candidiasis. Antimicrob Agents Chemother 2002;46(8):2554–63.

53. Schmitt C, Perel Y, Harousseau JL, et al. Pharmacokinetics of itraconazole oral solution in neutropenic children during long-term prophylaxis. Antimicrob Agents Chemother 2001;45(5):1561–4.

54. Greenstone LLC. Voriconazole. Available at: https://dailymed.nlm.nih.gov/dailymed/ drugInfo.cfm?setid=b8de04a0-238d-4e0b-b0d9-7f7878b149d4. Accessed March 2, 2017.

55. Girmenia C, Micozzi A, Gentile G, et al. Clinically driven diagnostic antifungal approach in neutropenic patients: a prospective feasibility study. J Clin Oncol 2010;28(4):667–74.

56. Driscoll TA, Frangoul H, Nemecek ER, et al. Comparison of pharmacokinetics and safety of voriconazole intravenous-to-oral switch in immunocompromised adolescents and healthy adults. Antimicrob Agents Chemother 2011;55(12):5780–9.

57. Neely M, Rushing T, Kovacs A, et al. Voriconazole pharmacokinetics and pharmacodynamics in children. Clin Infect Dis 2010;50(1):27–36.

58. Nett JE, Andes DR. Antifungal agents spectrum of activity, pharmacology, and clinical indications. Infect Dis Clin North Am 2016;30(1):51–83.

59. Cornely OA, Maertens J, Winston DJ, et al. Posaconazole vs. fluconazole or itraconazole prophylaxis in patients with neutropenia. N Engl J Med 2007;356(4): 348–59.

60. Maertens J, Cornely OA, Ullmann AJ, et al. Phase IB study of the pharmacokinetics and safety of posaconazole intravenous solution in patients at risk for invasive fungal disease. Antimicrob Agents Chemother 2014;58(7):3610–7.

61. Merck Sharp & Dohme Corp. Posaconazole. Available at: https://dailymed.nlm. nih.gov/dailymed/drugInfo.cfm?setid=b073b082-7b57-4423-8c06-4fd4263d6f84. Accessed March 2, 2017.

62. Jancel T, Shaw PA, Hallahan CW, et al. Therapeutic drug monitoring of posaconazole oral suspension in paediatric patients younger than 13 years of age: a retrospective analysis and literature review. J Clin Pharm Ther 2017;42(1):75–9.

63. Krishna G, Sansone-Parsons A, Martinho M, et al. Posaconazole plasma concentrations in juvenile patients with invasive fungal infection. Antimicrob Agents Chemother 2007;51(3):812–8.

64. Mullard A. 2014 FDA drug approvals. Nat Rev Drug Discov 2015;14(2):77–81.

65. Miceli MH, Kauffman CA. Isavuconazole: a new broad-spectrum triazole antifungal agent. Clin Infect Dis 2015;61(10):1558–65.

66. Kofla G, Ruhnke M. Pharmacology and metabolism of anidulafungin, caspofungin and micafungin in the treatment of invasive candidosis: review of the literature. Eur J Med Res 2011;16(4):159–66.

67. Walker SS, Xu Y, Triantafyllou I, et al. Discovery of a novel class of orally active antifungal beta-1,3-D-glucan synthase inhibitors. Antimicrob Agents Chemother 2011;55(11):5099–106.

68. Ernst EJ, Klepser ME, Pfaller MA. Postantifungal effects of echinocandin, azole, and polyene antifungal agents against Candida albicans and Cryptococcus neoformans. Antimicrob Agents Chemother 2000;44(4):1108–11.

69. Merck Sharp & Dohme Corp. Caspofungin. Available at: https://dailymed.nlm.nih.gov/dailymed/drugInfo.cfm?setid=3bad23a6-09a6-4194-9182-093ed61bc71c. Accessed March 3, 2017.

70. Groll AH, Gullick BM, Petraitiene R, et al. Compartmental pharmacokinetics of the antifungal echinocandin caspofungin (MK-0991) in rabbits. Antimicrob Agents Chemother 2001;45(2):596–600.

71. Stone JA, Holland SD, Wickersham PJ, et al. Single- and multiple-dose pharmacokinetics of caspofungin in healthy men. Antimicrob Agents Chemother 2002;46(3):739–45.

72. Saez-Llorens X, Macias M, Maiya P, et al. Pharmacokinetics and safety of caspofungin in neonates and infants less than 3 months of age. Antimicrob Agents Chemother 2009;53(3):869–75.

73. Zaoutis T, Lehrnbecher T, Groll AH, et al. Safety experience with caspofungin in pediatric patients. Pediatr Infect Dis J 2009;28(12):1132–5.

74. Smith PB, Walsh TJ, Hope W, et al. Pharmacokinetics of an elevated dosage of micafungin in premature neonates. Pediatr Infect Dis J 2009;28(5):412–5.

75. Hope WW, Mickiene D, Petraitis V, et al. The pharmacokinetics and pharmacodynamics of micafungin in experimental hematogenous Candida meningoencephalitis: implications for echinocandin therapy in neonates. J Infect Dis 2008;197(1):163–71.

76. Hope WW, Smith PB, Arrieta A, et al. Population pharmacokinetics of micafungin in neonates and young infants. Antimicrob Agents Chemother 2010;54(6):2633–7.

77. Arrieta AC, Maddison P, Groll AH. Safety of micafungin in pediatric clinical trials. Pediatr Infect Dis J 2011;30(6):e97–102.

78. Astellas Pharma US Inc. Micafungin. Available at: https://dailymed.nlm.nih.gov/dailymed/drugInfo.cfm?setid=bc234dd7-5221-4a68-b153-aa0393c75bbf. Accessed March 3, 2017.

79. Benjamin DK Jr, Driscoll T, Seibel NL, et al. Safety and pharmacokinetics of intravenous anidulafungin in children with neutropenia at high risk for invasive fungal infections. Antimicrob Agents Chemother 2006;50(2):632–8.

80. Warn PA, Livermore J, Howard S, et al. Anidulafungin for neonatal hematogenous Candida meningoencephalitis: identification of candidate regimens for humans using a translational pharmacological approach. Antimicrob Agents Chemother 2012;56(2):708–14.

81. Roerig. Anidulafungin. Available at: https://dailymed.nlm.nih.gov/dailymed/drugInfo.cfm?setid=a88d9010-55fb-4a02-baff-042cd27688ea#s12.4. Accessed March 3, 2017.

# Antiviral Drugs in Newborn and Children

Claudette L. Poole, MD*, David W. Kimberlin, MD

## KEYWORDS

- Influenza • Herpes simplex virus • Cytomegalovus • Hepatitis

## KEY POINTS

- Recommendations for the use of antivirals to treat herpetic diseases in neonates and children, including herpes simplex virus, varicella zoster virus, and cytomegalovirus, are based on randomized controlled trials.
- Guidelines for the treatment of influenza, including prophylaxis in neonates and children, also are evidence based.
- Food and Drug Administration– approved antivirals for the treatment of hepatitis B virus and hepatitis C virus in children are limited, but there are multiple agents in current phase III trials in the pediatric population.
- Antiretroviral agents for the treatment of HIV are beyond the scope of this article.

## INTRODUCTION

The availability of safe and effective antiviral medications is a recent addition to the antimicrobial armamentarium. Knowledge of viral pathogenesis and development of enhanced diagnostics coalesce with the development and application of novel antiviral agents to make this an exciting time for advancements in the treatment of viral infections in children.

## ANTIVIRAL CATEGORIES

Antiviral agents can be classified into a few broad categories based on their mechanism of action. These include the following.

### Nucleotide/Nucleoside Analogues

The nucleotide/nucleoside analogue agents are similar in structure to naturally occurring nucleotides/nucleosides. Once these are incorporated in the growing nucleic acid chain during transcription, they either result in chain termination, because their

Department of Pediatrics, University of Alabama at Birmingham, 1600 6th Avenue South, CHB 308, Birmingham, AL 35233, USA
* Corresponding author.
*E-mail address:* cpoole@peds.uab.edu

Pediatr Clin N Am 64 (2017) 1403–1415
http://dx.doi.org/10.1016/j.pcl.2017.08.014
0031-3955/17/© 2017 Elsevier Inc. All rights reserved.

structure does not allow for another nucleotide to be added, or in impaired function of the polymerase, which is the enzyme involved in translation.

These are by far the largest group of antiviral agents in clinical use. Their toxicity relates to their specificity to being incorporated into the growing viral nucleic acid chain versus the host cell DNA.[1,2]

### Neuraminidase Inhibitors

The neuraminidase inhibitor agents are directed to a viral specific enzyme that is involved in the process of release of the newly formed viral particles from the host cell. This enzyme is present in influenza viruses.[3]

### Interferons

Interferons are naturally occurring products of the cellular immune response targeting viruses. Interferons currently are used with other agents to treat hepatitis B virus (HBV) and hepatitis C virus (HCV) in children. They have many side effects and are used less frequently as safer and highly effective small molecules active against hepatitis viruses come to market.[4]

## ANTIVIRAL RESISTANCE

The viral replication process in general has low fidelity, resulting in a high mutation rate. In any given host there are many different mutant viral populations. In the presence of an antiviral agent, viruses that have developed a mutation conferring resistance to the present antiviral then replicate more efficiently and become the predominant virus present in the host, resulting in treatment failure. These resistant viruses usually are less virulent than wild-type virus but can still cause significant disease. Resistant viruses require an alternate agent that targets a different mechanism. Antiviral resistance testing often identifies these genetic mutations.[5]

---

**Patient categories**

In presenting antiviral therapies in pediatrics, 4 specific scenarios are focused on:

1. Treatment and prophylaxis of influenza
2. Neonatal herpes simplex virus (HSV) infection and congenital cytomegalovirus (CMV) disease
3. Treatment of herpes viral diseases beyond the neonatal period, including in immunocompromised hosts, together with other viral infections specific to an immunocompromised child
4. Approved antiviral treatments for HBV and HCC chronic infections in children

---

## INFLUENZA

- Oseltamivir, administered orally, is the only drug currently Food and Drug Administration (FDA) approved for both the treatment and the prophylaxis of influenza in children less than 5 years of age.
- Inhaled zanamivir is FDA approved for prophylaxis for children 5 years and older and for treatment of children 7 years and older. (Intravenous [IV] zanamivir is currently undergoing clinical trials and data on pediatric dosing have recently been published.)
- IV peramivir is only licensed for use in those 18 years and older.

Oseltamivir, zanamivir, and peramivir are neuraminidase inhibitors. Neuraminidase is an enzyme specific to the influenza viruses. It is required to cleave the newly formed viral progeny from the surface of the infected cell, enabling their release.[3,6]

### Oseltamivir (Tamiflu)

Dosing of oseltamivir has been established for infants 2 weeks of age and older (**Table 1**).

| Table 1 Oseltamivir treatment dosing | |
|---|---|
| For infants born prematurely dose adjust according to the postmenstrual age | • 28–38 wk postmenstrual age: 1 mg/kg per dose oral twice daily <br> • 38–40 wk postmenstrual age: 1.5 mg/kg per dose orally twice daily <br> • >40 wk postmenstrual age: 3 mg/kg per dose orally twice daily |
| For infants born at term to 8 mo of age | 3 mg/kg per dose orally twice daily |
| Babies 9–11 mo of age | 3.5 mg/kg per dose orally twice daily |
| 12–23 mo | 30 mg orally twice daily[7] |
| 12 months and older (weight based dosing) | • ≤15 kg: 30 mg orally twice daily <br> • 16–23 kg: 45 mg orally twice daily <br> • 24–40 kg: 60 mg orally twice daily <br> • >40 kg: 75 mg orally twice daily |
| Adults | 75 mg orally twice daily |

*Data from* Jonas, M.M., et al., Antiviral therapy in management of chronic hepatitis B viral infection in children: A systematic review and meta-analysis. Hepatology, 2016. 63(1): p. 307–18.

Prophylaxis dosing is the same weight-based dosing as indicated in **Table 1** but given once daily.[8,9] Prophylaxis in infants younger than 3 months of age generally is not recommended due to variability in pharmacokinetics in these youngest of children.

Oseltamivir is an ethyl ester prodrug that has very good oral bioavailability. After absorption, it is metabolized to its active form by the liver. It has a plasma half-life of 6 hours to 10 hours and is excreted by the kidney. It does require dose adjustment in renal impairment.

The main side effect includes gastrointestinal complaints, such as nausea, vomiting, and diarrhea.[10]

Following reports from Japan of neuropsychiatric events with fatal outcomes in children less than 19 years of age, the FDA conducted a comprehensive review of neuropsychiatric events and posted their findings and recommendations in 2007. There have been reports of neuropsychiatric events in children in the United States taking oseltamivir, but causality is inconclusive because these events are seen also in children with influenza who are not receiving oseltamivir. The FDA determined that there was insufficient evidence to restrict the use of oseltamivir but recommended a highlighted precaution to closely monitor for unusual behavior, especially in children on the first day of initiating treatment.[11]

Resistance to oseltamivir occurs due to mutations in the neuraminidase gene. A recent study documented a resistance rate of 4.4% among young infants in the United States.[7]

### Zanamivir (Relenza)

Treatment dosing is 10 mg inhaled twice daily for 5 days.[12]

Prophylaxis dosing is 10 mg inhaled daily for 10 days in household settings and up to 28 days in community outbreaks.[13]

Only approximately 13% of the dose distributes to the airways and lungs, where it exerts a local antiviral effect.[14] Approximately 4% to 17% of the dose is systemically absorbed and then excreted by the kidney. Dosing adjustment is not required in renal impairment.[15,16]

The main side effect is bronchospasm for which the risk is increased in patients with underlying pulmonary disease and should not be used in these patients.[17]

IV zanamivir is an investigational product and is only available by enrolling in an ongoing clinical trial or under an emergency investigational new drug request to the manufacturer for the use in hospitalized adult and pediatric patients with severe influenza.[18] Results from a phase II open-label, multicenter, single-arm study have provided data on dosing and pharmacokinetics for IV zanamivir in children. Doses of 14 mg/kg per dose 12 hourly for children ages 6 months to 6 years and 12 mg/kg per dose 12 hourly for children 6 years to 18 years (maximum dose of 600 mg) adjusted for renal function were administered for 5 days to 10 days. The mean serum areas under the curve were consistent with those seen in adults and there were no safety events reported.[19]

## NEONATAL DISEASES
### Neonatal Herpes Simplex Virus Disease

#### Acyclovir (Zovirax)
High-dose IV acyclovir decreases mortality and improves neurologic outcomes among survivors of neonatal HSV disease.[20] Six months of suppressive therapy with oral acyclovir after completion of parenteral therapy in acute disease further improves neurologic outcomes and prevents recurrent disease.[21]

- Initial treatment dosing with parenteral acyclovir: IV 20 mg/kg per dose given 8 hourly (for every low birthweight infants that are less than 2 weeks of age would recommend 20 mg/kg per dose given 12 hourly (**Table 2**)
- Subsequent suppressive dosing after neonatal HSV disease with oral acyclovir: 300 mg/m$^2$ body surface area per dose given 3 times a day for 6 months from end of IV treatment course (need to adjust dose monthly as infant gains weight)[21]

| Table 2 | |
|---|---|
| **Duration for initial treatment of neonatal HSV disease** | |
| Skin, eye, mouth disease | 14 d |
| Disseminated | 21 d |
| Central nervous system[a] | 21 d |

[a] Continue longer if CSF at 21 d is still positive for HSV by polymerase chain reaction; continue with weekly CSF HSV polymerase chain reaction testing until documented clearance.[20]

Given the devastating consequences of neonatal HSV disease, neonates born to women with active primary genital lesions should be treated with preemptive parenteral acyclovir for 10 days in an effort to prevent exposure from progressing to diseases.[22]

Acyclovir is a nucleoside analogue that preferentially is taken up by cells infected with HSV and requires thymidine kinase, a viral specific enzyme for the first step in phosphorylation to convert to its active triphosphate form. Once incorporated into the viral DNA chain by viral polymerase, it results in chain termination. As a consequence, acyclovir is highly effective against HSV with a good safety profile.[1]

IV acyclovir is widely distributed to all tissues throughout the body, and levels in the cerebrospinal fluid (CSF) are approximately 50% of serum levels. Oral acyclovir has poor bioavailability with only 15% to 30% of the dose absorbed.[1]

Resistant HSV has been described in neonates, presumably due to resistance that has developed in their mothers due to use of suppressive antiviral therapy.[23,24]

### Valacyclovir (Valtrex)

Valacyclovir (Valtrex) is the L-valyl ester form of acyclovir that dramatically increases the oral absorption and once absorbed is converted to the active drug after first-pass metabolism in the liver.[25] Studies have not yet been conducted for dosing recommendations for the use of valacyclovir for the suppressive treatment of neonatal HSV disease, and the recommended drug for this indication remains oral acyclovir. Pediatric dosing for valacyclovir beyond the neonatal period is 20 mg//kg per dose given twice daily or 3 times daily.[26] A recipe for making a liquid formulation of valacyclovir is found in the package insert.

The serum half-life of acyclovir is between 2 hours and 3 hours but can be as long as 5 hours in neonates. It is excreted by the kidneys and needs to be dose adjusted for renal compromise.[1]

Side effects and recommended monitoring

1. Nephrotoxic: can precipitate as crystals in the renal tubules causing tubular necrosis and acute renal failure. Ensuring adequate hydration reduces the risk.[27,28]
2. Extravasation from IV can result in tissue necrosis.
3. Neutropenia: high dose and prolonged use can result in myelosuppression. On initiation of acyclovir therapy, the absolute neutrophil count should be monitored at 2 weeks and at 4 weeks and, if stable, then monthly for the duration of the treatment course. If the absolute neutrophil count reproducibly decreases to below 500 cells/mm$^3$, consideration should be to treat with granulocyte colony-stimulating factor rather than discontinue acyclovir.[20]

### Keratoconjunctivitis

#### Topical ophthalmic 1% trifluridine or topical ophthalmic 0.15% ganciclovir
All neonates with neonatal HSV disease and evidence of eye disease (eg, lesions around the eye or conjunctival erythema) should be evaluated by an ophthalmologist and treated with topical agents in addition to systemic acyclovir.[29]

### Treatment failure on acyclovir
Progression of disease with the development of new lesions while on acyclovir therapy should prompt clinicians to consider an acyclovir-resistant virus. An isolate should be sent for confirmatory testing for mutations in the thymidine kinase gene. The agent of choice in this circumstance in foscarnet.[24]

## CONGENITAL CYTOMEGALOVIRUS

CMV is the most common congenital infection, with approximately 0.5% of live births affected. Approximately 10% of infants are born with clinically symptomatic disease.[30] A recent study established that 6 months of oral valganciclovir, if treatment was initiated within the first month of life, improved both neurologic and hearing outcomes for these moderately and severely symptomatic infants at birth.[31]

### Ganciclovir (Cytovene) and Valganciclovir (Valcyte)

Ganciclovir is a nucleoside analogue and has a similar mechanism of action to acyclovir but with varying activity against herpes viruses. It is preferentially taken up by virally infected cells and requires the first step of phosphorylation to be done by the virally encoded enzyme. For this reason, it cannot be used as an alternate treatment in the case of acyclovir resistance. In cases of CMV, this phosphorylase is coded for by the UL97 gene. Although the drug has a greater affinity for viral polymerase, it can be incorporated into cellular DNA, which results in its mutagenic properties. It has been shown to be both carcinogenic and teratogenic and to cause irreversible infertility in animal models. Given these concerns, the use of the drug is reserved for situations where the benefit of treatment is considered to outweigh the risks.[2]

Valganciclovir is the L-valyl ester prodrug of ganciclovir, with enhanced oral bioavailability compared with oral ganciclovir. Once absorbed, it is metabolized by the liver to the active form.[32]

Ganciclovir is widely distributed throughout the body. It has an intracellular half-life of 24 hours and an elimination half-life of 2 hours to 3 hours. It is eliminated by the kidney and requires dose adjustment in renal impairment.[2]

Parenteral ganciclovir improves audiologic outcomes when administered for 6 weeks to babies with symptomatic congenital CMV disease.[33] A recent comparison of 6 weeks and 6 months of oral valganciclovir in this same population demonstrated that the longer course of therapy further improved hearing outcomes and also improved developmental outcomes.[31] Recent international consensus recommendations concluded that babies with moderately and severely symptomatic congenital CMV disease should be treated with the 6-month duration of oral valganciclovir.[34]

The dose for treatment of symptomatic congenital CMV
Oral valganciclovir: 16 mg/kg per dose given twice daily for 6 months
IV ganciclovir: 6 mg/kg per dose given twice daily[31]

Side effects and recommended monitoring
1. Neutropenia is a particular concern and requires close monitoring throughout the treatment course. It occurs in one-fifth of infants treated with oral valganciclovir and in two-thirds of infants treated with IV ganciclovir. An absolute neutrophil count should be monitored weekly on the initiation of therapy for the first 6 weeks and, if stable, at 8 weeks and then monthly for the remainder of the treatment course.[31]
2. Transaminitis occurs less frequently and serum aminotransferase levels should be monitored monthly throughout therapy.[35]

## HERPETIC DISEASES BEYOND THE NEONATAL PERIOD
### Herpes Simplex Viral Infections

Acyclovir IV is the treatment of choice for these more severe conditions, and oral valacyclovir can be used for suppressive therapy for patients suffering from recurrent orolabial or genital infection or at risk for severe disease (**Table 3**).

| Table 3 Herpes simplex virus recommended dosing | |
| --- | --- |
| HSV encephalitis for children older than 4 mo | IV acyclovir 10–15 mg/kg per dose given 8 hourly[36] |
| Mucocutaneous HSV treatment | • Immune-competent hosts: oral acyclovir 20 gm/kg per dose given 4 times daily (maximum 800 mg per dose) for 5–7 d[37]<br>• Immunocompromised hosts: IV acyclovir 5–10 mg/kg per dose given 8 hourly[38] |
| Mucocutaneous HSV suppressive therapy | Oral valacyclovir 20 mg/kg per dose given 3 times a day (maximum 400 mg per dose) for 6–12 mo[26] |

### Varicella-zoster Viral Infections

Prior to vaccination, varicella was a common childhood illness. Severe disease can occur in neonates whose mothers developed varicella around the time of delivery and immunocompromised children. The treatment of choice in these neonates is IV acyclovir because perinatal acquisition is associated with a 30% mortality rate (**Table 4**).

| Table 4 Varicella-zoster viral infections treatment dosing | |
|---|---|
| Varicella-zoster in an immune competent host | • Oral acyclovir 20 mg/kg per dose given divided 4 times a day for 5 days (maximum 800 mg per dose)<br>• Oral valacyclovir (approved for children 2 y and older) 20 mg/kg per dose given 3 times a day (maximum dose of 1 g).[39,40] |
| Severe primary chickenpox, disseminated infection, or infection in an immunocompromised host | 10–15 mg/kg per dose given. Duration is typically 7–14 d depending on clinical response[41,42] |

### Cytomegaloviral Infections

CMV can result in severe, even fatal disease in immunocompromised patients, such as those post-transplant and in patients with HIV, in whom CMV retinitis is of particular concern.[43,44]

Ganciclovir and valganciclovir are the drugs of choice in these circumstances (**Table 5**).

| Table 5 Cytomegaloviral infections: treatment and prevention | |
|---|---|
| Treatment of CMV disease in immunocompromised host | Induction: ganciclovir 5 mg/kg per dose IV given 12 hourly for 2–3 wk<br>Maintenance: ganciclovir 5 mg/kg IV daily for 5–7 d/wk—duration determined by degree of immunosuppression |
| Prevention of CMV disease in immunocompromised host (AIDS/transplant patients) | • Ganciclovir 5 mg/kg IV daily or 3 times/wk OR<br>• Valganciclovir total milligram dose calculated by 7 × body surface area × creatine clearance with a maximum daily dose of 900 mg orally given once daily |

*Data from* Boeckh M, Nichols WG, Papanicolaou G, et al. Cytomegalovirus in hematopoietic stem cell transplant recipients: Current status, known challenges, and future strategies. Biol Blood Marrow Transplant 2003;9(9):543–58; and Griffiths P, Whitley R, Snydman DR, et al. Contemporary management of cytomegalovirus infection in transplant recipients: guidelines from an IHMF workshop, 2007. Herpes 2008;15(1):4–12.

Ganciclovir resistance has been documented in immunocompromised patient populations, primarily due to mutations in the UL97 gene. Viral resistance is most frequently encountered in immunocompromised patients who have been treated with antivirals for extended periods of time.

The recommended treatment of resistant HSV or CMV infections is foscarnet.

### Foscarnet (Foscavir)

Foscarnet is the drug of choice to treat acyclovir-resistant strains of HSV, varicella-zoster virus (VZV), and CMV. Resistance is suggested by worsening disease while receiving acyclovir or ganciclovir and is confirmed by testing viral isolates for mutations in the thymidine kinase gene, UL97 gene, or, less frequently, the viral DNA polymerase gene.

Foscarnet is an inorganic pyrophosphate analogue that directly inhibits DNA polymerase and is approximately 100-fold more active against viral polymerase than host cellular enzymes.[45] It can only be administered IV and has a long serum half-life of approximately 48 hours, being excreted by the kidney and requiring dose adjustment in renal impairment.

Foscarnet is a very nephrotoxic agent, with approximately half of patients having increased serum creatinine levels by the second week of therapy that is reversible for most patients on discontinuation of therapy; however, some develop frank acute kidney injury either from acute tubular necrosis or interstitial nephritis.[46]

In addition, foscarnet can cause multiple electrolyte disturbances and require close monitoring. Serum ionized calcium is chelated by foscarnet and can result in a rapid drop in ionized calcium resulting in parasthesias, tetany, seizures, and cardiac arrhythmias.[47]

Less commonly, foscarnet can result in elevated liver enzymes, granulocytopenia, and anemia (**Table 6**).[48]

| Table 6 Foscarnet dosing recommendations | |
| --- | --- |
| CMV infections | 60 mg/kg per dose given every 8 hours for 14–21 d followed by a maintenance dose of 90–120 mg/kg per dose given once daily[48] |
| HSV/VZV infections | 40 mg/kg per dose given 8 hourly—continued until disease resolved[49] |

### Cidofovir (Vistide)

Cidofovir is approved for the treatment of CMV retinitis in adult patients with AIDS who have failed other treatments.[50] It has a wide antiviral spectrum and in addition to activity against CMV has demonstrated in vitro activity against HSV, VZV, Epstein-Barr virus, human herpesvirus 6, human herpesvirus 8, polyomaviruses, orthopoxviruses, adenovirus, BK virus, and human papillomavirus.[51] There have been no prospective clinical trials to study the safety and efficacy of cidofovir in pediatric patients. Case reports and small case series suggest that cidofovir may be beneficial in the management of adenovirus[52,53] and BK virus[54,55] in immunocompromised patients. The dosing schedules that have been used in these clinical settings are

- 5 mg/kg per dose IV once weekly
- 1 mg/kg per dose to 1.5 mg/kg per dose IV 3 times per week

Cidofovir is a nucleotide analogue that already has a single phosphate attached and thus does not require viral enzyme for the first step in phosphorylation. It has a greater affinity for viral DNA polymerase over host cellular polymerase, thereby selectively inhibiting viral DNA replication.[56,57]

Cidofovir is administered IV and has a short plasma half-life but a long intracellular half-life of 17 hours to 48 hours.[58,59]

Clinical use of the drug is limited due to its near universal nephrotoxicity. The drug concentrates in the proximal tubules, manifesting initially as proteinuria and glycosuria and then decreased creatinine clearance. The drug should not be used in patients with baseline elevated serum creatinine or proteinuria and requires aggressive IV prehydration and coadministration of probenecid with each dose.[58–60]

## HEPATITIS B AND HEPATITIS C CHRONIC INFECTIONS IN CHILDREN

Both hepatitis B and hepatitis C can be acquired perinatally, resulting in congenital infection, or can be acquired later in adolescents through sexual activity or IV drug use. Both infections can result in chronic infection, liver cirrhosis, and hepatocellular carcinoma.[61]

Currently the treatment options for children with chronic infections to prevent development of cirrhosis and hepatocellular carcinoma are as follows (**Tables 7** and **8**):

Lamivudine, adefovir, telbivudine, entecavir, and sofosbuvir are all nucleoside analogues that interfere with the growing viral chain and viral polymerase.

Ledipasvir, which is administered in combination with sofosbuvir, blocks the action of an HCV-specific protein crucial for viral replication.[62]

Table 7
**Hepatitis B virus: age for indication and drug for treatment**

| Age for Indication | Drug |
| --- | --- |
| ≥3 mo | Lamivudine |
| ≥1 y | Interferon |
| ≥12 y | Adefovir |
| ≥16 y | Telbivudine and entecavir |

*From* Jonas MM, Lok AS, McMahon BJ, et al. Antiviral therapy in management of chronic hepatitis B viral infection in children: a systematic review and meta-analysis. Hepatology 2016;63(1):307–18.

Table 8
**Hepatitis C virus: age for indication and drug treatment**

| Age for Indication | Drug |
| --- | --- |
| 3 y to 12 y | Pegylated interferon and oral ribavirin |
| ≥12 y | Sovaldi (sofosbuvir) and Harvoni (ledipasvir and sofosbuvir) |

*From* Balistreri WF, Murray KF, Rosenthal P, et al. The safety and effectiveness of ledipasvir-sofosbuvir in adolescents 12 to 17 years old with hepatitis C virus genotype 1 infection. Hepatology 2017;66(2):371–8.

## REFERENCES

1. Wagstaff AJ, Faulds D, Goa KL. Aciclovir. A reappraisal of its antiviral activity, pharmacokinetic properties and therapeutic efficacy. Drugs 1994;47(1):153–205.
2. Faulds D, Heel RC. Ganciclovir. A review of its antiviral activity, pharmacokinetic properties and therapeutic efficacy in cytomegalovirus infections. Drugs 1990; 39(4):597–638.
3. Treanor JJ, Hayden FG, Vrooman PS, et al. Efficacy and safety of the oral neuraminidase inhibitor oseltamivir in treating acute influenza: a randomized controlled trial. US Oral Neuraminidase Study Group. JAMA 2000;283(8): 1016–24.
4. Arnaud P. The interferons: pharmacology, mechanism of action, tolerance and side effects. Rev Med Interne 2002;23(4):449s–58s [in French].
5. Kimberlin DW, Whitley RJ. Antiviral resistance: mechanisms, clinical significance, and future implications. J Antimicrob Chemother 1996;37(3):403–21.

6. Hayden FG, Osterhaus AD, Treanor JJ, et al. Efficacy and safety of the neuramin-idase inhibitor zanamivir in the treatment of influenzavirus infections. GG167 Influenza Study Group. N Engl J Med 1997;337(13):874–80.

7. Kimberlin DW, Acosta EP, Prichard MN, et al. Oseltamivir pharmacokinetics, dosing, and resistance among children aged <2 years with influenza. J Infect Dis 2013;207(5):709–20.

8. Welliver R, Monto AS, Carewicz O, et al. Effectiveness of oseltamivir in preventing influenza in household contacts: a randomized controlled trial. JAMA 2001; 285(6):748–54.

9. Hayden FG, Belshe R, Villanueva C, et al. Management of influenza in households: a prospective, randomized comparison of oseltamivir treatment with or without postexposure prophylaxis [see comment]. J Infect Dis 2004;189(3): 440–9.

10. FDA. Oseltamivir [package insert]. 2004. Available at: http://www.fda.gov/downloads/Drugs/DrugSafety/InformationbyDrugClass/ucm147992.pdf.

11. Tamiflu (oseltamivir) – Safety Update on Neuropsychiatric Events; Review of Neuropsychiatric Events with other antiviral products 2007 November 9, 2007. Available at: https://www.fda.gov/ohrms/dockets/ac/07/briefing/2007-4325b_02_04_Tamiflu%20Adverse%20Event%20Review%202007.pdf.

12. Hedrick JA, Barzilai A, Behre U, et al. Zanamivir for treatment of symptomatic influenza A and B infection in children five to twelve years of age: a randomized controlled trial. Pediatr Infect Dis J 2000;19(5):410–7.

13. Hayden FG, Gubareva LV, Monto AS, et al. Inhaled zanamivir for the prevention of influenza in families. Zanamivir Family Study Group. N Engl J Med 2000;343(18): 1282–9.

14. Cass LM, Brown J, Pickford M, et al. Pharmacoscintigraphic evaluation of lung deposition of inhaled zanamivir in healthy volunteers. Clin Pharmacokinet 1999; 1:21–31.

15. Cass LM, Efthymiopoulos C, Bye A. Pharmacokinetics of zanamivir after intravenous, oral, inhaled or intranasal administration to healthy volunteers. Clin Pharmacokinet 1999;36(Suppl 1):1–11.

16. Cass LM, Efthymiopoulos C, Marsh J, et al. Effect of renal impairment on the pharmacokinetics of intravenous zanamivir. Clin Pharmacokinet 1999;1:13–9.

17. Cass LM, Gunawardena KA, Macmahon MM, et al. Pulmonary function and airway responsiveness in mild to moderate asthmatics given repeated inhaled doses of zanamivir. Respir Med 2000;94(2):166–73.

18. CDC Considerations Related to Investigational Use of Intravenous Zanamivir for 2016-2017 Influenza Season. 2016 November 3, 2016; Available at: https://www.cdc.gov/flu/professionals/antivirals/intravenous-antivirals.htm. Accessed May 8, 2017.

19. Blumer J, Bradley JS, Romero JR, et al. Safety, tolerability and pharmacokinetics (PK) of intravenous zanamivir (IVZ) treatment in hospitalized pediatric and adolescent patients with influenza: a phase II open-label, multicenter, single-arm study. IDWeek 2016 (national meeting of the Infectious Diseases Society of America, the Pediatric Infectious Diseases Society, and the Society for Healthcare Epidemiology of America), New Orleans, Louisiana, October 26-30, 2016; [abstract: 57391].

20. Kimberlin DW, Lin CY, Jacobs RF, et al. Safety and efficacy of high-dose intravenous acyclovir in the management of neonatal herpes simplex virus infections. Pediatrics 2001;108(2):230–8.

21. Kimberlin DW, Whitley RJ, Wan W, et al. Oral acyclovir suppression and neurodevelopment after neonatal herpes. N Engl J Med 2011;365(14):1284–92.
22. Kimberlin DW, Baley J, Committee on Infectious Diseases, Committee on Fetus and Newborn. Guidance on management of asymptomatic neonates born to women with active genital herpes lesions. Pediatrics 2013;131(2):e635–46.
23. Field AK, Biron KK. "The end of innocence" revisited: resistance of herpesviruses to antiviral drugs. Clin Microbiol Rev 1994;7(1):1–13.
24. Laufer DS, Starr SE. Resistance to antivirals. Pediatr Clin North Am 1995;42(3):583–99.
25. Lai L, Xu Z, Zhou J, et al. Molecular basis of prodrug activation by human valacyclovirase, an alpha-amino acid ester hydrolase. J Biol Chem 2008;283(14):9318–27.
26. Kimberlin DW, Jacobs RF, Weller S, et al. Pharmacokinetics and safety of extemporaneously compounded valacyclovir oral suspension in pediatric patients from 1 month through 11 years of age. Clin Infect Dis 2010;50(2):221–8.
27. Rao S, Abzug MJ, Carosone-Link P, et al. Intravenous acyclovir and renal dysfunction in children: a matched case control study. J Pediatr 2015;166(6):1462–8.e1-4.
28. Steinberg I, Kimberlin DW. Acyclovir dosing and acute kidney injury: deviations and direction. J Pediatr 2015;166(6):1341–4.
29. Carmine AA, Brogden RN, Heel RC, et al. Trifluridine: a review of its antiviral activity and therapeutic use in the topical treatment of viral eye infections. Drugs 1982;23(5):329–53.
30. Britt WJ. Cytomegalovirus. Infectious diseases of the fetus and newborn infant. In: Remington JS, Klein JO, editors. Philadelphia: Elsevier Saunders; 2011.
31. Kimberlin DW, Jester PM, Sánchez PJ, et al. Valganciclovir for symptomatic congenital cytomegalovirus disease. N Engl J Med 2015;372(10):933–43.
32. Brown F, Banken L, Saywell K, et al. Pharmacokinetics of valganciclovir and ganciclovir following multiple oral dosages of valganciclovir in HIV- and CMV-seropositive volunteers. Clin Pharmacokinet 1999;37(2):167–76.
33. Kimberlin DW, Lin CY, Sánchez PJ, et al. Effect of ganciclovir therapy on hearing in symptomatic congenital cytomegalovirus disease involving the central nervous system: a randomized, controlled trial. J Pediatr 2003;143(1):16–25.
34. Rawlinson WD, Boppana SB, Fowler KB, et al. Congenital cytomegalovirus infection in pregnancy and the neonate: consensus recommendations for prevention, diagnosis, and therapy. Lancet Infect Dis 2017;17(6):e177–88.
35. Cocohoba JM, McNicholl IR. Valganciclovir: an advance in cytomegalovirus therapeutics. Ann Pharmacother 2002;36(6):1075–9.
36. Whitley RJ, Alford CA, Hirsch MS, et al. Vidarabine versus acyclovir therapy in herpes simplex encephalitis. N Engl J Med 1986;314(3):144–9.
37. Aoki FY, Law BJ, Hammond GW, et al. Acyclovir (ACV) suspension for treatment of acute herpes simplex virus (HSV) gingivostomatitis in children: a placebo(PL) controlled, double blind trial. in 33rd Interscience Conference on Antimicrobial Agents and Chemotherapy. New Orleans (LA), October 17–20, 1993.
38. Rubin RH, Tolkoff-Rubin NE. Antimicrobial strategies in the care of organ transplant recipients. Antimicrob Agents Chemother 1993;37(4):619–24.
39. Balfour HH Jr, Rotbart HA, Feldman S, et al. Acyclovir treatment of varicella in otherwise healthy adolescents. The Collaborative Acyclovir Varicella Study Group. J Pediatr 1992;120(4 Pt 1):627–33.

40. Dunkle LM, Arvin AM, Whitley RJ, et al. A controlled trial of acyclovir for chicken-pox in normal children. N Engl J Med 1991;325(22):1539–44.

41. Whitley RJ, Gnann JW Jr, Hinthorn D, et al. Disseminated herpes zoster in the immunocompromised host: a comparative trial of acyclovir and vidarabine. The NIAID Collaborative Antiviral Study Group. J Infect Dis 1992; 165(3):450–5.

42. Nyerges G, Meszner Z, Gyarmati E, et al. Acyclovir prevents dissemination of varicella in immunocompromised children. J Infect Dis 1988;157(2):309–13.

43. Miller W, Flynn P, McCullough J, et al. Cytomegalovirus infection after bone marrow transplantation: an association with acute graft-v-host disease. Blood 1986;67(4):1162–7.

44. Crumpacker CS, Heath-Chiozzi M. Overview of cytomegalovirus infections in HIV-infected patients: current therapies and future strategies. J Acquir Immune Defic Syndr 1991;4(1):S1–5.

45. Crumpacker CS. Mechanism of action of foscarnet against viral polymerases. Am J Med 1992;92(2A):3S–7S.

46. Deray G, Martinez F, Katlama C, et al. Foscarnet nephrotoxicity: mechanism, incidence and prevention. Am J Nephrol 1989;9(4):316–21.

47. Jacobson MA, Gambertoglio JG, Aweeka FT, et al. Foscarnet-induced hypocalcemia and effects of foscarnet on calcium metabolism. J Clin Endocrinol Metab 1991;72(5):1130–5.

48. Palestine AG, Polis MA, De Smet MD, et al. A randomized, controlled trial of foscarnet in the treatment of cytomegalovirus retinitis in patients with AIDS. Ann Intern Med 1991;115(9):665–73.

49. Balfour HH Jr, Benson C, Braun J, et al. Management of acyclovir-resistant herpes simplex and varicella-zoster virus infections. J Acquir Immune Defic Syndr 1994;7(3):254–60.

50. Lalezari JP, Stagg RJ, Kuppermann BD, et al. Intravenous cidofovir for peripheral cytomegalovirus retinitis in patients with AIDS. A randomized, controlled trial. Ann Intern Med 1997;126(4):257–63.

51. Williams-Aziz SL, Hartline CB, Harden EA, et al. Comparative activities of lipid esters of cidofovir and cyclic cidofovir against replication of herpesviruses in vitro. Antimicrob Agents Chemother 2005;49(9):3724–33.

52. Lenaerts L, De Clercq E, Naesens L. Clinical features and treatment of adenovirus infections. Rev Med Virol 2008;18(6):357–74.

53. Carter BA, Karpen SJ, Quiros-Tejeira RE, et al. Intravenous Cidofovir therapy for disseminated adenovirus in a pediatric liver transplant recipient. Transplantation 2002;74(7):1050–2.

54. Vats A, Shapiro R, Singh Randhawa P, et al. Quantitative viral load monitoring and cidofovir therapy for the management of BK virus-associated nephropathy in children and adults. Transplantation 2003;75(1):105–12.

55. Kadambi PV, Josephson MA, Williams J, et al. Treatment of refractory BK virus-associated nephropathy with cidofovir. Am J Transplant 2003;3(2):186–91.

56. Ho HT, Woods KL, Bronson JJ, et al. Intracellular metabolism of the antiherpes agent (S)-1-[3-hydroxy-2-(phosphonylmethoxy)propyl]cytosine. Mol Pharmacol 1992;41(1):197–202.

57. Yang H, Datema R. Prolonged and potent therapeutic and prophylactic effects of (S)-1-[(3-hydroxy-2-phosphonylmethoxy)propyl]cytosine against herpes simplex virus type 2 infections in mice. Antimicrob Agents Chemother 1991;35(8): 1596–600.

58. Cundy KC, Petty BG, Flaherty J, et al. Clinical pharmacokinetics of cidofovir in human immunodeficiency virus-infected patients. Antimicrob Agents Chemother 1995;39(6):1247–52.
59. Lalezari JP, Drew WL, Glutzer E, et al. (S)-1-[3-hydroxy-2-(phosphonylmethoxy)propyl]cytosine (cidofovir): results of a phase I/II study of a novel antiviral nucleotide analogue. J Infect Dis 1995;171(4):788–96.
60. Lalezari JP, Drew WL, Glutzer E, et al. Treatment with intravenous (S)-1-[3-hydroxy-2-(phosphonylmethoxy)propyl]-cytosine of acyclovir-resistant mucocutaneous infection with herpes simplex virus in a patient with AIDS. J Infect Dis 1994;170(3):570–2.
61. El-Shabrawi M, Hassanin F. Treatment of hepatitis B and C in children. BMC Infect Dis 2014;14(Suppl 6):S5.
62. German P, Mathias A, Brainard D, et al. Clinical pharmacokinetics and pharmacodynamics of ledipasvir/sofosbuvir, a fixed-dose combination tablet for the treatment of hepatitis C. Clin Pharmacokinet 2016;55(11):1337–51.

# Drug Dosing in Obese Children

## Challenges and Evidence-Based Strategies

Ye Xiong, PhD[a], Tsuyoshi Fukuda, PhD[a,b],
Catherijne A.J. Knibbe, PharmD, PhD[c,d],
Alexander A. Vinks, PharmD, PhD, FCP[a,b],*

## KEYWORDS

- Pharmacokinetics • Pharmacodynamics • Obese children • Model-informed doing
- Prediction in pharmacology

## KEY POINTS

- Pathophysiologic alterations associated with obesity can predict changes in the pharmacokinetics and pharmacodynamics of drugs, but drug-specific properties, disease progression, and other comorbidities also need to be considered.
- Appropriate weight-based descriptors serve as important factors for estimating critical pharmacokinetic parameters as part of dose calculations.
- Future research should focus on pediatric population pharmacokinetic/pharmacodynamic studies to allow evidence-based dosing in obese children.

## INTRODUCTION

The incidence of overweight and obesity is rising at an alarming rate around the world. Within the United States, the prevalence of obesity increased from less than 15% in the 1990s to more than 36% in 2010 according to the data obtained from the US Centers for Disease Control and Prevention (CDC). An estimated 1.1 billion individuals will be obese worldwide by 2030 if the current trend persists.[1] In 2013, the American Medical Association officially redefined obesity as a disease.

Disclosure Statement: None of the authors declared a conflict of interest.
[a] Division of Clinical Pharmacology, Cincinnati Children's Hospital Medical Center, 3333 Burnet Avenue, MLC 6018, Cincinnati, OH 45229-3039, USA; [b] Department of Pediatrics, University of Cincinnati College of Medicine, Cincinnati, OH, USA; [c] Department of Clinical Pharmacy, St Antonius Hospital, PO Box 2500, Nieuwegein 3430 EM, The Netherlands; [d] Division of Pharmacology, Leiden Academic Center for Drug Research, Faculty of Science, Leiden University, PO Box 9502, 2300 RA, Leiden, The Netherlands
* Corresponding author. Cincinnati Children's Hospital Medical Center, 3333 Burnet Avenue, MLC 6018, Cincinnati, OH 45229-3039.
E-mail address: sander.vinks@cchmc.org

Obesity is associated with a variety of pathophysiologic changes and has an etiology that encompasses behavioral and genetic factors. Childhood obesity often continues into adulthood, because it is greatly impacted by environment and habit. Obesity in children is commonly defined as a body mass index (BMI) above the 95th percentile of specific age and sex according to CDC growth charts. This classification differs slightly from the current definition by the World Health Organization, which states a BMI of greater or equal than 2 times the standard deviation of the average BMI for age and sex (equal to approximately the 97th percentile in the CDC charts). Per the 2014 CDC update, 1 in 6 children and adolescents in the United States is obese.

In recent years, specific pediatric drug information has been progressively implemented in drug labels under the initiatives of the Best Pharmaceuticals for Children Act and the Pediatric Research Equity Act. In 2012, the US Food and Drug Administration launched the New Pediatric Labeling Information Database, which simplifies the search of drugs with pediatric information based on trade and generic name or indication. At present, there are 684 drug labels with pediatric study data available, which include 619 labels of small molecule drugs and 65 of biologics.

Currently, US Food and Drug Administration labels lack information for appropriate use in obese children or obese patients in general. This is in part due to a limited number of obese children participating in clinical studies, and the lack of demand for inclusion of obese subjects in clinical trials, except for studies specifically addressing obesity related indications. However, owing to the high incidence of childhood obesity, it is increasingly common for clinicians to face important treatment and dosing decisions for this population.[2] The absence of studies or surveillance data in obese subjects not only impedes the ability of clinicians to appropriately dose, but also compromises the safety and efficacy of drug administration in this growing population.

Obesity is a complex, multifactorial disease that can be either primary or secondary. Besides the alteration in body composition, obesity-associated underlying conditions are causing changes in drug disposition and clinical responses, which compromise pharmacologic treatment in many diseases.[3–5] In this article, we discuss how the drug pharmacokinetics (PK) and disease-specific response to therapy are modified by obesity. In addition, evaluation and suggestions for the dosing of drugs in obese pediatric subjects including current evidence-based dosing strategies, are being discussed.

## OBESITY AND CHANGES IN DRUG DISPOSITION
### Obesity-Induced Physiologic and Pathologic Changes

Prominent changes as part of obesity are disproportional body weight gain with a significantly increased ratio of fat to lean body mass. These changes are highly and positively correlated with BMI.[6] Obesity is accompanied by numerous physiologic and pathologic alterations, such as increased cardiac output and circulating blood volume, reduced tissue perfusion, and altered liver and kidney function.[7–9] These changes are likely to influence drug disposition and pharmacologic effects. **Table 1** summarizes the potential effects of obesity related changes in body composition and physiology on drug PK and pharmacodynamics (PD). Changes in drug disposition can be characterized by a number of PK parameters, such as bioavailability ($F$), total body clearance (CL), volume of distribution ($V_d$), and absorption rate ($K_a$). These PK parameters, together with the maximum or peak ($C_{max}$) and minimum or predose trough concentrations ($C_{trough}$) and the area under the concentration-time curve characterize the extent and duration of drug exposure, and provide an indication whether obese patients are underexposed or overexposed compared with nonobese patients.

**Table 1**
Selected physiologic and pathologic changes in the obese population and their suggested effects on PK/PD as reported in the literature

| Body Composition | Expected Change | PK/PD Parameter Influenced | |
|---|---|---|---|
| Weight | ↑ | $V_d$ | Hydrophilic drugs are considered to exhibit moderate increases in $V_d$ |
| Lean mass | ↑ | $V_d$ | Lipophilic drugs typically exhibit increased $V_d$, except for drugs with high protein binding[12] |
| Fat mass | ↑ | $V_d$ | |
| Lean/fat ratio | ↓ | $V_d$ | |
| Physiology | | | |
| Cardiovascular | | | |
| Cardiac output (stroke volume) | ↑ | $V_d$ | Cardiac output will also impact clearance particularly medium to high extraction ratio drugs |
| Blood volume | ↑ | $V_d$ | |
| Plasma proteins | ↔, inconclusive | $V_d$ | |
| Plasma lipids | ↑ | $V_d$ | |
| Gut | | | |
| Gastric emptying | ↑ | F | Bioavailability has been reported as mostly unchanged after oral administration[12,13] |
| Gut blood flow | ↑ | F | |
| Gut wall permeability | ↑ | F | |
| Liver | | | |
| CYP enzyme activity | ↑, ↓, ↔ | $CL_{hepatic}$ | Hepatic clearance alters depending on the metabolic pathway |
| Phase II metabolic enzyme | ↑, ↔ | $CL_{hepatic}$ | Clearance increases for drugs with high hepatic extraction[14] |
| Hepatic blood flow | ↑ | $CL_{hepatic}$ | |
| Kidney | | | |
| Kidney size | ↑ | $CL_{renal}$ | Renal clearance mostly increases[14] |
| Glomerular filtration rate | ↑, ↓, ↔ | $CL_{renal}$ | |
| Tubular secretion | ↑ | $CL_{renal}$ | |
| Tubular reabsorption | ↑, ↓ | $CL_{renal}$ | |
| Renal blood flow | ↑ | $CL_{renal}$ | |
| Pulmonary | | | |
| Blood/gas partition | ↓ | $T_{max}$ | Mostly decrease[15] |
| Pathology | | | |
| Nonalcoholic fatty liver disease | | $CL_{hepatic}$ | Reported data are inconclusive[14] |
| Kidney impairment | | $CL_{renal}$ | Reported data are inconclusive[16,17] |
| Chronic inflammation | | PD | Resistance to medication effects[18] |
| Diabetes | | PD | Resistance to medication effects[19] |

*Abbreviations*: CL, total body clearance; CYP, cytochrome P; *F*, bioavailability; PD, pharmacodynamics; PK, pharmacokinetics; $V_d$, volume of distribution.

The changes in PK and PD parameters as summarized in Box 1 are general in nature and ordered according to pathophysiologic alterations in obese subjects. To assess the influence of physiologic and pathologic changes, PK and PD parameters need to be evaluated in a mechanistic way and for many drugs, drug/disease-specific pharmacologic changes should be investigated clinically.[10,11]

## Pharmacokinetic Changes Caused by Obesity

### Effects of obesity on drug absorption

The $F$ of medications is defined as the amount of drug that reaches the general circulation and $K_a$ reflects how fast the drug is absorbed from the site of extravascular administration. Both processes are influenced by the physiochemical properties of the drug and gastrointestinal milieu and motility. The most common route of drug delivery is oral administration. Factors including gut pH and permeability, gastric emptying, regional blood flow, first-pass metabolism, and the gut flora could be influenced by obesity and subsequently influence the rate and extent of absorption. Among these factors, the increase in intestinal permeability and splanchnic blood flow in obese subjects are thought to improve bioavailability.[13,27] Despite these changes, the rate and extent of absorption for a spectrum of drugs seems to be quite unaltered.[28–31] To date, midazolam is the only drug reported to exhibit greater bioavailability in obese subjects, which could be identified on a semisimultaneous oral and intravenous study design.[23] For this higher bioavailability, suppressed

---

**Box 1**
**Some cautionary tales when applying general principles for predicting pharmacokinetics/Pharmacodynamics in obese patients**

It should be emphasized that drug properties determine the ultimate effect. This is not limited to lipophilicity (although often mentioned as the most important factor), but it also applies to extraction ratio, and for instance the relative contribution of other elimination pathways involved.

- Although for hydrophilic drugs only moderate increases in $V_d$ are expected, the clinical consequences of such increases can be significant. For instance, Diepstraten and colleagues found that, for nadroparin (an example of a hydrophilic drug) in morbidly obese patients, TBW was the best predictor for clearance, whereas LBW proved the most predictive covariate for the central volume of distribution. These investigators showed that even small increases in $V_d$ (nadroparin $V_d$ was only 7 L) can still be very relevant clinically. Based on their findings, they suggested that individualized dosing of nadroparin should be based on LBW in morbidly obese patients.[20,21]
- Similarly for lipophilic drugs, it cannot be always assumed that $V_d$ will significantly increase with increases in TBW. For instance, propofol has a large $V_d$ that in obese patients further increases but that is not statistically significant to allow the use of TBW to estimate the propofol loading dose.[22] This is in contrast with midazolam, where a substantial increase in $V_d$ was observed that correlated well with increases in TBW in obese patients.[22,23]
- With respect to the kidney and hyperfiltration, renal clearance is expected to increase for renally cleared drugs but this does not always occur. For instance, for cefazolin no increase in clearance could be identified in morbidly obese patients,[24,25] indicating that there is more to it than just GFR for drugs that also undergo significant elimination via tubular secretion processes.
- Another issue to be anticipated is that prolonged obesity may lead to renal damage over time, thereby leading to reduced renal function and reduced drug clearance despite a large TBW.[26]

*Abbreviations:* GFR, glomerular filtration rate; LBW, lean body weight; TBW, total body weight; $V_d$, volume of distribution.

cytochrome P (CYP)3A protein expression in the gut, resulting in higher unchanged appearance of midazolam in the circulation, increased gut permeability, or an increase in splanchnic blood flow with obesity was hypothesized. Absorption in obese subjects has only been characterized in adults, which might overlook the ontogenic differences that could be at play in very young obese patients.

The time to reach $C_{max}$ ($T_{max}$) is important for conditions that require rapid onset of effect, for drugs such as analgesics, anesthetics, anticoagulants, antiasthma drugs, antihypertensives, antimicrobials, and antifungals. The rate of absorption is the primary determinant of $T_{max}$ when a drug is administered via the oral or extravascular route. For noninhalational agents, the absorption rate relies on the regional blood flow, which is anatomically regulated by cardiac output. Viscera receive about 73% of cardiac output, compared with 5% delivered to fat tissues, and 22% to lean tissues.[12] Absorption after oral administration occurs in the gut and is expected to be accelerated by increased splanchnic blood flow and gut permeability; however, the rate of absorption is reported as largely unchanged in obese subjects. However, owing to the substantial variability observed in nonobese control subjects, true differences might have been obscured.[8,13,32]

In the case of inhalation anesthetics, the absorption is determined by the oil/gas partition coefficient (extent of absorption), and the blood/gas partition coefficient (rate of absorption), with the latter being the key factor for drug action. The induction rate is inversely related to the blood/gas partition coefficient, because a large value means a higher proportion of drug entering the blood and, therefore, a slower equilibrium and a longer induction period.[33] Cardiac output negatively regulates the induction rate; high cardiac output accelerates drug removal and prolongs the equilibrium time in brain tissue. Obesity, despite increasing cardiac output, is associated with a shorter induction time for volatile anesthetics including enflurane, sevoflurane, and halothane, which is at least in part contributed by a reduced blood/gas partition.[15]

### Effect of obesity on drug distribution

Apparent volume of distribution is a theoretic parameter that reflects distribution of drug over the body. $V_d$ determines the magnitude of $C_{max}$, and is a practical parameter for calculating the loading dose of a drug. The magnitude of $V_d$ is influenced by the physiochemical properties of a drug, such as lipid solubility and plasma protein binding. $V_d$ can be greatly influenced by disease states of obesity, which alters body mass, blood volume, extracellular water, and tissue perfusion. The lipid partition coefficient generally predicts lipid solubility. Depending on lipophilicity and protein binding, drugs would either be more confined to the general circulation, or distribute to highly perfused organs and the periphery, specifically adipose tissues.

For hydrophilic drugs, distribution is relatively confined to the blood and extracellular water, and hence obese subjects exhibit a modest increase in their $V_d$. In such cases, $V_d$ is well-correlated with lean body weight (LBW).[34] In contrast, the distribution of lipophilic drugs is not predictable solely by lipophilicity. Theoretically, lipophilic drugs are considered to easily diffuse into fat, and obese patients are expected to have a larger $V_d$. This is the case for many of drugs with a high lipid partition coefficient value, such as benzodiazepine and opioids.[28] However, incomplete distribution into excessive fat often occurs, affected by lipid solubility or the absolute amount of unbound drug. Hence, drugs with moderate lipid affinity (ie, ranitidine) and/or high plasma protein binding (ie, cyclosporine or propofol) have a similar $V_d$ in obese subjects compared with nonobese subjects.[35–37]

Protein binding reduces the movement of free drug throughout the body and consequently restricts distribution. Acidic drugs are normally bound to albumin, whereas basic drugs mostly bind to acute phase $\alpha 1$-acid glycoprotein in plasma. Although albumin levels are not altered in moderate to morbid obesity, the changes in $\alpha 1$-acid glycoprotein are variably reported among studies in obese individuals. Elevated cholesterol and triglyceride concentrations in obese individuals are expected to affect lipoprotein binding of some drugs, but the overall impact of this binding on the $V_d$ is unclear. In summary, $V_d$ is influenced primarily by the differences in body composition, weight, and the extent of drug distribution into fat mass. Therefore, weight descriptors are commonly used to normalize $V_d$, and the one that best reconciles the differences in $V_d$ between obese and nonobese subjects is often chosen to calculate the loading dose of a drug in obese subjects, which is further illustrated in the Dosing in Obese Children section.

### Effect of obesity on metabolism and elimination

Drug clearance is an informative parameter in the design of maintenance dosing regimens. For small molecule drugs, CL primarily reflects drug metabolism in the gut and liver and/or renal elimination. Hepatic metabolic pathways are characterized by phase I reactions (oxidation, reduction, and hydrolysis of exogenous substances) and phase II reactions (conjugation of endogenous substituents, ie, glucuronidation, sulfation, methylation, and acetylation). Drugs that undergo metabolism are modified chemically to facilitate their elimination via the kidneys, the bile, and/or the feces. The majority of obese patients will develop nonalcoholic fatty liver disease with different degrees of severity, ranging from steatosis to nonalcoholic steatohepatitis, which correlates with BMI.[38] Owing to this condition, the enzymatic expression and activity of liver enzymes are likely influenced as a result of abnormal fat deposition and obesity-related chronic inflammation.

The main players in phase I metabolism are CYP-450 enzymes. Among the CYP family, CYP3A4 metabolizes approximately 50% of all drugs, and a lower enzymatic activity is observed in obese subjects. This reduced activity may potentially increase drug exposure as a result of a reduced first-pass effect and decreased metabolic clearance. Sometimes, the reduced CYP activity can be compensated by an increase in the size of the liver, liver blood volume, and/or bioavailability.[14] Data in the literature on other phase I enzymes (ie, CYPs other than CYP3A4, and xanthine oxidase) and phase II enzymes (ie, uridine diphosphate glucuronosyltransferase) show mixed results and studies sometimes report higher activity or no changes in obese patients.

For drugs with high hepatic extraction ratio, CL is largely dependent on liver blood flow. The impact of obesity on liver blood flow remains inconclusive owing to bidirectional modulation: a reduction of blood flow by nonalcoholic steatohepatitis–mediated sinusoidal narrowing, and an increase of liver blood flow owing to increased cardiac output and blood volume. Few studies report an increased clearance in obese subjects for drugs with high clearance (>1.5 L/min, close to liver blood flow of 2.0–2.5 L/min), implicating a dominant impact of increased cardiac output and blood volume.[14,22]

The kidneys are the primary organ for drug elimination, which includes 3 processes: glomerular filtration, tubular secretion, and tubular reabsorption. An overall increase in renal clearance is found in obese patients for many drugs, which linearly correlates with lean body mass.[39] This increase is mainly contributed to an exacerbated glomerular filtration rate (GFR) owing to glomerular dysfunction rather than a change in kidney blood flow.[40] In addition, some drugs, such as procainamide and lithium, exhibit increased renal clearance in obese subjects as a result of increased tubular secretion and reduced tubular reabsorption, respectively.[14,41] Notably, unlike what has been observed in adults, renal clearance in children does not seem to differ in the presence or absence of obesity.[42]

## Pharmacodynamic Changes Caused by Obesity

Obesity is accompanied by chronic inflammatory responses to adipokines and cytokines, thereby impacting the homeostasis of the immune system. Treatments that are associated with immune modulation include vaccinations, primary immune deficiency therapy such as immunoglobulin, and antiasthma agents such as inhaled corticosteroids. In children with asthma, IgE and eosinophilia are elevated in obesity and increase the resistance to treatment; the highest dose of the biologic agent omalizumab over the shortest duration is, therefore, needed in obese subjects to achieve a good response.[43,44] In contrast, immunoglobulin treatment for immunocompromised patients does not require dose adjustment in the obese population.[45] Response to immunization by vaccines is also altered in obese subjects and depends on the type of vaccination. For example, immunogenicity to flu vaccine is enhanced in the obese population, whereas response to hepatitis B or tetanus vaccine seems to be unchanged with no specific dose adjustment recommended.

A common complication of obesity is alteration in insulin sensitivity and its downstream signaling molecules, which are in part caused by chronic inflammation. This change ultimately compromises the response to exogenously administered insulin, and typically requires dose escalation, specifically in patients who developed type 2 diabetes.[19] Changes in target expression or affinity, or organ dysfunction also contribute to disease specific resistance to therapy, thereby affecting drug effects.[8] Hence, the dose–concentration effect and safety relationships should be further studied for dose individualization in the obese population, specifically for drugs with narrow therapeutic ranges.

## DOSING GUIDELINES IN PEDIATRICS

Owing to the relative lack of age-appropriate dosing information for the use of drugs in children in general, off-label use of drugs is common in pediatric practice. In a recent prospective observational study investigators showed that 27% of pediatric emergency department visits were due to medication-related adverse events in the absence of dosing guidelines. This also resulted in a significantly higher probability of hospitalization than non–medication-related emergency department visits.[46] The issue of drug safety could be even more compelling in obese patients, because this population tends to use multiple prescriptions while at the same time evidence-based dosing guidelines are lacking.

Several strategies have been proposed to derive appropriate dosage regimens for children. Most commonly, this strategy involves extrapolation of dosing information from adult patients. This leveraging of existing clinical data from a studied adult population can be divided into 2 general categories: (1) approaches that use a size descriptor for dosing in children, and (2) approaches that encourage the use of scaled PK parameters or PK–PD models to identify the most appropriate pediatric doses. This latter strategy primarily addresses the effects of growth and maturation on body size and organ function, and the resultant changes in drug disposition, with the goal of achieving effective and safe drug exposures.[47]

## Body Weight–Based Dosing

### Weight measures

There have been multiple size descriptors proposed for the scaling of the dose of a drug in children. These include the direct measure of total body weight (TBW), as well as derived measures including body surface area (BSA), ideal body weight (IBW), adjusted body weight (ABW), LBW, fat-free mass, and BMI (**Table 2**).[7,13,48,49]

**Table 2**
General body size descriptors and their application

| Body Size Descriptor | Equation | Population | Application |
|---|---|---|---|
| BMI for age[55] | CDC BMI-for-age chart (boy or girl) | 2–20 y | Categorizes degree of obesity |
| BSA[56] | $BSA = \frac{TBW\ (kg) \times height\ (cm)}{3600}$ | Children and adults | Commonly used for antineoplastic drug[57] |
| FFM[34] | $FFM\ (male) = \frac{42.92 \times TBW\ (kg) \times height\ (cm)^2}{30.93 \times height\ (cm)^2 + TBW\ (kg)}$ <br> $FFM\ (female) = \frac{37.99 \times TBW\ (kg) \times height\ (cm)^2}{35.98 \times height\ (cm)^2 + TBW\ (kg)}$ | Adults | Accounts for sex differences, corresponds to lean mass (sum of vital organs, extracellular fluid, muscle, bone) <br>• Suggested for dosing of biologics and hydrophilic drugs[53] <br>• Not applicable for patients with BMI > 30 |
| LBW[52] | $LBW\ (male) = 1.1 \times TBW(kg) - 0.0128 \times \frac{TBW\ (kg)^2}{height\ (m)^2}$ <br> $LBW\ (female) = 1.07 \times TBW(kg) - 0.0148 \times \frac{TBW\ (kg)^2}{height\ (m)^2}$ <br> $LBW\ (child) = 0.0817 \times TBW\ (kg)^{0.5469} \times height\ (cm)^{0.7236}$ | ≤13 y | |
| IBW[50] | $IBW = [50\text{th percentile BMI for the child's age} \times height\ (cm)]^2$ | 2–20 y | Accounts for sex differences <br>• Suggested for hydrophilic drugs and biologics[58] <br>• Suggested for determining maintenance dose[57,58] |
| ABW[54] | $ABW = IBW + factor \times (TBW - IBW)$ <br> Typical value of factor: 0.3–0.4 | Adults mostly | Accounts for body composition <br>• Suggested for lipophilic drugs with partial fat distribution <br>• Used for dosing of aminoglycosides[59] |

*Abbreviations:* ABW, adjusted body weight; BMI, body mass index; BSA, body surface area; CDC, Centers for Disease Control and Prevention; FFM, fat-free mass; IBW, ideal body weight; LBW, lean body weight; TBW, total body weight.

Among these descriptors, TBW is generally applied for calculating doses in children. BSA is a more empirical scaler that is commonly used in oncology for the dosing of antineoplastic medication. Fat-free mass and LBW both estimate lean body mass (the total of vital organs, extracellular fluid, bones, and muscles), except that LBW also includes fat accumulated in cell membranes, the bone marrow, and the central nervous system. IBW in adults is derived from life insurance tables that indicate the optimal adult body size associated with life expectancy; in children, IBW can be obtained using the BMI method as described in **Table 2**.[50] Notably, LBW, fat-free mass, and IBW are predictors that take gender into account, and are considered to be robust for predicting the limited distribution of hydrophilic drugs over the body.[34,51–53] ABW is another measure mentioned in the literature that uses a correction factor (0.3 or 0.4) to account for a proportion of the excessive fat (extra fluid in adipose tissue), but is not commonly used.[54] These weight descriptors are generally selected in relation to drug distribution and clearance. BMI is rarely used as a scaler for dosing, but is a commonly used descriptor to classify people into normal, obese, and morbidly obese categories. For pediatric LBW calculation as described by Peters and colleagues,[52] BMI is used to set a cap on the estimation, because the formula cannot be reliably used for patients with BMI of greater than 30 kg/m$^2$.

### Allometric scaling

Apart from these body size scalers, the dose in children can be also predicted by applying principles of allometry, in which dose is calculated as an exponential function of weight. This methodology assumes that the physiologic processes that dictate drug disposition, such as blood flow, GFR, and liver/kidney size, increase with weight in a nonlinear manner.[60] Dose in children is predicted from the adult dose using the equation below[61–63]:

$$\text{Dose in children} = \text{adult dose} \times (\text{TBW of a child}/70)^{0.75} \tag{1}$$

The fixed exponent of 0.75 (theoretic allometry), which correlates with basal metabolic rates, can reasonably predict dose in children as young as 2 years of age depending on the properties of the drug such as fraction unbound in adults, extraction ratio, elimination pathway, and binding proteins.[60,62,64] It is noteworthy that the choice of exponent in dose prediction, for most small molecule drugs, is tightly linked to clearance predicted by weight allometry from adults; the rationale is illustrated below in a description of clearance based dosing.

### Clearance-Based Dosing

From a PK perspective, drug dosing regimens are determined by volume of distribution and clearance. Dosage in children is specifically reliant on the ability to predict the effects of growth and maturation on volume and clearance. The ontogeny of renal function and metabolic enzymes are considered to be the most influential factors impacting drug elimination in children and determines the pharmacologic responses.[65] Hence, a predicted or estimated CL in children can be used to calculate the age-appropriate dose.[61] Similar to equation (1), the following equation has been suggested to calculate the dose in children [61]:

$$\text{Dose for the child} = \text{adult dose} \times (\text{CL in the child}/\text{CL in adults}) \tag{2}$$

If an estimated pediatric clearance is available, then this formula provides an accurate prediction for clinical application. When pediatric population PK or individual data are not available, clearance can be extrapolated from adult data using allometric scaling, and then applied in equation (2) for dose calculation, according to[61,63]:

$$CL\ in\ the\ child = CL\ in\ adults \times (TBW\ of\ a\ child/70) \tag{3}$$

This fixed exponent of 0.75 is commonly used and predicts reasonably well for children older than 2 years of age.[64,66,67] However, this scaling method leads to increasing prediction errors as the age decreases, and becomes unreliable for children aged 1 year and younger.[61,64]

## DOSING IN OBESE CHILDREN

The doses of drugs used in obese patients are largely based on empiricism and experience of prescribers rather than based on clinical evidence. The incorporation of pediatric PK information becomes critical to guide weight-appropriate dose selection. In a consensus document on Medication Dosing in Overweight and Obese Children by the PPAG Advocacy Committee authors proposed guidelines of how to apply PK data for dosing decisions and adjustment in obese children.[68] A summary of the guidelines is shown as a flow diagram in **Fig. 1**. As general guidelines, these authors indicated that, for obese children exceeding a weight of 40 kg, the regular adult dose should be considered. Furthermore, the estimated pediatric dose should not be greater than the adult maximum dose.

### Determining the Appropriate Dose for Obese Subjects

#### When prior pharmacokinetic information is available
Obese pediatric populations explored in clinical studies are generally above the age of 6 years (approximately 75%).[7] For children under 6 years of age, the prevalence of obesity is relatively low (<10%), and safety in this age group outweighs efficacy. In general, drugs with wide therapeutic windows are used for patients of this age range, and the TBW-based dose is commonly recommended. Alternatively, dose titration to desired effect, use of loading doses, and sometimes dose prediction based on allometric scaling can be applied for treatment to minimize the risk of adverse events.

Anthropometry-based dosing, which includes dosing by weight and by allometric scaling, addresses the differences in body size and physiologic conditions that likely influence drug disposition. $V_d$ and CL as the most important PK parameters do not always increase linearly with weight increases. Green and colleagues[69] reviewed more than 30 small molecule drugs and concluded that TBW was the best size descriptor for $V_d$ and LBW was for CL. The latter would imply an important influence of gender besides weight, because men have a higher LBW than women, even when they have the same TBW. Given that $V_d$ and CL are critical for attaining target concentration initially and during steady state, independent assumptions were made for loading and maintenance dose estimation, as described below.

For therapy that demands a rapid onset of effect, achieving an effective concentration as soon as possible is critical and likely necessitate an adjustment of loading dose for obese patients. $V_d$ correlates with the total amount of drug distributed in the body. Thus, the best weight descriptor to be used for loading dose can be identified by comparing $V_d$ corrected for weight (the values expressed per kg of TBW, IBW, or LBW) between obese and nonobese cohorts. A similar $V_d$/TBW indicates that excess weight markedly affects distribution, in which case TBW should be applied for dose calculation. If volume of distribution/TBW of obese subjects is smaller to nonobese subjects, but the volume of distribution/IBW or volume of distribution/LBW is comparable, a limited impact by excess mass is suggested, and dose based on IBW or LBW

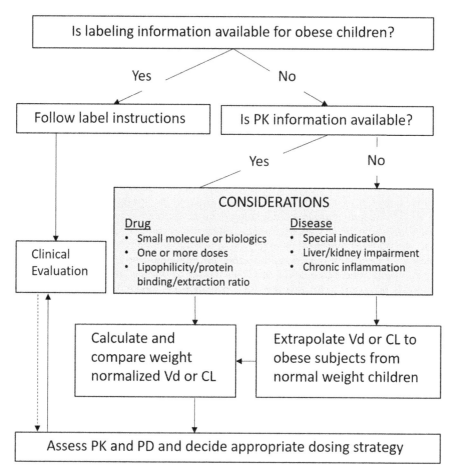

**Fig. 1.** Flow diagram for dosing decisions in obese children. Flow diagram structured according to guidelines published by PPAG Advocacy Committee. CL, total body clearance; PD, pharmacodynamics; PK, pharmacokinetic; Vd, volume of distribution. (*Data from* Matson KL, Horton ER, Capino AC. Advocacy committee for the pediatric pharmacy advocacy G. medication dosage in overweight and obese children. J Pediatr Pharmacol Ther 2017;22(1):81–3.)

could be a better approach.[70] In case $V_d$ divided by TBW, IBW, or LBW does not seem comparable with nonobese subjects, $V_d$ should be plotted against these parameters to establish the exact relationship.

For chronic therapies that dose repeatedly, maintenance dose may also need to be adjusted for obese subjects. Because clearance is key to maintain effective plasma concentration during steady state, a similar comparison of this parameter between obese and nonobese cohorts can be made to predict the appropriate weight metric dosing. If CL/TBW is the same in obese and normal weight subjects, then TBW should be used for determining maintenance dose. If CL/TBW is lower in obese subjects, and CL/LBW or CL/IBW is comparable, LBW- or IBW-based dosing may be applicable, such as for midazolam and carbamazepine.[7,14,48,71] In any case, the relationship between weight descriptors and clearance should be explored via plotting and population modeling to provide analyzable details. Take propofol as an example: clearance has been suggested to increase linearly or nonlinearly with weight by different research groups. Diepstraten and colleagues[72] summarize that, although linear function oan oufficiontly doooribc oubjcoto with low or normal woighto, tho nonlinoar (allo metric) relation fits better for obese subjects. They conclude that dosing regimen by TBW using 0.75 allometry should be applied for obese children (**Box 2**).[7]

### When prior pharmacokinetic information is not available

When no PK information in obese children is available, extrapolation from other data sources could be considered. For instances where PK data for obese children are absent, but there are pediatric PK data, extrapolation of PK parameters from normal weight children could be used with allometric scaling to address the differences in body size between obese and nonobese subjects,[61,77] even though there is as yet no evidence with this approach.

In situations where no pediatric PK data are available, adoption of the weight metric used for dosing in obese adults could be considered for dosing in obese children.[57] One thing to keep in mind is extrapolating dose from obese adults to obese children is not always scientifically sound for dose prediction given differences in PK between obese and normal cohorts relate to growth, development, and disease progression of obesity.[71,78] Clinicians may consider other approaches. For instance, the starting dose can be divided into a series of smaller doses to quickly attain therapeutic concentrations followed by therapeutic drug concentration monitoring for assessment if available.[79] Alternatively, dose titration could include escalating doses until the therapeutic target is achieved. Ideally, these strategies are combined with therapeutic drug concentration monitoring, which would help to reduce the risk of toxicity and manage long-term efficacy and adverse events.[80]

### Other Considerations

#### Body surface area–based dosing in oncology

Dosing chemotherapeutic agents based on BSA is common practice in oncology,[81] and several protocols apply dose capping for instance at 2.0 m$^2$ based on concerns of adverse effects such as neurotoxicity. As a result, in morbidly obese patients, underexposure to the drug may occur, which could lead to cancer recurrence or even death. Cancer is one of the therapeutic areas where the need for adequate response outweighs the risk of toxicity, because the goal of the treatment is to cure.[82] Thus, achieving comparable exposure to normal weight patients is essential for remission and overall survival. TBW-based dosing or BSA without capping delivers better

---

**Box 2**

**A lesson learned from dosing of heparin in children**

UFH is a commonly used anticoagulant in children. It is dosed based on total body weight and administered via continuous infusion. In a retrospective study, investigators found that a significantly lower amount of unfractionated heparin was needed to achieve the same effect in obese subjects.[73] This is because heparin has a relatively small volume of distribution (not correlated with total weight/kg), and hence a modest increase in $V_d$ disproportionate to weight in obese objects. Therefore, when dose is given by total body weight, the concentrations of UFH (related to dose divided by $V_d$) are higher in obese subjects and likely result in over-exposure and subsequently adverse events, such as bleeding. A maximal initial dose is suggested for patients that are morbidly obese.[74] Given that the degree of adiposity can be markedly different within morbidly obese population, a capped dose could result in underexposure.[75] A recent report suggests that obese subjects require dose adjustment based on LBW to guarantee adequate clinical response.[76]

*Abbreviations:* LBW, lean body weight; $V_d$, volume of distribution; UFH, unfractionated heparin.

responses and survival in obese subjects. Furthermore, increasing risk of toxicity with TBW based dosing has not been identified definitively. Thus, TBW or BSA calculated by TBW without capping is now propagated as the preferred method for dosing of most antineoplastic drugs in obese patients with close monitoring for toxicity.[82] An example of an oncology drug that needs to be dosed in obese children without capping is busulfan, because the model that was developed predicted well in underweight, overweight, and obese children of different ages.[83]

### Obesity and related comorbidities
Kidney disease is one of the comorbidities linked to prolonged obesity and its influence on drug clearance should be considered for drugs that are primarily cleared via kidney. In obese children with renal impairment, changes in the GFR were not consistent among studies.[16,17] These discrepancies could be attributed to complex etiology and the state of obesity such that GFR is distinctively influenced by hyperfiltration or kidney dysfunction.[26] In case of reduced renal clearance, a dose decrease or lengthening of the dosing interval is recommended to minimize the risk for overexposure.[84] Last, for morbidly obese children who undergo bariatric surgery, several factors such as changes in gastric emptying time, lipid homeostasis, and metabolic enzyme expression and activity, affect drug PK behavior.[85]

### Gut microbes
Obesity is found to be influence the microbiome. Not only does the microbiome play an important role in processing food, several recent studies highlight the involvement of commensal gut microbiota in the metabolism of drugs, with some identifying the specific strains that are involved in altering the expression of CYP enzymes and transporters.[86–88] Incorporation of this type of information may be insightful when integrated with techniques such as physiologically based PK modeling and pharmacometabolomics.[89,90] Although research in this area is just starting, there are high expectations for its eventual clinical applicability.

### Biologics
The PK of biologics such as peptides and proteins differs from conventional small molecular drugs. Owing to their low oral bioavailability, biologics are mostly given via parenteral administration. The extravascular route of administration (ie, intramuscular or subcutaneous) is common, after which the biologic is slowly taken up by blood capillaries or the lymphatic system, depending on molecular weight. Given the poor diffusion of large molecules, distribution is usually limited to circulation. Many biologics exhibit target-mediated drug disposition, which corresponds with the special situation where a significant proportion of a drug (relative to dose) is bound with high affinity to the pharmacologic target, such that this interaction is reflected in the PK characteristics of the drug. This phenomenon is highly dynamic depending on the target level and occupancy.[91] The chronic inflammation triggered by obesity can provoke changes in clearance that are related to rapid proteolysis and antibody neutralization by "antigen sink" (an enriched reservoir of inflammatory cytokine that is the target antigen). A particular challenge has been described with anti-tumor necrosis factor therapy in treating autoimmune disease, such as inflammatory bowel disease, in which a sizable percentage of patients being treated (up to 40%) is obese. Obesity has been identified as an independent risk factor that is associated with reduced responses and remissions, which has been attributed to a failure to maintain minimally effective concentrations above the target concentration during long-term treatment.[18] In this respect, particularly drugs that are labeled as fixed dose, as opposed to drugs dosed per kilogram, are at risk for reduced responses.

Dose regimens in drug labels are proposed pertinent to phase II and III clinical trials of a relatively homogenous population. In postapproval practice, the suggested dose regimens could lead to highly variable clinical responses as a result of diversity in patients' population, disease conditions, comorbidities, concurrent medications, and so on. These considerations could provide insights of what strategies and tools to use when facing this challenge. Collectively, the obese population as a specific population should be implemented in clinical trials or studies to validate dosing recommendation and adjustment.[8]

## FUTURE PERSPECTIVES
### Individualization

Dose prediction based on weight is a preliminary means of individualization, where the selection of the appropriate weight metric is critical in achieving target concentration. Apart from that, precision medicine is advocated in the past few years aiming to improve clinical outcomes. The model-informed precision dosing will propel clinical data gathering upon which a tight collaboration between health providers and research institutes forms, and prospectively move study in special populations forward.

### Model-informed precision dosing model

A common approach of individualization is model-informed dosing. Two algorithms frequently used are population based PK and physiologically based PK.[92] With a priori PK modeling, the interpolation of posterior observations, and information of physiology and drug properties to PK models will not only validate the identified covariates, but also further guide dosing in special populations where clinical evidence is lacking.[93]

**Population-based pharmacokinetics** An individual prediction is often derived from Bayesian post hoc estimation based on a population model constructed in the specific population. The demographic information, laboratory values, and genetic information, if determined as covariates during modeling processes, will be used as the factors that generate individual predictions of PK parameters. Loading and maintenance doses for the special populations, obese subjects in our case, is subsequently deduced. In the process of personalization, therapeutic drug concentration monitoring is the pivotal tool to provide feedback into a population model for an on-target dosing adjustment. This feedback supplies observations to update individual PK parameters using Bayesian methodology, ensuring safety and efficacy during chronic therapy. It also monitors potential temporal change of PK profile influenced by disease progression, comorbidity, and drug coadministered.

**Physiology-based pharmacokinetics** A physiologic-based PK approach is increasingly used for dose development. This approach uses physiologic and biochemical data to mechanistically predict PK behavior and drug–drug interaction before the selection of the first in human dose. A physiologically based PK model can also implement pathologic conditions to envision PK alteration. However, this method requires an in-depth understanding of physiology and biochemistry to reliably calibrate each factor that can influence PK profile; thus, a large amount of system information, time, and expertise is needed for the building and validation of the model. A simplified physiologically based PK model has been developed for predicting PK and dose in obese subjects during steady state. This approach incorporates a noncompartmental model with the physiochemical property of the drug (adipose tissue–plasma partition) and physiologic parameters of the body (fat fraction), and predicts with fair precision even in cases of inaccurate terminal concentration measurements.[94] With limited applications, a physiologically based PK model predicts reasonably well for adults, but poorly for younger children.[95] Nonetheless, this strategy has its unparalleled advantage in PK profiling in special populations given a robust prediction made by a small number of subjects and invaluable mechanistic insights.

### Pharmacometabolomics integration

Pharmacometabolomics is recently implicated to be useful for personalizing drug therapy. This technique incorporates high-definition analytical instruments to discover clinically relevant biomarkers by referencing to baseline metabolomics, and predicts exposure via quantitating changes of biomarkers. The identified biomarkers can potentially be integrated into model-informed dosing as a Bayesian priori or serves as a PD marker for clinical evaluation. However, the baseline information is relatively chaotic and identification of biomarkers for each disease indication in routine clinical practice requires great amount of work; hence, it is currently at its infancy. As a novel tool, further research is vital to formulate the database for application and validation.[90,96]

### Labeling Information

Pursuant to Best Pharmaceuticals for Children Act, implementation of pediatric studies has resulted in labeling changes in safety, efficacy, PK, PK–PD, tolerability, and immunogenicity of 140 drugs covering 54 therapeutic categories. Although obesity is listed as a risk factor for cardiovascular and thromboembolic adverse events for many drugs in the *Physician's Desk Reference*, the correspondent dose recommendation remains absent. Interestingly, weight, as the most influential covariate for the 2 main PK parameters that determine the dose, can often not be rigorously investigated in PK study of clinical trial because of insufficient coverage of weight range, or a lack of inclusion criteria related to weight or BMI in trial protocol. Therefore, the application on such a patient population remains more empirical than data driven, and warrants further retrospective investigation. The inclusion of wide weight distribution, especially in diseases common in obese individuals, will thus refine the current protocol and foster labeling change to better the clinical practice.

### What's Next?

Advocates continuously strive for improving pediatric care. Anderson and Holford recently proposed the use of normal fat mass calculated as the fraction of fat influencing key PK parameters that could be likely applied for dosing in obese patients.[92] This size metric corresponds with the ABW, but further refines body composition by substituting IBW with fat-free mass. As a comprehensive strategy, Brussee and colleagues[97] urged the prospective application of PK–PD modeling as a systems-level approach for precision dosing in pediatric patients. This strategy encompasses both PK and PD assessment, hence truly leveraging efficacy in model development.[97] Although no commentary is made in this article, the introduction of new concepts and tools will undoubtedly reduce the knowledge gap and allow the application of evidence-based designs in clinical trials and the use of model-based precision dosing in clinical practice.

## AN EXAMPLE OF PROOF-OF-CONCEPT DOSE ESTIMATION IN OBESE CHILDREN

Propofol is widely used for induction and maintenance of anesthesia in both pediatrics and adults. The PK information is available for both obese and nonobese subjects in adults and pediatrics.[22] We demonstrate dose prediction by assuming 2 conditions: without prior information or with prior information. CL in normal and obese age-matched pediatric population is either directly obtained or with simple calculation and then applied for decision making of maintenance dose.

### Extrapolating Clearance in Obese Pediatrics on the Basis of a Previously Published Model

**Step 1: Obtain key information—exponent for weight allometry**

$$CL = \text{population } CL_{pediatrics} \times (TBW/70 \text{ kg})^x$$

Where population CL is 1.75 mL/min in a 70-kg pediatric subject; exponent $x = 0.73$.[22]

**Step 2: Apply the weight exponent to calculate obese pediatric CL**

- Normal pediatrics [median TBW = 54 kg]

$$CL_{normal} = 1.75 \text{ mL/min} \times (54/70 \text{ kg})^{0.73} = 1.45 \text{ mL/min}$$

- Obese pediatrics [median TBW = 125 kg]

$$CL_{obese} = 1.75 \text{ mL/min} \times (125/70 \text{ kg})^{0.73} = 2.66 \text{ mL/min}$$

After estimating the CL in a typical normal and obese patient, weight-normalized CL will be calculated and compared as illustrated in the steps 1 and 2 below.

### Compare Clearance Between Normal and Obese Pediatrics

**Step 1: Calculate weight normalized CL in these 2 populations**

- Normal pediatrics [$CL_{normal}$ = 1.45 mL/min]
  TBW = 54 kg, IBW = 55 kg, LBW = 37 kg, ABW (factor of 0.4) = 55 kg
  $CL_{normal}$/TBW = 0.027
  $CL_{normal}$/IBW = 0.026
  $CL_{normal}$/LBW = 0.039
  $CL_{normal}$/ABW = 0.027
- Obese pediatrics [$CL_{obese}$ = 2.66 mL/min]
  TBW = 125 kg, IBW = 59 kg, LBW = 63 kg, ABW (factor of 0.4) = 85 kg
  $CL_{obese}$/TBW = 0.021
  $CL_{obese}$/IBW = 0.045
  $CL_{obese}$/LBW = 0.042
  $CL_{obese}$/ABW = 0.031

**Step 2: Compare CL, weight normalized CL between normal and obese subject**

- $CL_{normal} < CL_{obese}$
- $CL_{normal}$/TBW > $CL_{obese}$/TBW
- $CL_{normal}$/IBW < $CL_{obese}$/IBW
- $CL_{normal}$/LBW ≈ $CL_{obese}$/LBW
- $CL_{normal}$/ABW ≈ $CL_{obese}$/ABW

### Recommendation for Dosing in Obese Pediatrics

LBW-normalized CL is comparable between the normal and obese populations. Therefore, an LBW-based maintenance dose may be appropriate for propofol in obese subjects, which agrees to linear function of LBW in CL. An ABW-based dose may also be applicable and it has been applied for obese patients previously for propofol maintenance.[72,98] We emphasize that, in this case, the ABW-based linear dosing (or LBW linear dosing) leads to similar results as the use of TBW with an allometric exponent of 0.73.[22]

## REFERENCES

1. Kelly T, Yang W, Chen CS, et al. Global burden of obesity in 2005 and projections to 2030. Int J Obes (Lond) 2008;32(9):1431–7.
2. Johnson PN, Miller JL, Hagemann TM, et al. Assessment of inpatient admissions and top 25 medications for obese pediatric patients at two academic hospitals. Am J Health Syst Pharm 2016;73(16):1243–9.
3. Kloiber S, Ising M, Reppermund S, et al. Overweight and obesity affect treatment response in major depression. Biol Psychiatry 2007;62(4):321–6.
4. Hamzavi Abedi Y, Perkins AM, Morales MB. Childhood obesity in pediatric patients with difficult-to-control asthma in a tertiary pediatric subspecialty clinic. Allergy Asthma Proc 2017;38(1):63–9.
5. Navarro WH. Impact of obesity in the setting of high-dose chemotherapy. Bone Marrow Transplant 2003;31(11):961–6.
6. Demerath EW, Schubert CM, Maynard LM, et al. Do changes in body mass index percentile reflect changes in body composition in children? Data from the Fels Longitudinal Study. Pediatrics 2006;117(3):e487–495.
7. Mulla H, Johnson TN. Dosing dilemmas in obese children. Arch Dis Child Educ Pract Ed 2010;95(4):112–7.
8. Jain R, Chung SM, Jain L, et al. Implications of obesity for drug therapy: limitations and challenges. Clin Pharmacol Ther 2011;90(1):77–89.
9. Cho SJ, Yoon IS, Kim DD. Obesity-related physiological changes and their pharmacokinetic consequences. J Pharm Invest 2013;43:161–9.
10. Beavers CJ, Heron P, Smyth SS, et al. Obesity and antiplatelets-does one size fit all? Thromb Res 2015;136(4):712–6.
11. Sankaralingam S, Kim RB, Padwal RS. The impact of obesity on the pharmacology of medications used for cardiovascular risk factor control. Can J Cardiol 2015;31(2):167–76.
12. Blouin RA, Warren GW. Pharmacokinetic considerations in obesity. J Pharm Sci 1999;88(1):1–7.
13. Knibbe CA, Brill MJ, van Rongen A, et al. Drug disposition in obesity: toward evidence-based dosing. Annu Rev Pharmacol Toxicol 2015;55:149–67.
14. Drill MJ, Diepstraten J, van Rongen A, et al. Impact of obesity on drug metabolism and elimination in adults and children. Clin Pharmacokinet 2012;51(5):277–304.
15. Luc EC, De Baerdemaeker EPM, Struys MMRF. Pharmacokinetics in obese patients. Contin Educ Anaesth Crit Care Pain 2004;4(5):152–5.
16. Koulouridis E, Georgalidis K, Kostimpa I, et al. Metabolic syndrome risk factors and estimated glomerular filtration rate among children and adolescents. Pediatr Nephrol 2010;25(3):491–0.
17. Correia-Costa L, Afonso AC, Schaefer F, et al. Decreased renal function in overweight and obese prepubertal children. Pediatr Res 2015;78(4):436–44.
18. Singh S, Dulai PS, Zarrinpar A, et al. Obesity in IBD: epidemiology, pathogenesis, disease course and treatment outcomes. Nat Rev Gastroenterol Hepatol 2017;14(2):110–21.
19. Schmid C, Krayenbuhl P, Wiesli P. Increased insulin dose requirement of long-acting insulin analogues in obese patients with type 2 diabetes. Diabetologia 2009;52(12):2668–9.

20. Diepstraten J, Janssen EJ, Hackeng CM, et al. Population pharmacodynamic model for low molecular weight heparin nadroparin in morbidly obese and non obese patients using anti-Xa levels as endpoint. Eur J Clin Pharmacol 2015; 71(1):25–34.

21. Diepstraten J, Hackeng CM, van Kralingen S, et al. Anti-Xa levels 4 h after sub-cutaneous administration of 5,700 IU nadroparin strongly correlate with lean body weight in morbidly obese patients. Obes Surg 2012;22(5):791–6.

22. Diepstraten J, Chidambaran V, Sadhasivam S, et al. An integrated population pharmacokinetic meta-analysis of propofol in morbidly obese and nonobese adults, adolescents, and children. CPT Pharmacometrics Syst Pharmacol 2013; 2:e73.

23. Brill MJ, van Rongen A, Houwink AP, et al. Midazolam pharmacokinetics in morbidly obese patients following semi-simultaneous oral and intravenous administration: a comparison with healthy volunteers. Clin Pharmacokinet 2014; 53(10):931–41.

24. van Kralingen S, Taks M, Diepstraten J, et al. Pharmacokinetics and protein bind-ing of cefazolin in morbidly obese patients. Eur J Clin Pharmacol 2011;67(10): 985–92.

25. Brill MJ, Houwink AP, Schmidt S, et al. Reduced subcutaneous tissue distribution of cefazolin in morbidly obese versus non-obese patients determined using clin-ical microdialysis. J Antimicrob Chemother 2014;69(3):715–23.

26. Palatini P. Glomerular hyperfiltration: a marker of early renal damage in pre-diabetes and pre-hypertension. Nephrol Dial Transplant 2012;27(5):1708–14.

27. Rainone V, Schneider L, Saulle I, et al. Upregulation of inflammasome activity and increased gut permeability are associated with obesity in children and adoles-cents. Int J Obes (Lond) 2016;40(6):1026–33.

28. Greenblatt DJ, Abernethy DR, Locniskar A, et al. Effect of age, gender, and obesity on midazolam kinetics. Anesthesiology 1984;61(1):27–35.

29. Bowman SL, Hudson SA, Simpson G, et al. A comparison of the pharmacoki-netics of propranolol in obese and normal volunteers. Br J Clin Pharmacol 1986;21(5):529–32.

30. Flechner SM, Kolbeinsson ME, Tam J, et al. The impact of body weight on cyclo-sporine pharmacokinetics in renal transplant recipients. Transplantation 1989; 47(5):806–10.

31. Cheymol G, Weissenburger J, Poirier JM, et al. The pharmacokinetics of dexfen-fluramine in obese and non-obese subjects. Br J Clin Pharmacol 1995;39(6): 684–7.

32. Rowland TW. Effect of obesity on cardiac function in children and adolescents: a review. J Sports Sci Med 2007;6(3):319–26.

33. Preckel B, Bolten J. Pharmacology of modern volatile anaesthetics. Best Pract Res Clin Anaesthesiol 2005;19(3):331–48.

34. Janmahasatian S, Duffull SB, Ash S, et al. Quantification of lean bodyweight. Clin Pharmacokinet 2005;44(10):1051–65.

35. Hanley MJ, Abernethy DR, Greenblatt DJ. Effect of obesity on the pharmacoki-netics of drugs in humans. Clin Pharmacokinet 2010;49(2):71–87.

36. Gardier AM, Mathe D, Guedeney X, et al. Effects of plasma lipid levels on blood distribution and pharmacokinetics of cyclosporin A. Ther Drug Monit 1993;15(4): 274–80.

37. Davis RL, Quenzer RW, Bozigian HP, et al. Pharmacokinetics of ranitidine in morbidly obese women. DICP 1990;24(11):1040–3.

38. Harnois F, Msika S, Sabate JM, et al. Prevalence and predictive factors of non-alcoholic steatohepatitis (NASH) in morbidly obese patients undergoing bariatric surgery. Obes Surg 2006;16(2):183–8.

39. Han PY, Duffull SB, Kirkpatrick CM, et al. Dosing in obesity: a simple solution to a big problem. Clin Pharmacol Ther 2007;82(5):505–8.

40. Ribstein J, du Cailar G, Mimran A. Combined renal effects of overweight and hypertension. Hypertension 1995;26(4):610–5.

41. Reiss RA, Haas CE, Karki SD, et al. Lithium pharmacokinetics in the obese. Clin Pharmacol Ther 1994;55(4):392–8.

42. Savino A, Pelliccia P, Giannini C, et al. Implications for kidney disease in obese children and adolescents. Pediatr Nephrol 2011;26(5):749–58.

43. Grotta MB, Squebola-Cola DM, Toro AA, et al. Obesity increases eosinophil activity in asthmatic children and adolescents. BMC Pulm Med 2013;13:39.

44. Kwong KY, Jones CA. Improvement of asthma control with omalizumab in 2 obese pediatric asthma patients. Ann Allergy Asthma Immunol 2006;97(3):288–93.

45. Shapiro R. Subcutaneous immunoglobulin (16 or 20%) therapy in obese patients with primary immunodeficiency: a retrospective analysis of administration by infusion pump or subcutaneous rapid push. Clin Exp Immunol 2013;173(2):365–71.

46. Zed PJ, Black KJ, Fitzpatrick EA, et al. Medication-related emergency department visits in pediatrics: a prospective observational study. Pediatrics 2015;135(3):435–43.

47. Holford N. Dosing in children. Clin Pharmacol Ther 2010;87(3):367–70.

48. Natale S, Bradley J, Nguyen WH, et al. Pediatric obesity: pharmacokinetic alterations and effects on antimicrobial dosing. Pharmacotherapy 2017;37(3):361–78.

49. Shank BR, Zimmerman DE. Demystifying drug dosing in obese patients. 1st edition. Bethesda (MD): American Society of Health-System Pharmacists; 2016.

50. Phillips S, Edlbeck A, Kirby M, et al. Ideal body weight in children. Nutr Clin Pract 2007;22(2):240–5.

51. Devine BJ. Gentamicin therapy. Drug Intell Clin Pharm 1974;8:650–5.

52. Peters AM, Snelling HL, Glass DM, et al. Estimation of lean body mass in children. Br J Anaesth 2011;106(5):719–23.

53. Morgan DJ, Bray KM. Lean body mass as a predictor of drug dosage. Implications for drug therapy. Clin Pharmacokinet 1994;26(4):292–307.

54. Krenitsky J. Adjusted body weight, pro: evidence to support the use of adjusted body weight in calculating calorie requirements. Nutr Clin Pract 2005;20(4):468–73.

55. Centers for Disease Control and Prevention (CDC). Data Table of BMI-for-age Charts. 2000. Available at: https://www.cdc.gov/growthcharts/clinical_charts.htm.

56. Mosteller RD. Simplified calculation of body-surface area. N Engl J Med 1987;317(17):1098.

57. Kendrick JG, Carr RR, Ensom MH. Pharmacokinetics and drug dosing in obese children. J Pediatr Pharmacol Ther 2010;15(2):94–109.

58. Erstad BL. Dosing of medications in morbidly obese patients in the intensive care unit setting. Intensive Care Med 2004;30(1):18–32.

59. Pai MP, Bearden DT. Antimicrobial dosing considerations in obese adult patients. Pharmacotherapy 2007;27(8):1081–91.

60. Anderson BJ, Holford NH. Tips and traps analyzing pediatric PK data. Paediatr Anaesth 2011;21(3):222–37.

61. Mahmood I. Dosing in children: a critical review of the pharmacokinetic allometric scaling and modelling approaches in paediatric drug development and clinical settings. Clin Pharmacokinet 2014;53(4):327–46.

62. Emoto C, Fukuda T, Johnson TN, et al. Development of a pediatric physiologically based pharmacokinetic model for sirolimus: applying principles of growth and maturation in neonates and infants. CPT Pharmacometrics Syst Pharmacol 2015;4(2):e17.

63. Vinks AA, Emoto C, Fukuda T. Modeling and simulation in pediatric drug therapy: application of pharmacometrics to define the right dose for children. Clin Pharmacol Ther 2015;98(3):298–308.

64. Calvier EA, Krekels EH, Valitalo PA, et al. Allometric scaling of clearance in paediatric patients: when does the magic of 0.75 fade? Clin Pharmacokinet 2017; 56(3):273–85.

65. Kearns GL, Abdel-Rahman SM, Alander SW, et al. Developmental pharmacology–drug disposition, action, and therapy in infants and children. N Engl J Med 2003;349(12):1157–67.

66. Edginton AN, Shah B, Sevestre M, et al. The integration of allometry and virtual populations to predict clearance and clearance variability in pediatric populations over the age of 6 years. Clin Pharmacokinet 2013;52(8):693–703.

67. Momper JD, Mulugeta Y, Green DJ, et al. Adolescent dosing and labeling since the food and drug administration amendments act of 2007. JAMA Pediatr 2013; 167(10):926–32.

68. Matson KL, Horton ER, Capino AC. Advocacy committee for the pediatric pharmacy advocacy G. medication dosage in overweight and obese children. J Pediatr Pharmacol Ther 2017;22(1):81–3.

69. Green B, Duffull SB. What is the best size descriptor to use for pharmacokinetic studies in the obese? Br J Clin Pharmacol 2004;58(2):119–33.

70. Shi R, Derendorf H. Pediatric dosing and body size in biotherapeutics. Pharmaceutics 2010;2(4):389–418.

71. Harskamp-van Ginkel MW, Hill KD, Becker KC, et al. Drug dosing and pharmacokinetics in children with obesity: a systematic review. JAMA Pediatr 2015; 169(7):678–85.

72. Diepstraten J, Chidambaran V, Sadhasivam S, et al. Propofol clearance in morbidly obese children and adolescents: influence of age and body size. Clin Pharmacokinet 2012;51(8):543–51.

73. Taylor BN, Bork SJ, Kim S, et al. Evaluation of weight-based dosing of unfractionated heparin in obese children. J Pediatr 2013;163(1):150–3.

74. Barletta JF, DeYoung JL, McAllen K, et al. Limitations of a standardized weight-based nomogram for heparin dosing in patients with morbid obesity. Surg Obes Relat Dis 2008;4(6):748–53.

75. Joncas SX, Poirier P, Ardilouze JL, et al. Delayed efficient anticoagulation with heparin in patients with a weight of 110 kg and more treated for acute coronary syndrome. Obesity (Silver Spring) 2013;21(9):1753–8.

76. Rachel Park SC, Varghese J, Leddy C, et al. Assessing safety and efficacy of lean body weight-based intravenous heparin dosing in obese and morbidly obese patients. Chest 2015;148(4):1010A.

77. Mahmood I. Application of allometric principles for the prediction of pharmacokinetics in human and veterinary drug development. Adv Drug Deliv Rev 2007; 59(11):1177–92.

78. Sampson M, Cohen-Wolkowiez M, Benjamin D Jr, et al. Pharmacokinetics of antimicrobials in obese children. GaBI J 2013;2(2):76–81.

79. Erstad BL. Which weight for weight-based dosage regimens in obese patients? Am J Health Syst Pharm 2002;59(21):2105–10.
80. Huttner A, Harbarth S, Hope WW, et al. Therapeutic drug monitoring of the beta-lactam antibiotics: what is the evidence and which patients should we be using it for? J Antimicrob Chemother 2015;70(12):3178–83.
81. Baker SD, Verweij J, Rowinsky EK, et al. Role of body surface area in dosing of investigational anticancer agents in adults, 1991-2001. J Natl Cancer Inst 2002; 94(24):1883–8.
82. Griggs JJ, Mangu PB, Anderson H, et al. Appropriate chemotherapy dosing for obese adult patients with cancer: American Society of Clinical Oncology clinical practice guideline. J Clin Oncol 2012;30(13):1553–61.
83. Bartelink IH, van Kesteren C, Boelens JJ, et al. Predictive performance of a busulfan pharmacokinetic model in children and young adults. Ther Drug Monit 2012;34(5):574–83.
84. Munar MY, Singh H. Drug dosing adjustments in patients with chronic kidney disease. Am Fam Physician 2007;75(10):1487–96.
85. Brocks DR, Ben-Eltriki M, Gabr RQ, et al. The effects of gastric bypass surgery on drug absorption and pharmacokinetics. Expert Opin Drug Metab Toxicol 2012; 8(12):1505–19.
86. Khalsa J, Duffy LC, Riscuta G, et al. Omics for understanding the gut-liver-microbiome axis and precision medicine. Clin Pharmacol Drug Dev 2017;6(2): 176–85.
87. Chiaro TR, Soto R, Zac Stephens W, et al. A member of the gut microbiota modulates host purine metabolism exacerbating colitis in mice. Sci Transl Med 2017; 9(380) [pii:eaaf9044].
88. Clayton TA, Baker D, Lindon JC, et al. Pharmacometabonomic identification of a significant host-microbiome metabolic interaction affecting human drug metabolism. Proc Natl Acad Sci U S A 2009;106(34):14728–33.
89. Xie L, Ge X, Tan H, et al. Towards structural systems pharmacology to study complex diseases and personalized medicine. PLoS Comput Biol 2014;10(5): e1003554.
90. Kantae V, Krekels EH, Esdonk MJ, et al. Integration of pharmacometabolomics with pharmacokinetics and pharmacodynamics: towards personalized drug therapy. Metabolomics 2017;13(1):9.
91. Peletier LA, Gabrielsson J. Dynamics of target-mediated drug disposition: characteristic profiles and parameter identification. J Pharmacokinet Pharmacodyn 2012;39(5):429–51.
92. Anderson BJ, Holford NH. Getting the dose right for obese children. Arch Dis Child 2017;102(1):54–5.
93. Darwich AS, Ogungbenro K, Vinks AA, et al. Why has model-informed precision dosing not yet become common clinical reality? lessons from the past and a roadmap for the future. Clin Pharmacol Ther 2017;101(5):646–56.
94. Derezhkovskiy LM. On the accuracy of estimation of basic pharmacokinetic parameters by the traditional noncompartmental equations and the prediction of the steady-state volume of distribution in obese patients based upon data derived from normal subjects. J Pharm Sci 2011;100(6):2482–97.
95. Mahmood I. Prediction of drug clearance in children: a review of different methodologies. Expert Opin Drug Metab Toxicol 2015;11(4):573–87.
96. Kohler I, Hankemeier T, van der Graaf PH, et al. Integrating clinical metabolomics-based biomarker discovery and clinical pharmacology to enable precision medicine. Eur J Pharm Sci 2017. http://dx.doi.org/10.1016/j.ejps.2017.05.018.

97. Brussee JM, Calvier EA, Krekels EH, et al. Children in clinical trials: towards evidence-based pediatric pharmacotherapy using pharmacokinetic-pharmacodynamic modeling. Expert Rev Clin Pharmacol 2016;9(9):1235–44.
98. Servin F, Farinotti R, Haberer JP, et al. Propofol infusion for maintenance of anesthesia in morbidly obese patients receiving nitrous oxide. A clinical and pharmacokinetic study. Anesthesiology 1993;78(4):657–65.

Printed and bound by CPI Group (UK) Ltd, Croydon, CR0 4YY

03/10/2024

01040495-0007

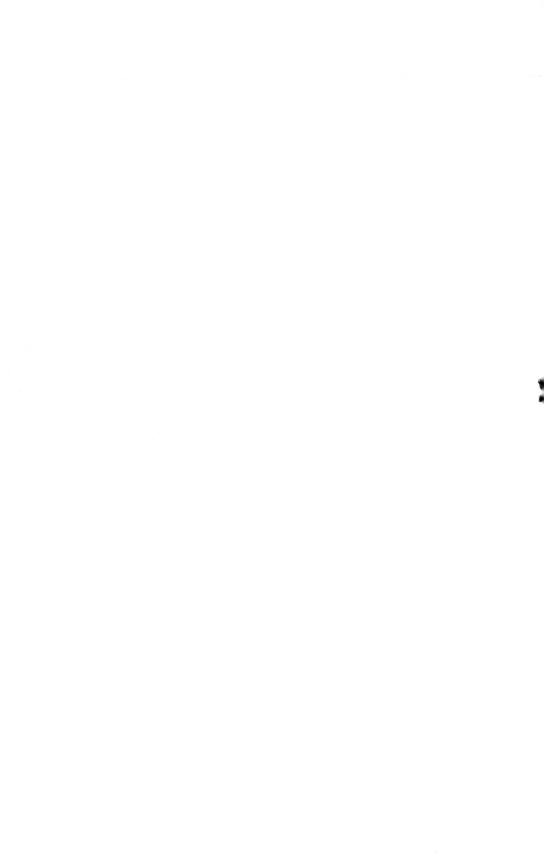